EXERCISES in ORAL RADIOLOGY and INTERPRETATION

5th Edition

ROBERT P. LANGLAIS, BA, DDS, MS, PhD, FRCD(C)

Diplomate, American Board of Oral and Maxillofacial Radiology
Professor Emeritus, Department of Dental Diagnostic Science
University of Texas Health Science Center Dental School
San Antonio, Texas
CEO, Emeritus Enterprises
San Antonio, Texas

CRAIG S. MILLER, DMD, MS

Diplomate, American Board of Oral Medicine
Professor of Oral Diagnosis, Oral Medicine, and Oral Radiology
Department of Oral Health Practice
College of Dentistry
University of Kentucky
Lexington, Kentucky

ELSEVIER

ELSEVIER

3251 Riverport Lane
St. Louis, Missouri 63043

EXERCISES IN ORAL RADIOLOGY AND INTERPRETATION, FIFTH EDITION

ISBN: 978-0-323-40063-3

Notices

Library of Congress Cataloging-in-Publication Data
Names: Langlais, Robert P., author. | Miller, Craig S., author.
Title: Exercises in oral radiology and interpretation / Robert P. Langlais, Craig S. Miller.
Description: 5th edition. | St. Louis, Missouri : Elsevier, [2017] | Includes index.
Identifiers: LCCN 2016021052 | ISBN 9780323400633 (pbk. : alk. paper)
Subjects: | MESH: Radiography, Dental | Stomatognathic Diseases–radiography | Examination Questions
Classification: LCC RK309 | NLM WN 18.2 | DDC 617.6/07572076–dc23 LC record available at https://lccn.loc.gov/2016021052

Senior Content Strategist: Kristin Wilhelm
Content Development Manager: Luke Held
Content Development Specialist: Kelly Skelton
Publishing Services Manager: Jeffrey Patterson
Senior Project Manager: Tracey Schriefer
Design Direction: Patrick Ferguson

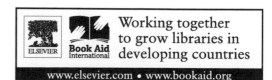

This book is dedicated to our students.
It is they who stimulate us to learn and therefore teach
us to be the best we can be.

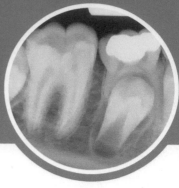

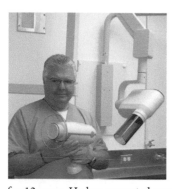

Dr. Bob Langlais is a Professor Emeritus at the University of Texas Health Science Center at San Antonio; is currently CEO of Emeritus Enterprises, a research company; consults and presents for Planmeca; and is a Board-Certified OMF Radiologist. He was the Secretary General of the International Association of Dento-Maxillo-Facial Radiology (IADMFR) for 12 years. He has presented some 600 courses and lectures in all continents except Antarctica, has over 120 scientific papers, and has written the first edition of eleven textbooks, two of which are being prepared for the 5th edition. Currently his presentations are on the subjects of common oral lesions, CBCT, and Pan Bite Wings. Dr. Langlais is also the former National Consultant in Dental Radiology to the Surgeon General of the United States Air Force with the civilian military equivalent rank of Brigadier General; upon his retirement he was awarded the Exceptional Service Award, the highest medal the USAF can award to a civilian. He also holds the line officer rank of Commander C.D. (ret.) in the Canadian Navy Reserve. In March 2014 he graduated with a PhD from the University of the Western Cape in South Africa; his thesis was to characterize a new Cadmium Telluride Photon Counting digital sensor for Pans and CBCT.

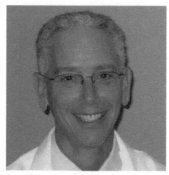

Dr. Craig Miller is a Professor at the University of Kentucky College of Dentistry in the Division of Oral Diagnosis, Oral Medicine, and Oral Radiology. He holds a joint appointment at the University of Kentucky College of Medicine in the Department of Microbiology, Immunology, & Molecular Genetics. He is a recipient of the University Provost Distinguished Service Professorship and has taught at the University of Kentucky for 28 years. He currently serves as Editor of the Oral Medicine Section of *Oral Surgery, Oral Medicine, Oral Pathology, Oral Radiology,* and for more than two decades has been funded by and serves as a consultant to the National Institutes of Health. He has authored more than 180 scientific articles, editorials, textbook chapters, and monographs regarding oral radiology, oral infections, dental pharmacology, dental management, and oral manifestations of systemic disease, and has co-authored four dental textbooks that have been used nationally and internationally. Dr. Miller served in the United States Air Force and United States Air Force Reserves as a Captain and was awarded a commendation medal for his service. He has received lifetime achievement awards from the American Academy of Oral Medicine and the Organization of Teachers of Oral Diagnosis.

PREFACE

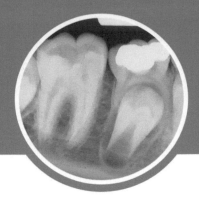

First and foremost I would like to welcome Dr. Craig Miller as my new coauthor of this book. I have been very closely associated with Craig for close to 30 years, including all five editions of our other textbook, *Color Atlas of Common Oral Lesions.* Without his ideas and hard work, this book in its present form and with its current content could never have been as complete. In keeping with tradition, we kept the "humorous asides" or "outtakes" such as "OK, now take a break" in which the authors speak to students directly. This book remains well known for this feature, which was pioneered by Dr. Langlais.

The order of the chapters has been changed to more closely reflect the scheduling of the courses and deliver a more orderly development of the contents. All of the chapters have been updated. Several chapters have been combined and new chapters have been added such as Basic Principles of Dental Radiology, Radiology Infection Control, Caries Detection and Panoramic Bite Wings, Cone Beam Computed Tomography (CBCT), and Implant Imaging.

Perhaps the biggest qualitative addition to the illustrations in this textbook is the feature of color. We have added many new diagrams in color along with new questions based on the diagrams. Many of our previous illustrations have been converted to color, and new clinical photos and questions have been added.

In the wording of some questions, we have maintained the feature of subtle clues to the answers to some of our cases. These might include a fictitious patient name, symptom, laboratory values, or background history of the case. The cases include questions with a color diagram or color clinical photo or radiograph, and the student should try to think of the correct response before consulting the answer in the back of the book. In each chapter, we have also added multiple choice questions in either one or both of the following formats:

- One set of questions is based on a figure, which could be a diagram, clinical photo or radiograph, or some combination of these.
- The second type involves the subject matter of the chapter; however, there is no related figure.

We hope these variable formats will help the student to obtain the knowledge contained herein. With this help, students can become "the best they can be" by generating high-quality radiographic images of all types as a part of the practice of dentistry, and wherever applicable, make assessments and/or diagnoses, which will ultimately be helpful to their patients.

The 4th edition was the 25th Silver Anniversary edition in 2004. We hope this 5th edition will be as welcome as in the past, and we wish all of our former, current, and future readers the best of success in their endeavors.

Here are a few quotes that the reader may find interesting:

"The eye cannot see what the mind does not know."

Sir William Osler, late 1800s

"You can't be good at what you don't know; you can only be good at being no good."

Robert P. Langlais, March 2003

**Robert P. Langlais and Craig S. Miller,
September 2015**

ACKNOWLEDGMENTS

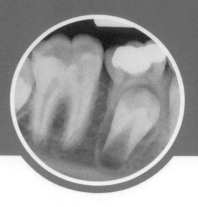

First, I would like to acknowledge my longtime coauthor, colleague, and friend Dr. Craig Miller who has consented to join me in this 5th edition of *Exercises in Oral Radiology and Interpretation*. His contributions have been invaluable. Second and as always: "un gros merci a mon épouse, Denyse. Je t'aime." Denyse Paré, who was my onetime dental assistant and office manager, remembers those first days in Montreal, Canada, working on the kitchen table of our apartment borrowed from my brother John Langlais. Our house was sold, and while we waited for our green cards, the first edition of the first book of 11 first-edition dental textbooks was being written. The title was: *Exercises in Dental Radiology volume 1: Intraoral Radiographic Interpretation*. Since then that book has evolved to its present title: *Exercises in Oral Radiology and Interpretation*, which reflects the expanded content of the present edition.

Some of the folks who have helped us include Dr. Diane Flint, Dr. John Preece, Dr. William "Doss" McDavid, Dr. Donald Nield, Dr. Paul Langlais, Denyse Langlais, Dr. Marcel Noujeim, and Dr. Peter Mah. Others who have contributed cases include the following representatives of the Planmeca USA company: Bob Pienkowski, CEO; Glen Kendrick, Sales Manager; Brett Hines, Sales Manager; Mark Langlais, Don Gowers, Matt Robson, Yanic Desrochers, Adam Winick, Brent Garvin, Arnaud Wauters, Blaine Atwater, Erin Holbrook, Jim Pienkowski, Jim Hooper, Jim Hughes, Joe Bell, Pete Kores, Rich Hoffman, Ron Tron, and Steve O'Neil; a special thanks to Robin Gathman who coordinated my various opportunities to work with these folks. A very special thank you goes to David Baker, Medical Illustrator Extraordinaire and artist to the Bush First Family of the United States and with whom Dr. Langlais has been working for the past 30-plus years. Dave was responsible for all of the new artwork, including the colorization of several of the old illustrations. His knowledge of anatomy and understanding of the principles we were trying to illustrate in a clear and simple way made the development of some of the unique artwork a great feature of this 5th edition and a boon to our readers. To Kristin R. Wilhelm, our publisher representative at Elsevier, we offer our grateful thanks for the much-needed support and guidance you provided in making this 5th edition a reality.

CONTENTS

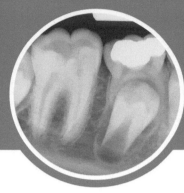

PART ONE

Principles and Interpretation

Chapter 1

Basic Principles of Dental Radiology

Goal

To learn the basic principles as they apply to dental radiographic imaging

Learning Objectives

1. Learn how dental radiation is generated
2. Learn the basic physical principles of how dental radiation is produced
3. Learn how dental x-radiation interacts with matter
4. Understand the factors affecting the projection geometry of the x-ray beam
5. Recognize the parts of a typical x-ray machine tube head
6. Understand the clinical significance of AC vs. DC x-ray generators

INTRODUCTION

The basic principles associated with dental radiology are traditional and have existed for more than 100 years. However, new ideas and technologies are creating an evolving field. For example, most dental x-ray machines have used alternating current (AC) to generate energy, and many of these remain in educational institutions and dental practices. However, newer dental x-ray generators are now usually based on direct current (DC) conversion from the AC power input into the machine. As we will see, there are distinct advantages to DC-powered x-ray generators. In addition, intraoral machines have traditionally been wall mounted and now portable handheld x-ray machines are available and safe to use.

It is probable that almost all institutional programs that train their dental assisting, dental hygiene, and dental students as well as most relevant dental graduate programs now utilize digital sensors. Because of this, we considered eliminating everything to do with film. However, we could not be certain of this as fact and could not confirm that everything to do with film is no longer required knowledge for the examination purposes of students at all levels. Undoubtedly digital imaging has not fully penetrated all dental practices, and some dentists use both digital- and film-based imaging. For example, the intraoral could be digitals, but the pan is still film based. Therefore we have left some film-related material in this edition. In any case, most of the physical principles as discussed here apply to both film and sensors, although radiation affects film differently than sensors. For example, too much radiation causes a dark image on film while on some sensors it causes "blooming." **Blooming** is a digital imaging artifact characterized by a blacking out of all or parts of the image, usually where structures are the least dense and therefore absorb the least amount of excess radiation.

Intraoral bitewing and **periapical imaging** are evolving with the development of panoramic bitewing images capable of displaying open interproximal contacts and well as all of the periapical regions of the involved teeth (pan bitewings). In addition, the panoramic device can capture a selected small area(s) of interest about the size of a single periapical image. The specific principles associated with this technology are covered in Chapter 6. This new technology is mentioned here as it may come to represent an alternative to most intraoral imaging as the field progresses.

Finally, cone beam computed tomography (CBCT) is also becoming more and more ubiquitous in both dental education programs and in dental practices and institutions such as hospital dental departments. Thus our chapter on CBCT focuses on some of the related specific principles as well as some cases to illustrate some of the advantages of CBCT imaging. That is to say, because CBCT allows us to study very thin slices of a selected anatomic region of interest in three dimensions, the technology can not only capture important diagnostic information that is absent in the intraoral, panoramic, or other images, but also linear, angular, and volumetric measurements are possible and are extremely accurate. For example, intraoral images have been used for endodontic procedures and for implant measurements; at present CBCT offers an alternative technology that is in many ways superior to intraoral imaging.

In spite of all of these recent advances, some of the basic principles regarding x-radiation remain unchanged while others have evolved depending on the technology in use. Thus we begin here with the most basic principles and will cover other more specific principles in the following chapters.

MULTIPLE CHOICE QUESTIONS WITH FIGURES

Instructions

Please select the best answer and check your selection with the correct answers in the Answer Key at the back of the book.

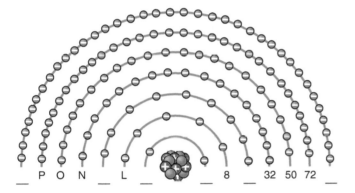

Figure **1-1**

1. This is a diagram showing the maximum number of electrons that can exist in each orbital shell. Which statement is incorrect?
   A. The K shell is closest to the nucleus and has 2 electrons
   B. The Q shell is outermost and has 96 electrons
   C. The M shell has 18 electrons
   D. The N shell has 32 electrons

2. The nucleus has:
   A. Positrons and electrons
   B. Protons and positrons
   C. Protons and neutrons
   D. A neutral charge

3. For tungsten the binding energy is usually:
   A. Greatest in the outer shell
   B. The same for each shell individually
   C. Greatest for the K shell
   D. A binding energy of 12 keV

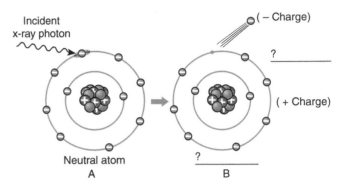

Figure **1-2**

1. In the above diagram, we have a neutral atom in diagram A. In diagram B an outer orbital electron is knocked out of the atom. Which statement is *not* true?
   A. An electron was knocked out by an x-ray photon
   B. This reaction is called decay
   C. An ion pair is formed
   D. This process is known as ionization

2. The ion pair in the above reaction consists of:
   A. The incident photon and the original atom
   B. The incident photon and the positively charged atom
   C. The original atom and the positively charged atom
   D. The free electron and the positively charged atom

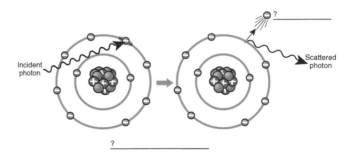

Figure **1-3**

1. As a result of knocking out the orbital electron, the original incident photon of radiation loses some energy and changes directions.
   A. This reaction is called Compton scattering
   B. This is an example of the braking reaction
   C. This effect is electron deceleration
   D. The free electron is called a photoelectric electron

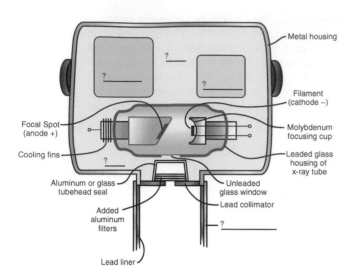

Figure **1-4**

1. The overall diagram of this part of an x-ray machine is called the:
   A. X-ray tube
   B. Yoke
   C. Generator
   D. Tube head

2. The components within this part of the machine, indicated in green, blue, and brown, consist of:
   A. A generator, a tube, and a portal
   B. Step-up and step-down transformers and the x-ray tube
   C. Two transformers, an x-ray tube, and a glass window
   D. Step-up and step-down transformers, x-ray tube, and oil

3. The part which helps to aim the x-rays is called the:
   A. Cone
   B. Beam indicating device
   C. BID
   D. All of the above

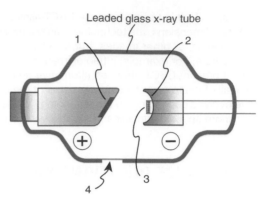

Figure **1-5**

1. This is a drawing of an x-ray tube. If we go clockwise starting with No. 1, the correct terms for each of the parts of the x-ray tube are:
   A. Molybdenum focusing cup, cathode/filament, anode/target, window/aperture
   B. Cathode/tungsten filament, anode/target, focusing cup, window/aperture
   C. Anode/target, cathode/filament, focusing cup, window/aperture
   D. Anode/target, focusing cup, cathode/filament, window/aperture

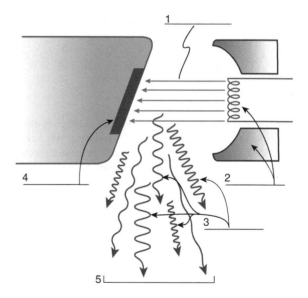

Figure **1-6**

1. This is a drawing of how x-rays are generated. If we go clockwise starting with No. 1 and ending with No. 5 in numerical order, the correct terms for each of the parts of this diagram are:
   A. 1. Electrons; 2. Focusing cup & cathode (-); 3. Homogeneous x-ray beam; 4. Anode (+); 5. X-ray beam with photons of different wavelengths
   B. 1. Electrons, anode (+); 2. X-ray beam; 3. Focusing cup & cathode (-); 4. X-ray photons of different wavelengths; 5. X-ray beam
   C. 1. Electrons; 2. X-ray photons of different wavelengths; 3. Focusing cup & cathode (-); 4. Heterogeneous x-ray beam; 5. Anode (+)
   D. 1. Electrons; 2. Focusing cup & cathode (-); 3. X-ray photons of different wavelengths; 4. Anode (+); 5. heterogeneous x-ray beam

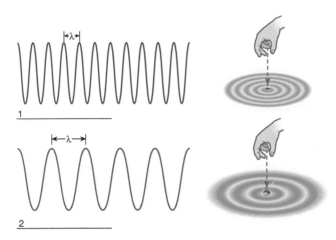

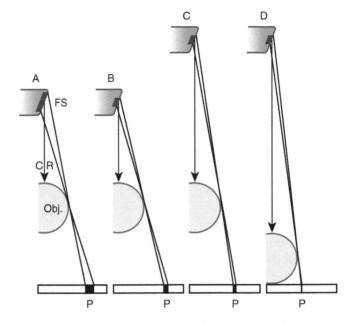

Figure **1-7**

1. This diagram has a Greek letter above the squiggly lines. This letter is:
   A. Alpha
   B. Beta
   C. Theta
   D. Lambda

2. The Greek letter indicates:
   A. The wavelength
   B. The frequency
   C. Alternating current
   D. None of the above

3. The upper example (1) in the diagram would be associated with:
   A. A more penetrating x-ray beam
   B. A higher frequency energy wave
   C. Particles called photons
   D. All of the above

4. The lower example (2) in the diagram would be associated with:
   A. A less penetrating x-ray beam
   B. A lower frequency energy wave
   C. A longer wavelength
   D. All of the above

Figure **1-8**   Here we see an illustration showing factors that increase the amount of "P" in the image.

1. What word does the letter "P" stand for?
2. In diagrams A and B what factor is the variable?
3. In diagrams C and D what factor is the variable?
4. What overall "message" does this figure convey?

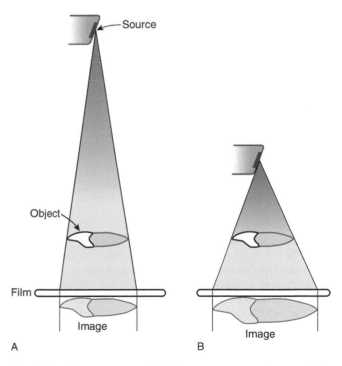

Figure **1-9**   Here we see a variable that causes magnification of the image.

1. What variable is being demonstrated here?
2. What is the effect of this variable on the image?

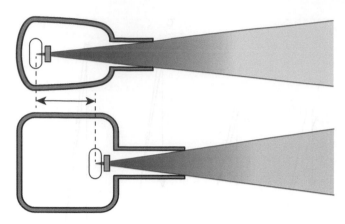

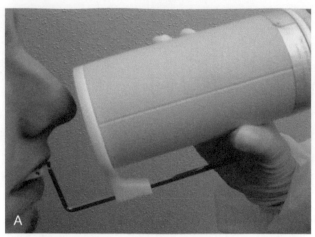

Figure **1-10**

1. What is the concept, as illustrated here, whereby the advantages in image quality of a long cone tube head can be combined with the convenience and advantages of a short cone tube head?

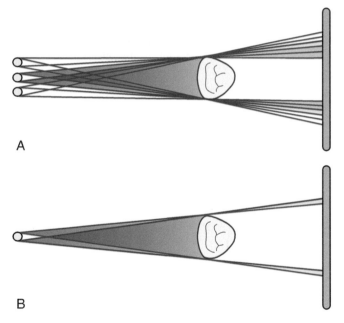

A

B

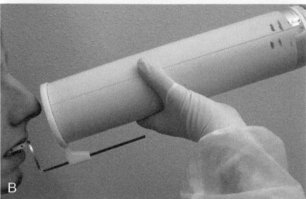

Figure **1-12**   Compare images A and B and answer the following question:

1. These photos of the short cone vs. the long cone demonstrate two identical principles when the two cone lengths are used to take radiographs. What are those two principles?

Figure **1-11**   Here we see exactly the same distance from the focal spot to the object and exactly the same distance between the object and the film or sensor. In the upper image the tube head of the machine is shaky (or moving), and the lower image shows the tube head is more stable.

1. What two effects do we see here relative to the tube head movement?

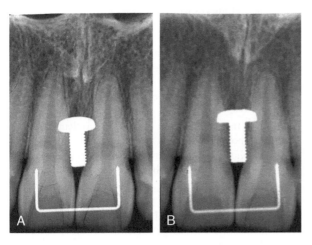

Figure **1-13** These are images of teeth on a dried skull; both were captured using a film/sensor positioning and alignment device.
1. Which image do you prefer?
2. List as many differences between these two images as you can.
3. Both were captured on the same capture device and tube head; this being the case what could be the cause of the differences between these two images?

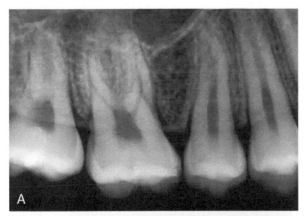

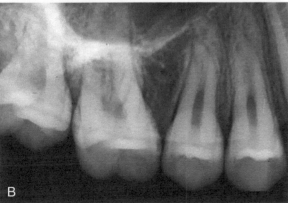

Figure **1-14** Image A was taken with the paralleling technique while image B was taken with the bisecting angle technique.
1. List as many differences as you can detect between the two images.
2. Which is the best image? State your reason(s) for your choice.

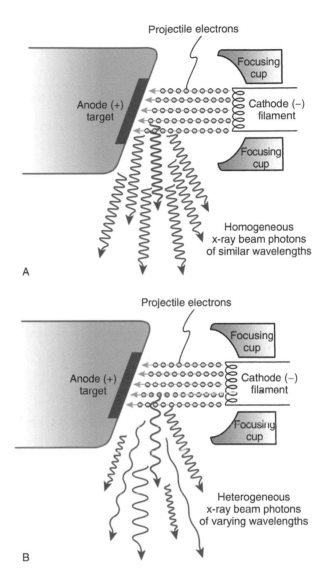

Figure **1-15** The above diagrams are similar.
1. Identify the one most important difference between the two diagrams.
2. If each diagram represents a type of x-ray unit, what would those be?
3. State the advantages of the best type of x-ray unit.

MULTIPLE CHOICE QUESTIONS WITHOUT FIGURES

Instructions

Please select the best answer and check your selection with the correct answers in the Answer Key at the back of the book.

1. Within an intraoral tube head, there is a filler substance or material. This material is:
   A. Oil
   B. Air
   C. Gel
   D. Foam

2. Within the x-ray tube there is a component that has much to do with the image quality. Which component is this?
   A. Focusing cup
   B. Filament
   C. Vacuum quality within the tube
   D. Focal spot (target) size

3. Which of the following digital sensor types requires scanning?
   A. CCD
   B. CMOS
   C. Super CMOS
   D. PSP

4. Which of the following electronic sensor types requires the least amount of power?
   A. CCD
   B. CMOS
   C. Super CMOS
   D. PSP

5. The Z number is:
   A. The number of protons in the nucleus
   B. Also referred to as the atomic number
   C. The number of electrons outside the nucleus
   D. All of the above

6. The type of x-ray tube that produces a homogeneous x-ray beam is:
   A. AC
   B. DC
   C. AC and DC
   D. Battery powered handheld only

7. When the target in the x-ray tube becomes pitted:
   A. Image quality degrades
   B. Image magnification occurs
   C. Longer exposure times are needed
   D. All of the above

8. The target usually consists of:
   A. Magnesium
   B. Carbide
   C. Hardened carbide
   D. Tungsten

9. The sharpest images will be produced by:
   A. The largest target
   B. The smallest target
   C. Small handheld x-ray machines
   D. Older AC machines

10. One of the characteristics of a heterogeneous x-ray beam is that:
    A. All of the photons are of the same wavelength
    B. The photons have two wavelengths
    C. The photons have multiple wavelengths
    D. The photons have variable wave forms but do not vary in wavelength

11. When the x-ray beam passes from the target to the cone, it goes through a filter usually made of:
    A. Aluminum
    B. Carbon carbide
    C. Tungsten
    D. Absorbable composite

12. All other factors being equal, which cone length will have the least penumbra?
    A. 4 inches
    B. 8 inches
    C. 12 inches
    D. 16 inches

13. All other factors being equal, which cone length will have the highest dose if the appropriate exposure time is used in each case?
    A. 4 inches
    B. 8 inches
    C. 12 inches
    D. 16 inches

14. According to the inverse square law, a 16-inch cone would need how much more exposure time than an 8-inch cone?
    A. 2 times more
    B. 4 times more
    C. 8 times more
    D. 16 times more

15. When converting from an 8-inch cone to a 16-inch cone, the exposure time must be increased. As a result, the patient exposure is _____ (if all other settings, such as mA or kV, remain unchanged).
    A. Less
    B. More
    C. The same
    D. Unpredictable due to variations in patient size

16. Increasing penumbra causes:
    A. Image clarification
    B. A sharper image
    C. No change in the image
    D. Blurring of the image

Chapter 2

Radiation Safety
Health and Protection

Goal

To know all aspects of radiation health according to current standards and practices

Learning Objectives

1. Recognize devices and supplies designed for protection of the patient
3. Know radiologic procedures for protection of the patient
4. Recognize operator radiation protection procedures

INTRODUCTION

The subject of radiation health includes the traditional concepts of patient and operator protection from biologic damage from radiation. These practices are currently under review by the National Council on Radiation Protection (NCRP), and new guidelines with significant changes are expected sometime in 2016.

> **NOTE TO STUDENTS:**
> The term *cone* and *beam indicating device* (BID) are used interchangeably. Another common term is *position indicating device* (PID).

SHORT ANSWER QUESTIONS WITH FIGURES

Instructions

Compare your answer to the correct answer in the Answer Key at the back of the book.

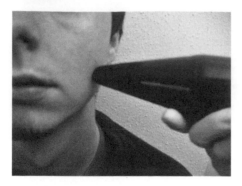

Figure **2-1**   Here you see an older BID design.
1. What is wrong in this picture? Explain.
2. What is the usual length of these BIDs?

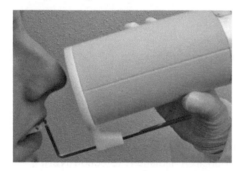

Figure **2-2**   Here you see a short, round, open-ended BID being used with the paralleling technique. Answer the following questions:
1. What size is the diameter of the open end of the BID limited to by law?
2. What is wrong in this picture?

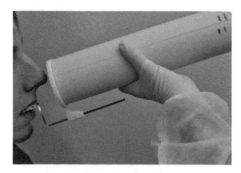

Figure **2-3**   Here you see a long, round BID being used. Answer the following questions:
1. Does the long, round BID design provide the lowest amount of radiation dose to the patient?
2. The long, 16-inch, round BID is said to expose the patient to less radiation than the short, 8-inch BID. Both BIDs have a diameter of 2¾ inches at the open end. If the short BID requires exposure times four times shorter than the long BID (this is true), how can the long BID result in less patient exposure? Explain.

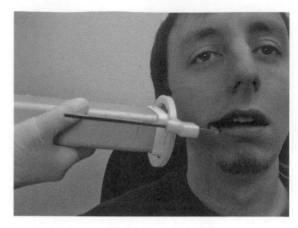

Figure **2-4**   Here you see a long, 16-inch, rectangular BID being used. Notice the locator ring is round. Remember also a retake doubles the dose to the patient for that exposure.
1. Why does the long rectangular BID provide less radiation exposure than the long round BID? Both use the same exposure time (true) as long as all other factors, such as machine type (AC vs. DC), kVp, mA, and film speed, are the same.
2. Will a cone cut occur if a rectangular locator ring is not used?
3. In terms of BID alignment (not shape), what unique feature does the rectangular BID always have that round BIDs never have?

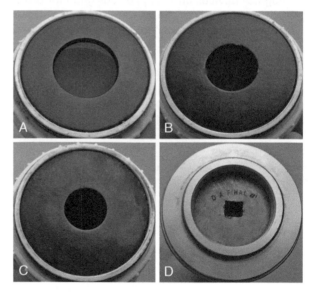

Figure **2-5**   Here you see four current collimators labeled A, B, C, and D. Answer the following questions; be sure to answer all of the questions before going to the answer page.
1. Where in the x-ray apparatus are the collimators located?
2. What material are the collimators made from?
3. Which of these is illegal for use on new equipment?
4. Which of these delivers the least amount of radiation to the patient?
5. Collimator size is matched up to BID length. Here we have the standard short BID and two long BIDs. What is the length of the associated BIDs for A, B, C, and D?
6. Which one is a rectangular BID?
7. Which one is the pointed cone?
8. Which two have the same exposure times?

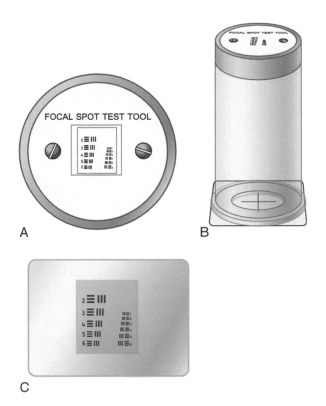

A   B

C

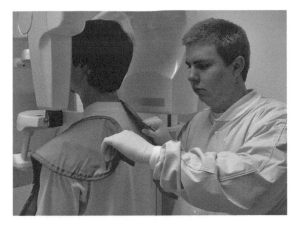

Figure **2-8** Here you see the patient being positioned in a digital panoramic machine.
1. What error(s) do you see in this picture?

Figure **2-6** This is an occlusal radiograph of a test object as seen above that is used to check the x-ray machine.
1. What is it used for (i.e., what function is being measured here)?
2. Explain how this test is performed and what term you used in answering part 1.
3. What causes the resolution to deteriorate?
4. Assess this test result and explain what resolution is clinically acceptable.
5. If the line pairs resolved (clinically visible as separate lines) is not clinically acceptable, what should be done?
6. When there are different brands and generations of machines in a clinic or dental office what other important function can this device be used for?

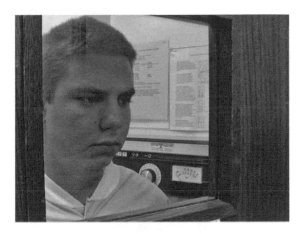

Figure **2-9** Here you see the operator behind a protective barrier while exposing an intraoral radiograph.
1. What material is usually incorporated in such barrier walls to protect the operator?
2. Why is the operator still protected in the area behind the patient observation window that is made of glass?

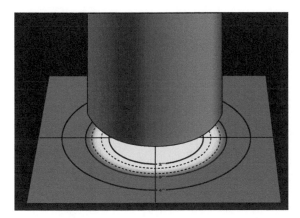

Figure **2-7** Here you can see the open end of a long, round cone and a piece of fluorescent screen material.
1. What part of the machine is being tested here?
2. What is the result of the test?

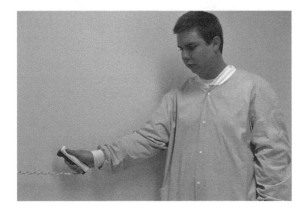

Figure **2-10** This student is about to take a panoramic radiograph. Appropriately, he is standing behind a protective wall.
1. What is wrong in this picture?
2. How must this be corrected?

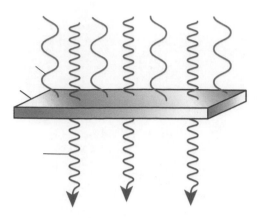

Figure **2-11** Here we see a diagram of photons of radiation of various wavelengths above a filter.
1. What can we say about the wavelength of the photons above the filter?
2. What type of material is this filter usually made of?
3. What do you notice about the wavelength of the photons below the filter?
4. In terms of radiation health, what does the filter do?
5. Are the photons of a DC-powered (vs. an AC-powered) x-ray machine pretty much the same in character? Explain your answer in one sentence if possible.

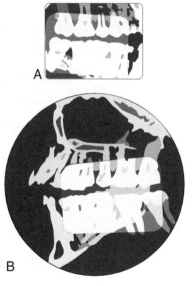

A

B

Figure **2-12** Here we see the exit radiation that exposed a panoramic radiograph for two intraoral radiographs taken on a skull on the opposite side. The intraoral film (similar for a PSP or electronic sensor) was positioned for an anterior bitewing exposure. A large film (or PSP plate), such as that used for a panoramic machine, was positioned on the opposite side of the skull. Both images were taken with the same mA, kVp, and exposure time. These were the resultant images as trimmed from the original panoramic size.
1. What type (shape) of cone was used for the top exposure?
2. What type (shape) of cone was used for the bottom exposure?
3. All the exposure factors being equal, did one patient get more exposure?
4. Explain your answer to question 3 in one sentence if possible.

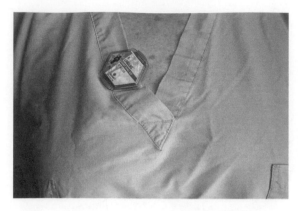

Figure **2-13** Here we see a badge pinned to the neckline of a scrub shirt.
1. What is this badge called?
2. What does the badge do?
3. What is the ultimate goal of wearing this badge?
4. Is the wearing of this badge required?

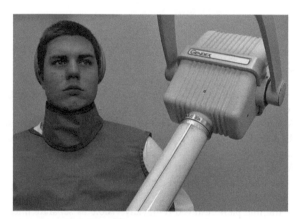

Figure **2-14** Here we see a patient wearing a lead apron and thyroid collar before having an intraoral radiograph taken.
1. Is the apron required?

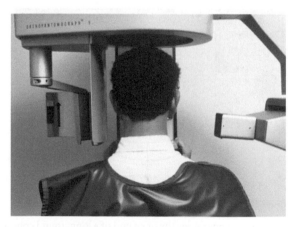

Figure **2-15** Here we see a patient about to have a panoramic radiograph taken.
1. Is the lead apron necessary?

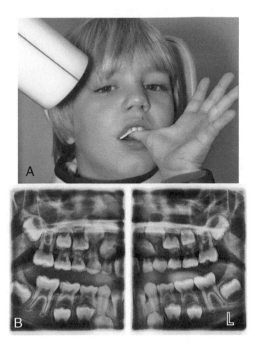

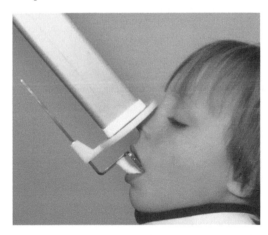

Figure **2-16** Here we see a child wearing a thyroid collar and about to have an intraoral periapical image taken as part of a full mouth survey including bitewings.
1. Is the thyroid collar necessary?
2. Is there some other way to obtain a similar set of images with more comfort, no thyroid collar, and a similar radiation dose?
3. Should patients hold the film or sensor?

Figure **2-17** Here we see the proper film positioning and beam alignment of a rectangular cone for the imaging of the upper centrals and parts of the laterals in a 6-year-old boy. Note the image receptor, which was film, must be placed back away from the teeth in order to obtain the apices in the image and remain parallel.
1. If there are no symptoms, no history of trauma, and no evidence of caries with transillumination, is this radiograph necessary?
2. Even though the thyroid collar is in place, is it possible that in this case there will be direct exposure of the thyroid gland with a portion of the exit beam?
3. If this image needs to be taken, is there a better way to do this with much less chance of exposing the thyroid gland?
4. If space analysis is to be performed, how accurate would the mesiodistal measurements of these teeth be?
5. What is the best method of accurately performing a space analysis?

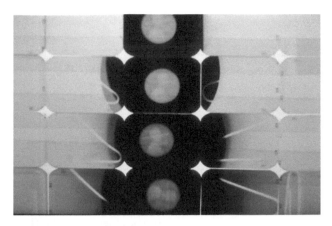

Figure **2-18** This is a figure that was created by Dr. John Preece, an eminent oral and maxillofacial radiologist, coauthor, and colleague. A Lincoln penny was placed on a film packet with no staples on a countertop. Beside this, two intraoral film packets were placed on each side. On each film packet, Dr. Preece affixed a large or small paper clip. The top image used a long, 16-inch, rectangular cone. The next image used a long, 16-inch, round cone. The third image used a short, 8-inch, round cone. The bottom image was exposed by a pointed cone. (Figure courtesy of Dr. John Preece).
1. Apart from use as an aiming device, what is the primary purpose of the cone?
2. In this example, which cone type fully collimated the beam?
3. If you compare the long, round cone to the short, round cone, was there any difference?
4. How about the long cones compared with the pointed cone?
5. Why do we see so few machines supplied with a long, round cone?
6. Which machine requires the least amount of space?

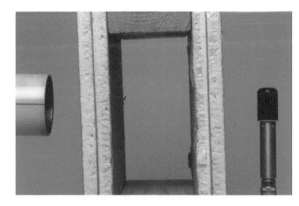

Figure **2-19** Here we see the tip of a round cone on the left, two thicknesses of ⅝-inch sheetrock on each side of a wall and an ionization chamber sensor on the other side of the wall. The ionization chamber measures the amount of radiation that strikes its sensor.
1. At the full range of normal exposures, how much radiation do you think will penetrate to the next room on the other side?
2. Under the above scenario is lead lining of the walls necessary?
3. In open clinics with x-ray machines in use, what is the safe distance from any of these sources of radiation at which you may stand?

LOSS OF LIFE EXPECTANCY DUE TO VARIOUS CAUSES			
CAUSE	DAYS	CAUSE	DAYS
Unmarried Male	3500	Firearms Accidents	11
Cigarette Smoking Male	2250	Natural Radiation	8
Unmarried Female	1600	Medical X-Rays	6
30% Overweight	1300	Coffee	6
< 8th-Grade Education	850	Oral Contraceptives	5
Cigarette Smoking Female	800	Accidents on Pedacycles	5
Cigar Smoking	330	Diet Drinks	2
Pipe Smoking	220	Ractor Accidents	0.02
Alcohol	130	Radiation from NUC Industry	0.02
Legal Drug Misuse	90	Air Bags in Car	-50

Figure **2-20**   Many such tables exist and are provided by various government agencies and other interested parties. The authors cannot vouch for the absolute accuracy of this table. (Table reprinted from Cohen BL, Lee I. A Catalog of Risks. Health Physics 1979; 36: 707–722, with permission from Health Physics Society).

1. What condition is purported to be the most major cause of loss of life expectancy in the United States?
2. If asked the question: Excluding male as a choice, which of the following three conditions has the greatest potential for loss of life expectancy: being an unmarried female, being 30% overweight, or having less than an 8th-grade education?

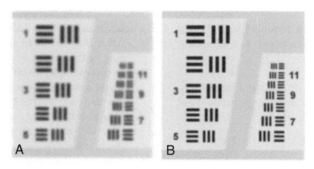

Figure **2-21**   Here we see the line pair test for two different intraoral machines.
1. Compare and contrast the left and right images.
2. Which of these two machines (A, Left or B, Right) produces the most acceptable intraoral images?

MULTIPLE CHOICE QUESTIONS WITHOUT FIGURES

Instructions

Please select the best answer and check your selection with the correct answer in the Answer Key at the back of the book.

1. When you are making an x-ray exposure, which of the following procedures will reduce your exposure to the x-rays?
   A. Positioning yourself outside the room or behind a barrier
   B. Never holding or stabilizing the tube head
   C. Standing at least 6 feet away from the tube head
   D. All of the above

2. In dental x-ray machines, filtration is used to remove:
   A. Long-wavelength photons
   B. Low-energy electrons
   C. Scatter radiation
   D. High-energy photons

3. To reduce the exposure to the patient, all of the following are recommended *except using:*
   A. "F"-speed film
   B. A CMOS vs. a CCD sensor
   C. An 8-inch BID
   D. Higher kilovoltage (kV) settings

4. Which of the following tissues is the most susceptible to radiation?
   A. Blood-forming tissue
   B. Brain tissue
   C. Muscle tissue
   D. Nerve tissue

5. Which of the following latent effects can be associated with whole-body, low-dose radiation?
   A. Epistaxis (bleeding nose)
   B. Epilation (hair loss)
   C. Leukemia
   D. Shock

6. The film badge service reports that the wearer was exposed to 5 mSv during the past month. The dental health care worker should:
   A. Immediately stop exposing x-ray images
   B. Report to the hospital for a blood count
   C. File the report as the reading is within normal acceptable limits
   D. Evaluate the x-ray procedures to avoid unnecessary radiation exposure

7. Collimation of the x-ray beam is the:
   A. Removal of most soft radiation from the beam
   B. Selective removal of hard radiation from the beam
   C. Reduction of the beam diameter
   D. Reduction of the beam intensity by 50%

8. At the cellular or nuclear level, the biologic effects of ionizing radiation may be significantly reduced by:
   A. Apoptosis
   B. Hormesis
   C. DNA damage-control biosystem
   D. A & B only
   E. All of the above

9. When a radiation-damaged cell passes along damage to offspring cells, this is a:
   A. Somatic effect
   B. Genetic effect
   C. Latent effect
   D. Indirect effect

10. During the exposure the dental health care worker should not hold:
    A. The film, PSP, or sensor
    B. The x-ray tube head, unless it is a portable machine
    C. A child during the exposure
    D. All of the above
    E. All of the above except B

11. The material used in the manufacture of x-ray filters is:
    A. Stainless steel
    B. Aluminum
    C. Lead
    D. Copper

12. The material used in the manufacture of x-ray collimators is:
    A. Stainless steel
    B. Aluminum
    C. Lead
    D. Copper

13. The average effective dose of ionizing radiation from natural background radiation to a person who lives in the United States is about:
    A. 3 mSv per year
    B. 6 mSv per year
    C. 10 mSv per year
    D. 50 mSv per year

(3) Radiology Infection Control

Goal

Know the dental radiology infection control steps as they relate to the appropriate clinical procedures

Learning Objectives

1. Recognize infection control procedures for patient protection
2. Identify infection control procedures for operator protection
3. Know the use of barriers for all aspects of radiology infection control
4. Understand infection control procedures for the transportation of contaminated materials from one part of the radiology area to another
5. Know infection control procedures for the processing of x-ray film or PSP scanning

INTRODUCTION

One must take note that radiology involves mainly contamination with saliva and rarely blood. Because of this, personnel must remember that saliva is considered a potentially infectious material and therefore specialized infection control procedures exist as they apply to dental radiology. Also these procedures are not optional. Guidelines for infection control are made by the **Centers for Disease Control**. The **Occupational Safety and Health Administration** (OSHA) also mandates regulations for protecting workers against transmission of infectious agents. Offices and institutions are subject to inspections and fines for a lack of compliance. In addition, there can be state and local requirements that must be followed. Accordingly, infection control is an important and integral part of dental radiology.

Intraoral Radiology

Intraoral radiology infection control consists of the following considerations: film-based imaging vs. digital imaging. Both technologies have infection control components: the preprocedural mouthwash, the x-ray machine, the patient chair, the nearby countertop, the film or sensor and its holding and aiming device, image processing such as the scanning of **photostimulable phosphor plates** (PSP) plates, and operator protection during and after the procedures.

Before starting, the patient may be given a preprocedural antiseptic mouthwash, such as chlorhexidine, to rinse with to reduce the microbial count in the mouth before taking intraoral radiographs. The x-ray machine requires that barrier material be used to wrap the tube head and cone, the yoke, the control panel, and the exposure switch. An optional foot exposure switch is available and does not normally require any infection control procedures. The arms of the chair and headrest may also be wrapped with barrier material, as well as any adjacent countertops that may become contaminated with saliva. Film is supplied prewrapped and therefore does not require additional barrier material. PSPs must be placed in a specially designed barrier envelope before each use. Electronic sensors

must first be isolated with a sleeve material, such as vinyl, approximately 12 inches long to protect the sensor and the electronic wire attached to the sensor. A rubber sleeve, which often consists of a finger cot, is slipped over the sensor and vinyl sleeve for further protection of the sensor from moisture and to secure the vinyl sleeve to the sensor and wire. After use most electronic sensors can be severely and terminally damaged by heat sterilization. Also most sensors cannot be soaked in disinfectant due to possible leakage that may cause internal damage. Therefore sensors are simply wiped with a disinfectant solution and aseptically wrapped for the next patient. The sensor holding and aiming device does not require barrier protection, although when used with an electronic sensor, the sensor barrier may also include parts of the sensor holder. The aiming instrument and sensor holder, both of which enter the patient's mouth, must be cleaned and then sterilized after each use. Because sensor holders are usually resistant to heat, this method is preferred over a liquid soaking (disinfection) process.

In the case of electronic sensors, no further procedures are needed because the image will be imported directly into the patient's file in the computer immediately after each exposure. Wireless electronic sensors are available, though they are bulkier than the already bulky standard electronic sensors. In general electronic sensors are 25% to

30% larger than film or PSPs, and the image area is about 25% to 30% smaller than film or PSPs. During the image capture phase, the operator will usually only need to wear gloves; a mask is not necessary as no spatter is usually created with this procedure. A mask may be worn if there is a danger of cross infection should the patient or operator be subject to sneezing or coughing or in some other way be exposed to potentially contaminated aerosols. Electronic sensors may be reused indefinitely.

In the case of digital PSPs, these will need to be transported aseptically, often in a clean paper cup, to the scanner area. Therefore a vinyl overglove or new glove should be worn because doorknobs and other items may be touched during this phase. The barrier envelope is then removed with clean gloved hands as aseptically as possible from each PSP and should be properly disposed of aseptically in the normal or contaminated waste container as required by local regulations. Unless the item contains blood or saliva or can release infectious agents it may be locally disposed of in the normal trash. Aseptic disposal into the normal trash means that the contamination of other items, countertops, or equipment should not occur as part of the disposal process. Each PSP plate is then placed into the laser scanner and, within several seconds, the image will be imported into the patient's file in the computer. The PSP scanner must be placed in a low-light area because bright light will cause effacement or degradation of the images on the PSPs. Finally the PSPs need to be erased by exposing them to a bright light and then stored in a reasonably dark place. The final erasure of the PSP is a function often incorporated in the scanner. Because PSPs are very subject to surface scratching, they may usually be reused about 50 times and then discarded. With care in handling the PSPs, a greater number of repeat uses are possible.

Film must also be aseptically transported to the darkroom or automatic processor for development. In the case of automatic processors with daylight loaders, the overgloves or new clean gloves must be worn before passing the hands through the sleeves into the daylight loader where the film packets are opened and the film loaded as aseptically as possible into the processor. Upon completion of film loading into the processor, both the contaminated film wrappers and the gloves must be removed from the daylight loader and properly disposed of according to local regulations. In the case of darkroom processing, the films must be unwrapped and placed onto the hanger clips with gloved hands and then placed into the processing solutions or fed into the automatic processor. Care must be taken if the contaminated gloves from film unwrapping have touched the handle part of the film rack(s) or other parts of the automatic processor. Both the contaminated film wrappers and the gloves must be properly disposed of according to local regulations. This usually means they may be disposed of in the normal trash.

Depending on individual office protocols, the clinical area where the images were taken must be decontaminated as soon as possible or before seating another patient. This means all wraps must be removed and properly disposed of, and other contaminated surfaces on the equipment and countertops must be disinfected. Personnel involved in these procedures must wash their hands thoroughly after degloving and dispose of all personal protective equipment according to the standard protocols (see http://www.cdc.gov/oralhealth/infectioncontrol/guidelines/).

Panoramic and Cephalometric Radiology

In terms of infection control, panoramic and cephalometric imaging require fewer steps compared with intraoral radiology. All panoramic machines have a chin rest and bite stick. A disposable sleeve is placed on the bite block part of the bite stick and barrier material may be placed on the chin rest. These are removed and disposed of by the patient after the exposure. In some offices multiple bite sticks are available such that the bite stick is removed and disinfected or sterilized after image acquisition. For cephalometric imaging, rubber sleeves may be placed on each of the ear rods and discarded after the procedure. The operator does not usually need to wear **personal protective equipment** (PPE) while operating a panoramic machine or taking a cephalometric image or both. PPE in the form of gloves may be worn in special circumstances, for example, if the patient has an infectious skin condition as the head and face may need to be contacted by the operator during the positioning of the patient in the machine. Other PPE, such as a mask, may be used if special problems, such as operator or patient sneezing or coughing, are likely to occur.

Because panoramic x-ray machines can now capture bitewing images with open contacts and include the periapical regions as well as individual periapical examinations, some doctors and staff may prefer this method for the x-ray examination of the patient. A simple bite sleeve and disinfection of the chin rest and side guides are all that are needed under normal circumstances. Also there is no real consideration with respect to decontamination or special handling of the cassette containing the film or PSP because most, if not all, of the panoramic machines capable of producing panoramic bitewing images are equipped with an electronic sensor, therefore no handling or contamination of the sensor is involved in the Pan BW technique.

Cone Beam Computed Tomography (CBCT)

Like panoramic imaging, **CBCT** does not require any special consideration in terms of infection control. Most of today's CBCT machines are either configured like panoramic devices or are on older separate imaging platforms. In either case there may be a bite block and/or a chin rest and head positioning rods that may contact the patient's skin and/or hair. Disposable sleeves may be used on the bite block, which will require gloves for their removal from the machine, or the patient can remove this item and discard it. Gloves can also be used to wipe down the chin rest and head positioning rods with a surface disinfectant. Because there will normally be no blood released from these items, they may be discarded aseptically as normal waste if permitted by local regulations.

Sometimes specially constructed single-use imaging guides are worn intraorally to locate the planned sites of implant placement. After the imaging procedure these may be discarded aseptically into the normal trash as they will not usually be contaminated with or release blood after removal from the mouth. If a saliva-contaminated imaging guide is to be placed on a countertop, a barrier such as a plastic-backed paper napkin may be placed on the countertop before the procedure and discarded with the imaging guide in the normal trash. Alternately, if the countertop becomes contaminated with saliva, surface disinfection can be carried out after the procedure. If the imaging guide is to be retained for later use as a surgical guide, it should be disinfected by soaking it in a liquid disinfectant and stored aseptically in a plastic bag for later reuse. Because most imaging/drilling guides have plastic as the major component, heat sterilization may not be possible. Ethylene oxide gas sterilization should be used for these guides. Ethylene oxide usually requires overnight sterilization. Because the gas is toxic, most doctors do not find it practical for use in their individual dental clinics; however, it is used in some larger clinics or institutions.

SHORT-ANSWER QUESTIONS WITH FIGURES
Instructions

Compare your answer to the correct answer in the Answer Key at the back of the book.

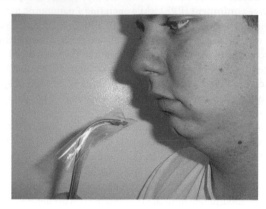

Figure **3-1**   Here we see the essential infection control needs for a healthy patient about to have a bitewing x-ray image taken by a healthy dental assistant. What type of bitewing is this?

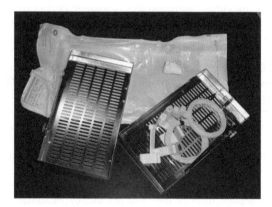

Figure **3-2**   Here we are preparing to have some instruments sterilized.
1. What instruments are these?
2. The instruments are in the bottom half of a specific type of infection control container; what is this container called?
3. In the background there is a plastic bag; most likely, what type of bag is this?
4. The instruments are being prepared for what type of infection control procedure?
5. For what specific type(s) of intraoral images are these instruments used?
6. What are the round rings called?
7. The plastic bag has a clear plastic front side; what is the purpose of this?
8. The plastic bag has a white paperlike material on the back; what is the purpose of this?

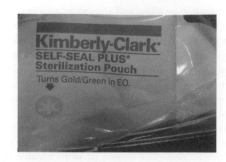

Figure **3-3**
1. This printing can be seen on a sterilization bag also called a pouch; there is an arrow pointing to a symbol. What is this symbol called and what is its purpose?
2. The printing says the following: "turns gold/green in EO." What does EO stand for?

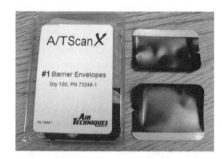

Figure **3-4**
1. On the left is a labeled plastic container. What does A/T stand for?
2. The label says: "#1 Barrier Envelopes"; what are these used for?
3. On the right we see two objects; what are they used for?
4. On the right the top object is smaller than the bottom one; what purpose does this size difference serve?
5. On the edge of the objects on the right what purpose does the "V"-shaped notch serve?
6. On one edge of each of these objects there is a white-colored strip; what purpose does this strip serve?
7. Are any components of this imaging system reusable?
8. Can the contents of these envelopes be sterilized or disinfected?

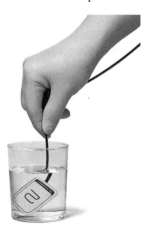

Figure **3-5**   (Figure courtesy of Planmeca USA, Roselle, IL.)
1. What imaging device do we see in this picture?
2. What is the cost range of one of these devices?
3. What is wrong with what this picture is illustrating?
4. Why is this generally wrong?

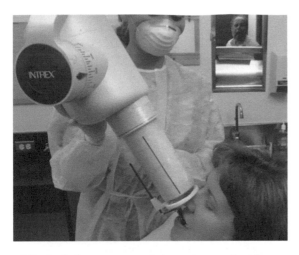

Figure **3-6**   Both the operator and the patient are healthy.
1. How many people are there in this illustration?
2. Identify what infection control elements are wrong in this picture.
3. What infection control liquid can you see in this picture?

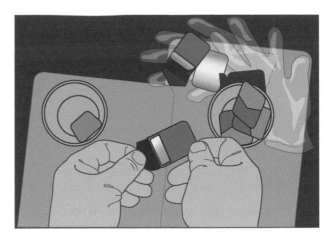

Figure **3-8**   This is a procedure that is being carried out under a safe-light either in a daylight loader or in the darkroom.
1. What procedure is being carried out?
2. What are the two paper cups for?
3. What personal protective equipment is being worn by the operator, if any?
4. Is this PPE contaminated at this stage of processing?

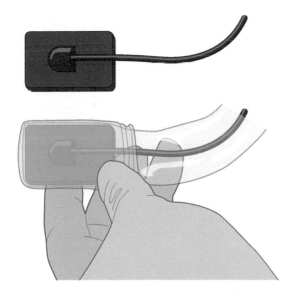

Figure **3-7**   Here we see a sensor with barriers in place.
1. What type of sensor is this?
2. What barriers are being used?

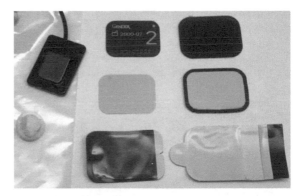

Figure **3-9**   Here we see the barrier needs for two different types of intraoral digital imaging technologies.
1. Left-to-right by vertical row, name the two types of intraoral imaging technologies.
2. On the left name the element(s) of the barrier system and describe the placement of these on the sensor.
3. On the right how many sensors are being illustrated?
4. What are the two objects on the bottom, middle, and right columns of the photo?
5. Which, if any, type of sensor produces the largest image?

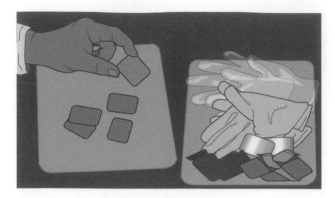

Figure **3-10**   Here we see two illustrations. On the left the hand is ungloved; on the right are discarded materials.

1. Name the correct image receptor technology:
    A. Film
    B. Photostimulable Phosphor Plate (PSP)
    C. Both A & B
    D. Other
2. On the left the ungloved hand is holding the unwrapped image receptor; name this receptor:
    A. Film
    B. PSP
    C. Both A & B
    D. Other.
3. On the right what personal protective barriers are illustrated?
    A. Latex glove
    B. Vinyl overglove
    C. Receptor wrap from the packet
    D. All of the above
    E. Only A and B
4. What location(s) does this set of two images represent?
    A. Daylight loader
    B. Darkroom
    C. Either A or B
    D. None of the above

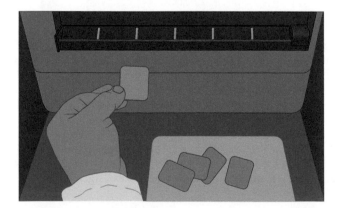

Figure **3-11**   This intraoral x-ray film is being developed in the darkroom.

1. What is the operator doing?
2. Is it appropriate to not be wearing gloves for this part of the procedure?
3. Why is your answer to Number 2 appropriate?
4. Why is the image red-orange in color?

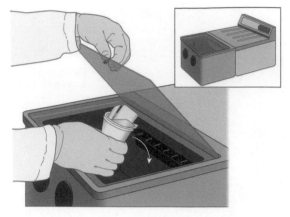

Figure **3-12**   This is a step in the development of intraoral film in an automatic processor outside of the darkroom.

1. What part of the automatic processor is this?
2. Why is the plastic cover orange colored? Won't the film get exposed?
3. How many paper cups are there? Why?
4. What does the operator have on his hands? Why?
5. There seems to be a barrier envelope on each of the film packets. Comment on this.

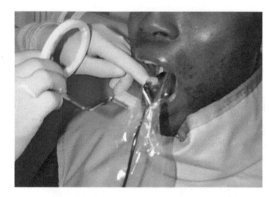

Figure **3-13**   Here we see a digital radiograph about to be placed in the mouth to capture an image.

1. What type of sensor is being used?
2. What is the apparatus attached to the sensor?
3. What does this apparatus do?
4. What region of the mouth is to be imaged?
5. What infection control error has been made here?

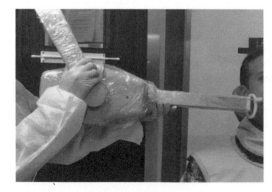

Figure **3-14**

1. What, if anything, is wrong with this image?

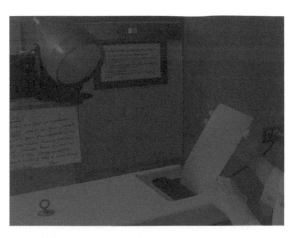

Figure **3-15** Here we see a panoramic film being loaded into an automatic processor.
What is the main problem seen here?

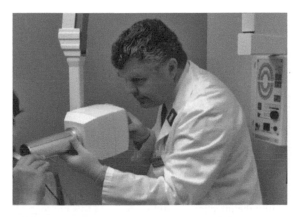

Figure **3-16** Here we see Dr. Langlais working with the first digital intraoral sensor manufactured in France and the supplied French DC-current x-ray machine. This image was taken before the current infection control guidelines. What infection control procedure is missing here?

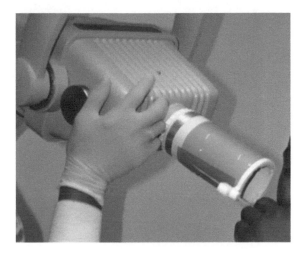

Figure **3-17** What infection control problem(s) do you see here?

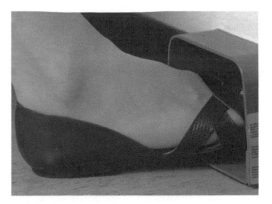

Figure **3-18** Here we see a foot-operated intraoral x-ray device.
1. What is it?
2. What is the advantage in infection control?

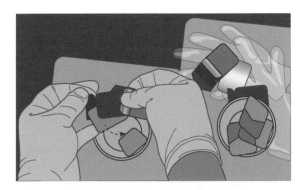

Figure **3-19** The setting here is inside the daylight loader of an x-ray film automatic processor.
1. Exactly what is happening here?
2. What is the shiny material in the left-hand and upper left-hand side of the photo?
3. Are gloves necessary for this step?
4. Is a similar step like this necessary if using PSPs?
5. What about electronic sensors? Are similar precautions needed?

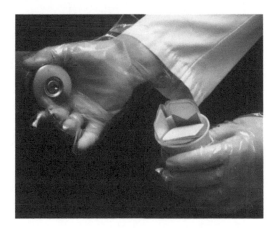

Figure **3-20** Here we see the intermediate step where packets are being transported from the exposure area to another part of the office for further processing.
1. Would this step be necessary if using an electronic sensor?
2. What does Dr. Langlais have on his hands?
3. What is in Dr. Langlais' left hand?
4. What is the colored band on Dr. Langlais' right wrist?

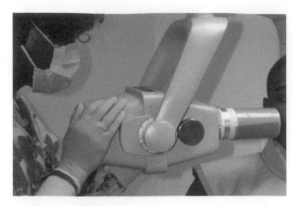

Figure **3-21**   Here we are again; we have a healthy operator and patient. We know the yoke, tube head, and parts of the cone need to be wrapped. What other infection control issue do we see here?

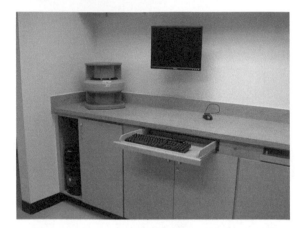

Figure **3-22**   Here we see some digital intraoral x-ray equipment.
1.   What is the item in the corner on the counter?
2.   What is its function?
3.   What is the purpose of the computer?

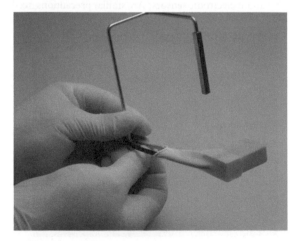

Figure **3-23**
1.   What is this?
2.   Name the infection control error.

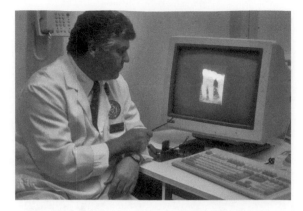

Figure **3-24**   This case is just for fun as it is the radiologic equivalent of looking at a picture of a Model "T" Ford, and I don't mean Dr. Langlais...though you may have thought so!!!
1.   Can you guess what is being viewed by Dr. Langlais in this image?

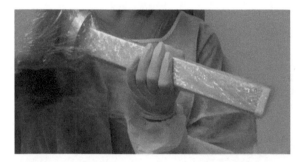

Figure **3-25**
1.   Identify the infection control elements in this photograph.
2.   Which infection control item shown is not normally necessary in this circumstance?

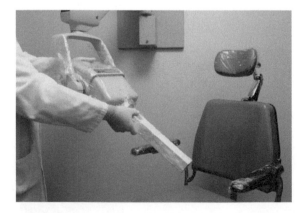

Figure **3-26**   Name the infection control items seen in this photograph.

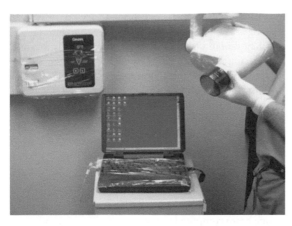

Figure **3-27** What is a laptop doing in this clinic scenario and is it adequately protected?

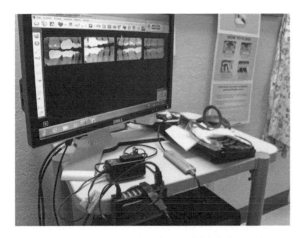

Figure **3-28** Here we see an intraoperatory imaging area that was prepared for the taking of a photographic display. Actually Dr. Langlais' bitewings can be seen on the monitor. The power plug for the power supply for the electronic sensor and other items are on the table for the picture and the capture computer is on the floor beneath the table. If we were to set up to take an x-ray, what infection control items would we need here?

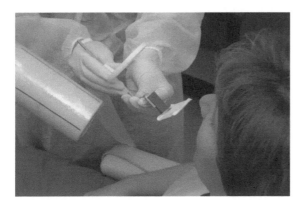

Figure **3-29** We are taking this periapical PSP image in the dental operatory, after which the patient is scheduled to have a periodontal procedure. As such are there any infection control omissions in this picture?

MULTIPLE-CHOICE QUESTIONS WITHOUT FIGURES

Instructions

Please select the best answer and check your selection with the correct answer in the Answer Key at the back of the book.

1. Regarding infection control, film-based intraoral imaging requires _____ precautions & procedures as digital imaging.
   A. The same
   B. Less
   C. More
   D. More or less

2. Before taking a series of intraoral radiographs, which patient-related procedure is recommended?
   A. Apply an aseptic bib or apron
   B. Don gloves
   C. Cover tube head parts
   D. An antiseptic mouthwash

3. Regarding intraoral x-ray procedures, which recommended infection control procedure(s) is (are) the *most* important?
   A. Placing barrier material on the yoke, tube head, and cone of the x-ray machine
   B. Covering the arm and headrest areas of the chair
   C. Using a disposable film/sensor-holding device
   D. Administering the preprocedural antiseptic mouthwash

4. In terms of intraoral x-ray imaging, which method requires the *most* infection control procedures?
   A. Digital imaging
   B. Analog film-based imaging
   C. Digital PSP-based imaging
   D. Infection control is the same for all intraoral imaging

5. Intraoral film is supplied prewrapped:
   A. However, applying an additional barrier, such as a finger cot, is recommended
   B. Therefore additional barriers over the film packets are not necessary
   C. Asking the patient to place the film and bite block in the mouth is a recommended precaution
   D. The film packet should be disinfected before opening it

6. When using electronic sensors it is recommended to:
   A. Apply a finger cot over the sensor
   B. Place a vinyl sleeve over the finger cot to protect the wire
   C. First place a vinyl sleeve over the sensor and wire, then slip a finger cot over the sensor
   D. Place barrier material on both the sensor and the sensor holding/aiming device

7. Which intraoral method requires the fewest infection control procedures?
   A. Film-based imaging
   B. Using an electronic sensor
   C. Using PSP plates
   D. All of the above require the same infection control procedures

8. In terms of bitewing imaging, which method requires the fewest infection control procedures?
   A. Film-based imaging
   B. Using an electronic sensor
   C. Using PSP plates
   D. Panoramic bitewings

9. If we are using intraoral film or PSP plates it will be necessary to:
   A. Aseptically transport the films or PSP plates to the processing area or scanner
   B. Aseptically remove the film or PSP plates from the supplied or added barrier envelopes
   C. Aseptically collect the film packets or barrier envelopes and place them in the trash
   D. All of the above

10. When acquiring a panoramic image, whether it is a full Pan image, a Pan BW, or a Pan periapical image, regardless whether it is a film-based analog or digital pan image using a pan PSP plate or an electronic pan sensor:
    A. Usually, the only infection control procedure is to apply a sleeve over the bite block and ask the patient to remove this after the exposure and place it in the trash
    B. Gloves should be worn if the patient has a potentially contagious skin condition
    C. A mask should be worn by the operator if there is coughing or sneezing
    D. All of the above

11. If an electronic sensor has been used to acquire an intraoral image, which of the following is true?
    A. It should he heat sterilized after use
    B. It may be disinfected by soaking in a disinfectant solution
    C. Barriers are removed and the sensor is wiped with a disinfectant solution
    D. All of the above

12. In order to transfer intraoral film and PSP sensors from the imaging area to the image processing area and into the processor, they should be transported aseptically. This means:
    A. Placing them in a clean paper cup or similar vessel
    B. Donning a vinyl over-glove to carry the film or PSP sensors
    C. Opening the film packets or barrier envelopes aseptically
    D. All of the above

13. Hands should be washed:
    A. Before gloving
    B. After degloving
    C. Upon discovery of a glove tear or perforation
    D. All of the above

14. If cone beam computed tomography (CBCT) is available in the office, under normal circumstances the infection control protocol is the same as for panoramic radiology except:
    A. Contaminated parts of a CBCT machine must be fully sterilized
    B. Greater machine contamination is possible due to the more elaborate bite block system
    C. Gloves are recommended when operating a CBCT device
    D. All of the above
    E. None of the above

15. If a CBCT scan is obtained with the patient wearing an imaging guide, the infection control protocol is:
    A. The operator must wear gloves as the imaging guide will need to be properly positioned in the mouth
    B. Countertops may be covered with plastic-backed paper or the surface disinfected if the contaminated imaging guide is to be placed here during or after the procedure
    C. Because the CBCT machine is often controlled by the computer, the operator must deglove and wash hands before making the exposure
    D. All of the above
    E. A and C only

Chapter 4

Digital Imaging

Goals

To understand digital image acquisition
To understand the basics of digital image processing

Learning Objectives

1. Explain basic sensor differences
2. Recognize clinical technique errors in digital image acquisition procedures
3. Know how to use ring locator devices with sensors
4. Learn how photostimulable phosphor plate (PSP) scanners are used
5. Explain PSP erasure procedures
6. Identify various digital image processing tools
7. Recognize the effects of image processing on the original image
8. Analyze digital image acquisition and processing errors

BASIC CONCEPTS OF DIGITAL IMAGING

1. **The computer:** A computer with digital imaging software is needed. Its function is to receive and view the digital image, identify the image as to orientation and patient/date data, process the image if needed, store the image, and transmit the image to other offices or third party payers. Safeguards must be in place to protect the patient's privacy as outlined by the **Health Insurance Portability and Accountability Act** (HIPAA) law that came into effect April 14, 2003. The computer can be a laptop, a wall-mounted type, a display-only monitor connected to a computer by a wire or wireless networking, or a full computer setup in the treatment room. To get a fast, flawless imaging setup, the computer will need at least 512 megabytes (Mb) of RAM (random access memory) and a fast processor with 2.5 gigahertz (GHz) speed, as well as adequate temporary storage in the 80-gigabyte (GB) range. Further high-capacity hard drive storage and a server will be needed for later storage, archiving, and retrieval of the images.

2. **The sensor:** Sensors are either wired or not wired. The wired type can be a CCD (charge coupled device) or a CMOS (complementary metal oxide sensor), which transfers the image instantaneously to the computer at the moment of image acquisition (analogous to exposing the film and developing it). The CMOS type is now available in a wireless format. The filmlike wireless type is called the PSP (photostimulable phosphor plate). The exposed plate or sensor (looks a lot like a piece of film) must then be scanned in a laser scanner, which then transfers the image into the computer.

3. **The scanner:** A laser scanner is needed only for PSP-type sensors. Depending on brand and model, some scanners may have faster scanning times.

4. **The imaging software:** Once the image is in the computer, the software allows the user to process the image. This means the original image can be altered. For security, most software systems do not allow the user to process the original image so it can be later retrieved if needed by third parties such as insurance carriers or courts of law.

5. **Image processing:** The original image can be copied and then altered by processing to enhance its appearance for diagnostics or to highlight a feature for patient education. Some basic processing options (algorithms) include: rotate or flip the image to get it properly oriented on the computer screen because the sensor cannot distinguish left, right, up, or down; lighten/darken the image (histogram shift); change the contrast (histogram stretch); use filters to sharpen the image, smooth edges, or remove noise; zoom, which magnifies a selected area; reverse the image so that it looks like a negative (everything black becomes white, and white become black) (histogram reverse); emboss, which produces a 3-D–like look; colorize all or a portion (e.g., a carious lesion or the inferior alveolar canal); and many other options, including some of those just mentioned that are known by different terms to make the individual brands appear different or unique.

6. **Image characteristics:**
   • **Spatial resolution** is really how clean and sharp the image is. It is a function of having small pixels in the 20- to

40-micron size range and lots of them (megapixels). Spatial resolution is expressed in line pairs per millimeter (lp/mm). Digital intraoral x-ray systems are capable of image resolution in excess of 20 lp/mm. The human eye can discern somewhere between 12 and 14 lp/mm. Most intraoral films are in the 11- to 12-lp/mm range. Most high-definition monitors are limited to 8 to 10 lp/mm. Most software systems keep only the best 8 lp/mm. The more lp/mm, the greater is the need for storage room in the computer or server. Resolution is limited to the lowest common denominator in the system; thus a system of 8 to 10 lp/mm represents the most current practical system.

- **Gray scale resolution** is how many shades of gray are in the image, also known as contrast or bit depth. The imaging system is capable of capturing and separating literally thousands of shades of gray. Contrast is expressed in bits. A 1-bit image has only two shades (pure black and white—the darkest and lightest shades of gray in the imaging scale) and is expressed as "1 to the power of 1." A 2-bit image is expressed as "1 to the power of 2," or $1 \times 2 = 2 \times 2 = 4$ shades of gray. A 3-bit image has 8 shades of gray, or $1 \times 2 = 2 \times 2 = 4 \times 2 = 8$. A 4-bit image has 16 shades of gray, and so on. In an 8-bit image, there are 256 shades of gray and this is the standard. However, systems capable of up to 12 bits, or 4098 shades of gray and more, presently exist. The more bits in the image, the greater are the storage needs for the images. The human eye of the person on the street can commonly separate 16 shades of gray; a photographer or radiologist can separate about 25 shades of gray; and under laboratory conditions, the maximum for the unaided eye to separate is somewhere around 64 shades of gray. The image itself usually does not occupy the entire gray scale as can be seen by viewing the histogram. The image may be confined to about 30 shades of gray. For best results it is desirable to have a system capable of at least 256 shades of gray. This way there is space on the scale to lighten or darken the image (histogram shift) or spread the shades of gray over a bigger part of the scale (histogram stretch). Remember, 8 bits or 256 shades of gray represents the limit of most monitors.

7. **Image viewing:** The image can be viewed on a monitor, a computer screen, printed on photo-quality paper, or printed on a filmlike acetate sheet.

8. **Sensor reuse:** All sensor types can be reused almost indefinitely. However, the PSP types need to be "erased" by exposing them to a bright light for a few moments or minutes before reuse.

9. **X-ray equipment:** Because of the shorter exposure times needed in digital imaging, the constant potential DC-type x-ray machine with exposure increments in 1/100 seconds is the most desirable. PSP sensors are the most adaptable to older AC machine designs because they are not very sensitive to exposure variations. CCD and CMOS sensors can also be used; however, noise from too little exposure and blooming from too much exposure will be more prone to occur as timer increments will be in impulses of 60 impulses per second. Sometimes the first one to three impulses produce varying amounts of radiation, especially in older machines, and older machines cannot have an exposure time in increments of less than ⅟₆₀ of a second.

10. **The next generation:** You saw it here first. There will be more use of wireless CCD or CMOS sensors than are currently on the market. These were first developed in Israel for gastrointestinal imaging with the so-called "pill cam." You will use a lightweight, handheld, miniature x-ray machine configured much like a digital camera. The wireless sensor will send the image to the back of the camera, as with current digital cameras, or to a palmheld computer or tablet to see if it is okay. The image will then either be saved in the portable x-ray machine itself or be sent electronically to a palmheld minicomputer or tablet currently on the market. At this point and using the wireless network, the image can be downloaded to any of the wall-mounted, flat computer screens, which will also display any photographs and the chart information, all of which are currently available. Further chart entries will be made by voice recognition software right in the operatory or anywhere else in the office where a microphone pick-up is installed … but of course you knew that. During all phases of treatment, the patient will have in place virtual reality goggles and will be able to choose from menus by locking on to an icon in the screen with the gaze of the retina of the eye; this feature exists right now in some video cameras. In this way, the patient can randomly access HIPAA chart information during treatment, or he or she can tune in to the video camera mounted on the handpiece or nearby to watch the procedure; watch a movie, a cartoon, or the news; or simply tune in to the virtual Carnegie Hall and listen to favorite music selections. Just about everything exists now, and it's coming soon to the dental office! Who can be anything but excited about these probabilities? Yep, it's great to be able to see into the future, though such writings may cause the author to be ridiculed and even publicly challenged by more nearsighted colleagues. Oh and by the way … **protective aprons** and "D" speed film will become a thing of the past!

> **NOTE TO STUDENTS:**
> You have just finished a grueling session on digital imaging. You may even have a headache or be tempted to quit and watch a little TV. Take a break, listen to a little music, get some exercise, or have a tasty snack, then come on back. We promise the rest is a lot easier.

DIGITAL IMAGING UPDATE

The development of digital imaging has gone through several phases since its introduction in dental offices. With the advent of electronic office management software, including appointment logs, patient reminders, and imaging equipment, many practitioners also adopted the electronic dental chart. Along with the existing chart records, clinical photos, and film-based x-ray images such as intraorals, pans, and cephalometric x-rays needed to be converted to a digital format such that these images could be stored in the electronic chart.

In order to accomplish this, an ordinary scanner could be used to digitize any printed paper or chart, printed clinical photos, or even existing *printed* x-rays or photos in color or in black and white formats as required. However, film-based color slides and radiographs needed to be scanned with a special type of scanner equipped with a transparency adapter, which is not normally a capacity of most printer-scanner-fax machines. In order to accomplish this special task, dental offices could choose to contract out the digitization of existing records or they could do it themselves, which could be a very time-consuming task and would require the purchase of a scanner with a transparency adapter. As a further option, dentists could keep the existing records in their original format and start anew with the digital records. Finally, an option was to digitize only the most recent or selected parts of the record and store the remaining nondigital records for a period of time as is dictated by state or provincial laws.

Once the initial digitization options were selected and accomplished, many offices continued with a kind of hybrid system. With this approach, the new digital imaging equipment was introduced in phases. For example, a digital camera could be first acquired so that clinical photos could be stored in the electronic chart, but the film-based radiographs continued to be stored in a physical chart. Sometime thereafter intraoral digital imaging could be introduced, and following that, the digital **panoramic and/or cephalometric x-rays** could be acquired. At this point all imaging would have been converted to a digital format and stored in the digital chart.

Meanwhile new practitioners could opt to buy an existing practice. Most likely the majority of new-graduate practice buyers would have been trained on digital equipment including the digital chart in the dental, hygiene, or assisting training program. Other practitioners seeking to buy existing practices may have retired from or left institutional positions such as corporate dental clinics, military service, educational institutions, or hospitals. In many of these instances, the buyer or new employee, such as a dentist associate, hygienist, or assistant, will have only worked with digital charts and/or imaging equipment. Thus any practitioner wishing to sell a practice or hire such individuals would be at an advantage if the office has already been converted to a digital format.

One of the problems with converting to digital format or installing digital equipment from the get-go is the cables. Essentially, the office will have to have its own internal electronic network. To accomplish, this CAT-5 or similar cables will need to be run invisibly to connect all of the digital equipment and computers to the network. The network not only delivers new information or images to the chart, but also allows almost instantaneous access to previous entries, photos, or radiographs. While the need for a network is something most folks understand, there can be real trouble if the cabling is not properly installed. For instance, cables cannot pass near fluorescent lights as they will generate interference; also cables cannot be bent at right angles as this may interfere with the streaming of data. Therefore while many may think it is better to hire an outside contractor to install the cables, it is much more desirable to have the dental dealer first custom design the cable network and second install it (Figure 4-1A). On the other hand, the wireless transmission of data is coming of age. Even now a digital panoramic image or panoramic bitewing, which is taken in one part of the office by a dental assistant or hygienist, can be immediately viewed by the dentist in another part of the office on a tablet or even on a cell phone. In addition, cable television can now be transmitted to any television set in the office within range of the cable or satellite receiver.

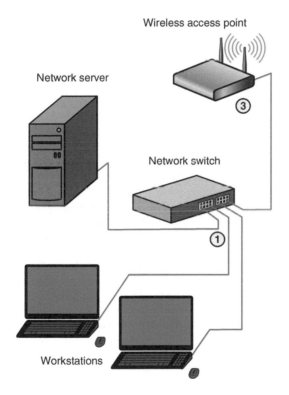
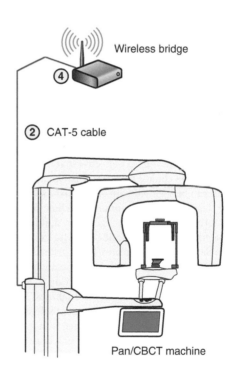

① All computers are networked using cables

② Pan/CBCT Ethernet is connected to a wireless bridge using CAT-5 cable supplied with x-ray

③ Wireless access point is connected to network switch

④ Pan/CBCT machine communicates wirelessly with network through bridge and access point

A

Figure **4-1A**   This is an example of a digital network with wired and wireless components.

One last problem that needs to be mentioned is where to safely store all of this digital data. Additionally, HIPAA requires that patient information be stored safely from robbery or vandalism, fire, flooding, or any other type of loss. Normally the electronic data will need to be stored in the office in a physical device, usually a server that can be expanded by adding more hard drives. At the end of each day, the office will need to send all of this data off site into a secure "cloud," which in reality, ends up being stored by a contractor or provider in at least three physical locations to ensure the safety, security, and retrieval of the data. The next day all of the electronic patient-related data is downloaded from the "cloud" for use. Another option is to download all of the patient data onto a "secure-encrypted" portable storage media.

At the time of publication of this text, all of the above types of dental practice exist with more and more offices being completely digital with each advancing year. In the following chapters, specific topics, including digital intraoral, panoramic, cephalometric and cone beam computed tomography (CBCT), will be discussed.

The Electronic Office

With the introduction of electronic office management software for appointments and billing, many practitioners have adopted the electronic dental chart. Along with the existing clinical photos, film-based x-ray images such as intraorals, pans, and cephalometric images can be converted to a digital format so that these images can be stored in the electronic chart. In order to do this an ordinary scanner could be used to digitize any clinical photos in color or even x-rays in black and white. However, as was previously stated, film-based color slides and all radiographs must be scanned with a special type of scanner equipped with a transparency adapter.

If we consider the intermediate stage between an analog office and offices with earlier digital imaging equipment, then several possibilities are actually still useful and very effective in today's practice. For example, Polaroid-type clinical pictures of patients and of the oral cavity and teeth can be scanned with an ordinary scanner into a digital patient file. The film-based panoramic machine can be converted to a digital format by simply changing the standard panoramic film cassette for a machine-specific cassette containing a reusable photostimulable phosphor plate (PSP). After the panoramic exposure, the PSP is scanned with a laser scanner and the resulting digital panoramic image can be viewed on a computer screen, be digitally processed (e.g., changing the brightness and contrast), and then the image can be stored in the patient's digital chart. The exposed PSP plate must then be erased either with a separate device consisting of a special light source, such as a laser scanner, or be erased by the same machine after the plate is scanned to obtain the digital image. In this way, panoramic PSP plates can be reused many times over if they are handled with care. For intraoral imaging, PSP plates are available in the same sizes as intraoral film, such as children's size "0" and adult sizes "1" and "2," as well as occlusal PSP plates. The intraoral PSP plates are subject to scratching and surface wear; thus they may only be reused about 40 to 50 times before discarding. In the case of cephalometric imaging, the cephalometric film cassettes can be replaced with PSP plates. All PSP plate formats can be scanned by a single scanner, which is designed to scan all PSP plate sizes. Smaller scanners are available if only smaller plate sizes are used.

At present most current digital x-ray equipment consists of electronic sensors for image capture. The advantage of these sensors is that the digital image can be viewed immediately without the need for scanning as is required for the PSP plates. Earlier on most of the sensors were charge coupled devices (CCDs). These were capable of producing very nice quality digital images. However, the manufacturing of CCD sensors was expensive, as was the purchase price. Furthermore, CCD sensors were very delicate and were subject to internal damage with rough or careless handling. Soon after the introduction of the CCD sensors, an older technology using the complementary metal oxide sensor (CMOS) was refined such that the manufacture was less costly and the image quality was comparable to CCD. One principle that applies to sensors is that the larger the sensor, the more expensive it is. Thus for panoramic and cephalometric imaging, the CMOS sensor was the most practical and is currently the most popular technology. The CMOS sensor is used on most current panoramic and pancephalometric machines. One problem with intraoral CCD and CMOS sensors is that they cannot be heat sterilized or soaked in a liquid disinfectant. Both of these procedures can result in damage to the internal components either due to heat damage or leakage of liquid disinfecting products. Thus these intraoral sensors need to be covered with a plastic sleeve to protect the wire, and on top of this, a rubber finger cotlike sheath is applied to the sensor itself. After use the sensor can be wiped carefully with alcohol or another disinfectant before reuse as was illustrated in Chapter 3.

The panoramic machine has become the base imaging unit for not only standard panoramic imaging but also for cephalometric (CEPH) and CBCT applications. The CBCT-equipped machines may have a flat panel silicone-type sensor for the CBCT function, which can also be used for the panoramic and cephalometric functions. (Note: Chapter 12 is devoted to CBCT imaging). In addition, the panoramic machine can now be programmed to capture panoramic bitewings (pan BWs) as well as panoramic-generated periapicals (pan PAs). The pan PAs generally consist of partial pan exposures whereby the user can select a small area only. In so doing, the four-bladed collimator in conjunction with the timing of the pan exposure at the selected anatomic region results in a partial pan exposure about as small as one or several periapical images or images of intermediate sizes between the small periapical size to the full pan exposure. Panoramic bitewings (pan BWs) is an incredible new technology that is described in detail in Chapter 9. Essentially, the pan BW is an image of the posterior teeth as well as the canines, sometimes the laterals with the corresponding periapical regions, and with the interproximal contacts open.

The newest panoramic sensor has been introduced in the United States on a limited number of machines and brands. This new sensor was the subject of Dr. Langlais' Ph.D. study completed in 2014 and represents a giant leap forward in terms of dental imaging potential. The sensor has been applied to standard panoramic imaging in Japan. It has been introduced for CBCT applications in the United States and other parts of the world. The new sensor is called a cadmium telluride photon-counting (CdTePC) sensor. The primary characteristic of this sensor is that it can capture and separate low, intermediate, and high energy photons into separate energy "bins" at a very fast rate. This means several things. First, the radiation doses will be significantly lower than for CCD, CMOS, and flat panel sensors. Currently digital sensors lower the dose by about 50% for most applications. The CdTePC sensor has the potential for further lowering of the doses of digital panoramic machines (i.e., several orders of magnitude) while having clinical utility for diverse image capture including Pans, pan BWs, pan PAs, pan CEPHs and pan CBCT imaging. Applications that address "imaging gently for children" will especially benefit from the significantly lower doses. In CBCT it is possible, and in fact probable, that hard and soft tissue windows will be available and bone density measurement applications may rival current methods including those of medical CT and DXA. For the pan BW equipped with tomosynthesis and operator usable software, any overlapped contacts will be capable of being opened after the exposure. WOW!!!

In summary, these new technologies will permit the dental practitioner to not only take advantage of new, improved versions of traditional dental radiographic applications, but we may also embrace these new functions that have the potential to truly expand the scope of dental x-ray imaging diagnostic information acquisition never seen or available before. Adopting these new developments will fully benefit our patients of all ages with their various routine and special needs, including the call for "imaging gently for children."

SHORT ANSWER QUESTIONS WITH FIGURES

Instructions

Compare your answer to the correct answer in the Answer Key at the back of the book.

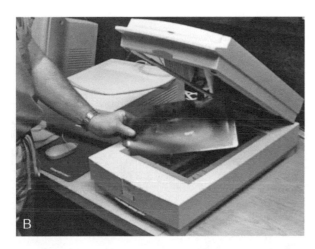

Figure **4-1B**   Here we see a panoramic radiograph being placed in a device in order to digitize it.
1.   How is the functioning of this device controlled?
2.   What is this device called?
3.   What unique feature must this device have in order to electronically reproduce this pan radiograph into the computer?
4.   Is this unique feature on the top or on the bottom of the device?
5.   Must this process be done in conditions of reduced light?

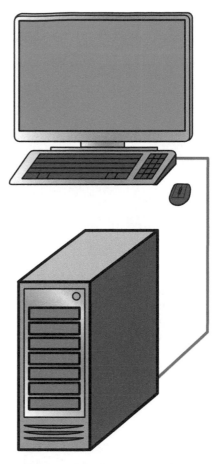

Figure **4-2**   The function of the device attached to the keyboard and monitor is to store all of the dental office digital information.
1.   What is this device called?
2.   Why is it needed?
3.   On the front of the device there are seven similar-appearing rectangular areas resembling drawers with slots. What exactly is in these drawers?

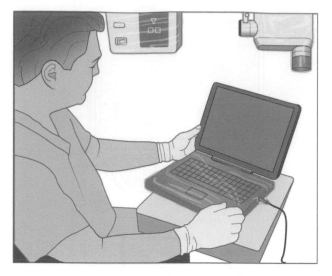

Figure **4-3**   Here we see Dr. Langlais with a laptop computer that is plugged into a nearby electrical receptacle. He is preparing to take a digital intraoral radiograph.
1.   What item of equipment appears to be missing?
2.   Does the infection control appear to be adequate?

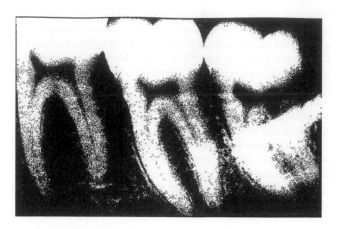

Figure **4-5**   This is a 2-bit image.
1.   How many shades of gray are there in this image?

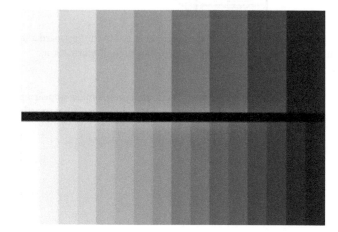

Figure **4-4**   These images are of two different aluminum step wedges.
1.   What term describes the number of shades of gray being displayed in an image?
2.   How would you express numerically the number of shades of gray in the top and bottom images?
3.   Which is more diagnostic?
4.   Which image involves the largest file size in the computer?

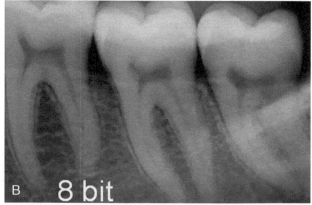
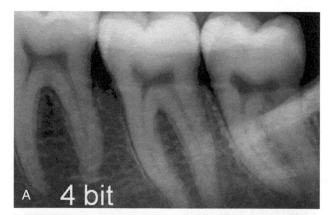

Figure **4-6**   The bit depths of these images are 4 bit and 8 bit as labeled.
1.   Can you see any difference(s) between these two images?

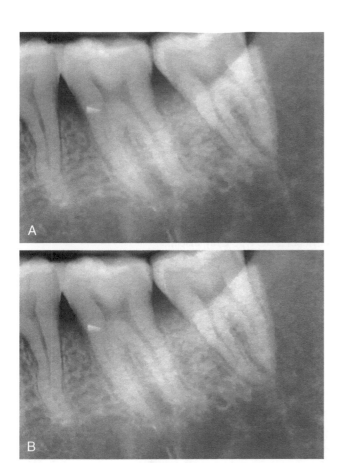

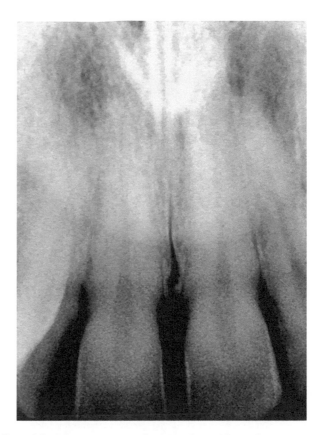

Figure **4-7**   If Figure A is an 8-bit image and B is a 24-bit image, what is the most important difference concerning these two images?

Figure **4-8**   This is a periapical image taken with an electronic sensor, and the image can be described as very "speckled-looking."
1.   What term used in digital imaging best describes the appearance of this image?
2.   What is the cause of this appearance?

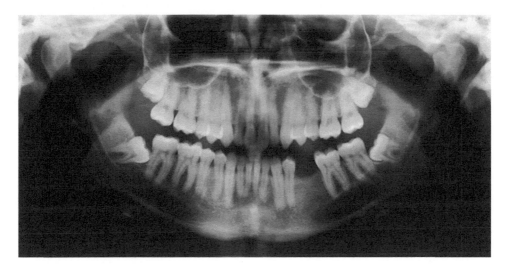

Figure **4-9**   This is an early digital panoramic image. In the image, areas of the ramus and mandibular body bilaterally appear "blacked out."
1.   What term used in digital imaging describes the appearance of this image?
2.   What is the cause of this appearance?

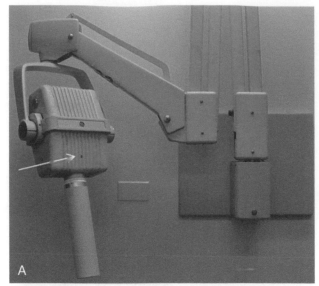

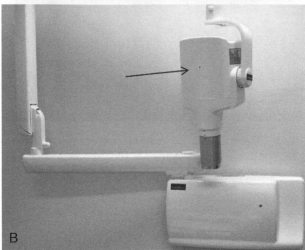

A

B

Figure **4-10** An alternating current (AC) machine is seen in A while B features a direct current (DC) model. Almost all newer machines are of the DC type.
1. List four major advantages of the DC type of intraoral x-ray machine.
2. A and B each have an arrow pointing to a small spot on the tube head; what does this small spot indicate?

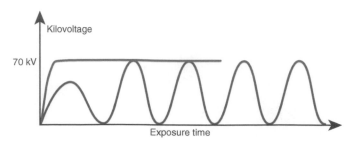

AC Time: 1/60 (1/50) sec. (1impulse (1/60 sec) = 16.6 ms)
DC Time: 1/100 & 1/1000 sec.

Figure **4-11** Looking at the diagram, answer the following questions.
Why does a DC-type x-ray machine:
1. Deliver about a 20%-less dose?
2. Result in less noise in the digital images?

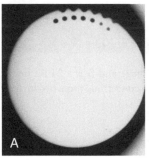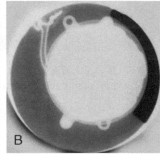

A

B

Figure **4-12** The object of this question is to demonstrate the differences in the way radiation is produced in AC units (A) vs. DC machines (B). In A, a metal spinning top with one hole and one groove at the edge is placed on a film or PSP and is exposed. In B, a battery-powered motorized spinning top is placed on a film or PSP and is exposed. The exposure times are eight impulses AC (A) and 0.330 sec DC (B).
1. What do these two images tell us about AC vs. DC technology and these two machines in particular?
2. Study the two images and see if you can identify the unit that is not working properly.

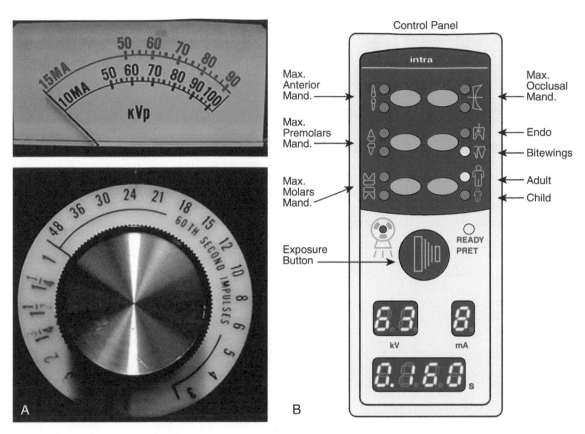

Figure **4-13**   Please study the pictures of the controls for each of two different types of intraoral x-ray units.
1.   What type of machine uses exposure times in 60ths of a second?
2.   For what type of patient and image is the DC machine set?
3.   Can the AC machine be set for 8 mA?
4.   If both machines were set at 63 kV and the same mA and exposure time, which one:
     A.   Would deliver the most radiation dose?
     B.   Would cause the most noise in the digital image?

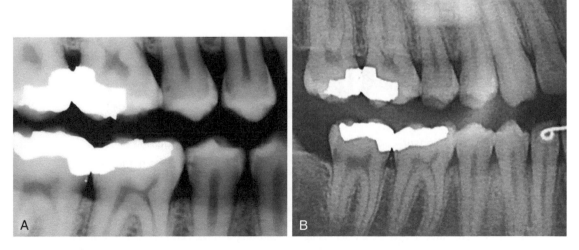

Figure **4-14**   Figure A is an electronic sensor bitewing and Figure B is a cropped panoramic bitewing, both of which were taken at the same appointment.
1.   Compare and contrast the interproximal caries lesions present or absent on the sensor bitewing vs. the pan bitewing
2.   Can you explain the reason for your findings?
Note: See Chapter 9 for more information on panoramic bitewings.

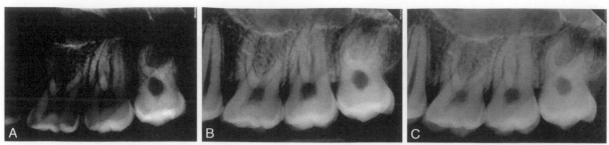

Figure **4-15**   A dental practice may own several brands or generations of intraoral x-ray machines and sensors of different brands, all of which have different effects on the digital image quality. Here we see examples of such possible differences in image quality. There are three factors that affect the ultimate diagnostic quality of the digital image.

1.   Can you name these three factors?

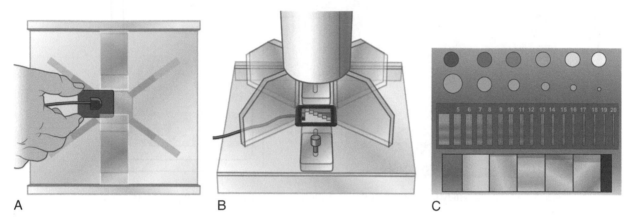

Figure **4-16**   Digital image quality assurance (QA) phantom (more info: dentalimagingconsultants. com). A: The sensor is positioned under the phantom; B: the QA imaging plate outlined in black within the phantom is being imaged; C: is an enlargement of the QA imaging plate. The goal is to obtain the most diagnostic image at the lowest x-ray dose for each machine-sensor combination in use.

1.   If there are three image quality factors consisting of: (1) dynamic range, (2) contrast detail, and (3) spatial resolution, how can each of these be determined using the appropriate row in the above phantom?

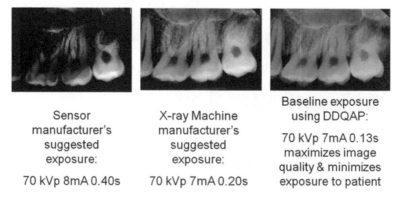

| Sensor manufacturer's suggested exposure: 70 kVp 8mA 0.40s | X-ray Machine manufacturer's suggested exposure: 70 kVp 7mA 0.20s | Baseline exposure using DDQAP: 70 kVp 7mA 0.13s maximizes image quality & minimizes exposure to patient |

Figure **4-17**   The three images were taken using the following settings: Left image: Sensor manufacturer's suggested exposure: 70 kVp, 8 mA, 0.40 sec. Middle image: X-ray tube head manufacturer's suggested exposure: 70 kVp, 7 mA, 0.20 sec. Right image: Dental Digital Quality Assurance Phantom (DDQAP) exposure setting: 70 kVp, 7 mA, 0.13 sec.

1.   Compare the baseline exposure using the DDQAP quality assurance device with the exposure settings suggested by the sensor manufacturer and x-ray tube head manufacturer then comment on the utility of the DDQAP tool.

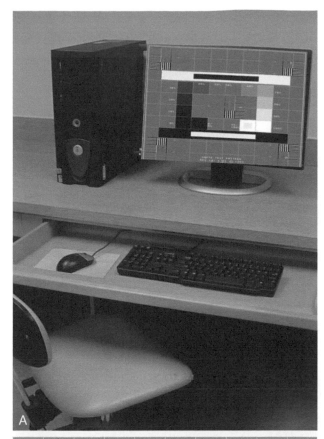

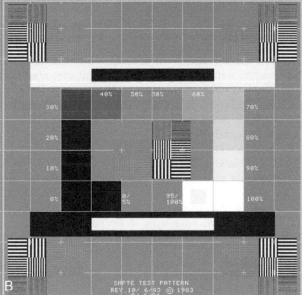

Figure **4-18** An important factor in digital imaging consists of monitor quality. After everything has been done relative to having x-ray machines and sensors optimally calibrated, the diagnostic yield of these devices can be affected by the ability of the monitor to optimally display fine image details as acquired by the sensor.
1. How can monitor image display quality be tested? Hint: The above two illustrations deal with this topic.

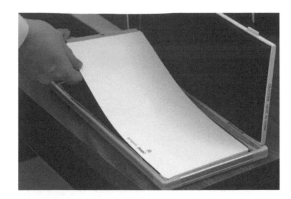

Figure **4-19** Here we see a type of digital imaging plate being loaded into a cassette.
1. What type of x-ray machine is this cassette assembly used for?
2. Exactly what object (device) is being loaded into the cassette?
3. What intermediate step is needed after the exposure before the image can be viewed?
4. Before taking another exposure with the above cassette assembly, what must be done to the object (device) being placed into the cassette?

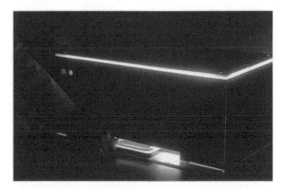

Figure **4-20** This is a photograph of a required procedure associated with a certain type of panoramic digital imaging.
1. What type of digital panoramic imaging does this photograph represent?
2. What procedure is being illustrated here?

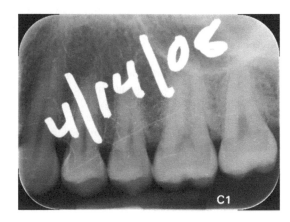

Figure **4-21** Here we see an intraoral image.
1. What standard size of image is this?
2. If this is a digital image, how was it acquired?
3. Why would a written date as seen here be placed in the image?
4. Why was all of the above done to this imaging device?

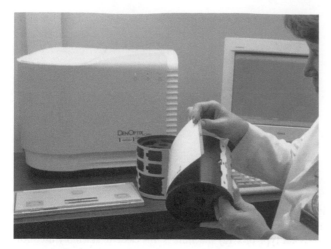

Figure **4-22**   Here we see a setup for viewing a digital image.
1. What type of digital imaging system is this?
2. Exactly what is happening in the picture?

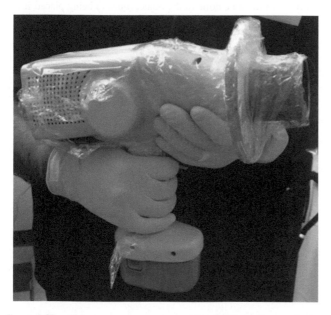

Figure **4-23**   Here we can see a newer type of intraoral x-ray device.
1. Because the device is not attached to the wall, by what term would you refer to this type of x-ray machine, keeping in mind this feature?
2. The blue part just below the handle is a rechargeable battery. Could such a low-powered x-ray machine be capable of properly exposing an intraoral image?
3. Because the operator holds this device while exposing the radiograph, is he or she subject to more exposure to radiation than by a wall-mounted unit with the exposure switch outside of the room or behind a barrier?
4. What is wrong with the setup of the machine in this picture?

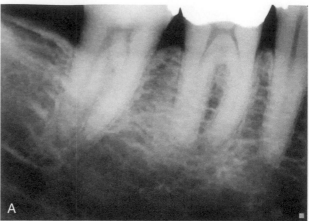

7/29/05, BL, Gendex GX-770, 70kVp, 7mA, 12 imp = 200 mS

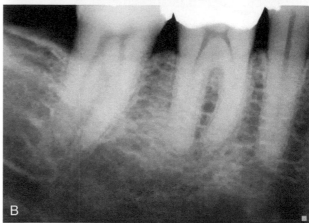

7/29/05, BL, Aribex Nomad, 60 kV, 2.3 mA, 120 mS

Figure **4-24**   As can be seen from the labeling under each image, A was taken with a wall-mounted AC-type intraoral x-ray machine; B was taken with a portable x-ray machine. The sensor in both cases was a complementary metal oxide sensor (CMOS). Each image is seen as acquired, except both were placed in a third-party software to increase the contrast.
1. Visually can you see any difference(s) between the two images?
2. Look at the labeling beneath each of the images. Compare the kV, mA, and exposure times expressed in milliseconds (ms); from this can you deduce which system provided the least x-ray dose to the patient?
3. Can you list some advantages of the portable type of x-ray machine?

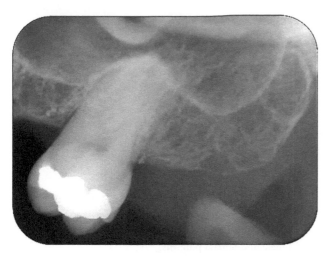

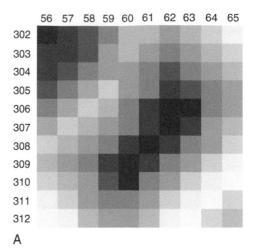

A

| | 56 | 57 | 58 | 59 | 60 | 61 | 62 | 63 | 64 | 65 |

86	87	89	95	110	110	105	110	115	120
87	87	89	105	110	105	95	105	110	115
87	89	95	105	105	95	89	95	105	110
89	95	110	115	105	95	87	89	95	105
95	110	115	110	95	87	86	86	95	105
105	115	110	105	95	87	86	87	105	110
115	110	105	95	87	86	87	95	105	115
110	105	95	87	86	87	95	105	115	120
115	110	105	89	86	95	105	115	120	135
120	115	105	95	95	105	115	120	135	115
135	120	110	105	105	110	120	135	115	110

B

Figure **4-25** Previously in this chapter, we have illustrated several examples of a step wedge for use to determine image quality, particularly with respect to the number of perceptible shades of gray (contrast). Ultimately there needs to be enough shades of gray to be able to distinguish differences between very dense tissues, such as enamel and dentin, but also subtle changes in density caused by demineralization of enamel as seen in early carious lesions or as seen in soft tissue shadows. Thus the shades of "gray" in an image might range from almost white to almost black with various shades of gray in between. The idea is that every patient has a "built-in" step wedge that the clinician can use in the evaluation of the image as a quick measure of the effectiveness of the machine settings. In general, the shades of gray increase with kV, although this is often not an adjustable factor; the density or overall lightness or blackness of an image relates to the mA in combination with the exposure time. Because most machines no longer have an adjustable mA setting, the exposure time can be adjusted for this factor. The bottom line is that every patient has a built-in step wedge, and the most diagnostic image will display the greater range of density differences in the tissues in the image. Look at Figure 4-25 and see how well it meets these criteria. Explain your answer.

Figure **4-27** This is a set of diagrams depicting features of a digital image.

1. In A we see the boxes containing shades of gray. Together what are the boxes called?
2. The numerical values in B and the shades of gray in A are arranged in squares. What are the squares called?
3. These squares are arranged horizontally and vertically. What two specific terms are used to describe these two arrangements?

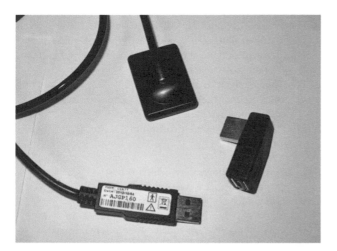

Figure **4-26** When a sensor is transported for use in different treatment rooms, it is possible that the pins on the USB connector on the sensor wire will wear such that a poor connection may cause the sensor to fail. What item illustrated here on the right side of the photo can be used to prevent this problem?

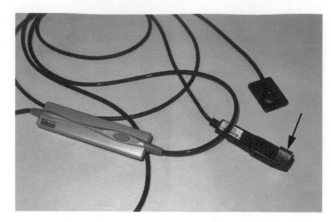

Figure **4-28** This is part of the same sensor setup we saw in Figure 4-26. In Figure 4-26 and in Figure 4-28 you can see a blue color associated with the USB male and female plug-ins.
1. What does this dark blue-black color indicate?
2. Also we see a gray rectangular part connected to the cabling. Generically, what does this part do?

MULTIPLE CHOICE QUESTIONS WITHOUT FIGURES

Instructions

Please select the best answer and check your selection with the correct answer in the Answer Key at the back of the book.

1. In order to digitize a radiograph, the following element should be on the scanner:
   A. A transparency adapter
   B. An opaque cover
   C. An opaque glass scanning plate
   D. The scanner need not be specially equipped

2. The main component of a server is:
   A. A computer
   B. A processor
   C. A series of hard drives
   D. All of the above

3. In a typical digital image, which of the following are arranged vertically?
   A. The rows
   B. The columns
   C. The image matrix
   D. Only the 3D image matrix in CBCT

4. In terms of the bit depth of a digital intraoral image, which bit depth is considered the most practical?
   A. 4-bit
   B. 8-bit
   C. 14-bit
   D. 16-bit

5. Let's say you had a 12-bit periapical image and a 12-bit pan image, which one would have the same number of shades of gray?
   A. The periapical
   B. The pan
   C. Both the intraoral and the pan
   D. Neither the periapical or the pan images

6. The production of noise in a digital radiograph:
   A. Is undesirable
   B. Is produced by low-energy x-ray photons
   C. Causes graininess in the image
   D. All of the above

7. In a digital image, whole areas of a fully exposed structure may be "blacked out" because:
   A. Too little radiation was used
   B. Too much kVp was used
   C. Too much mAs was used
   D. The sensor was inadvertently exposed to light

8. In terms of cone length, which one of the following will produce the sharpest image?
   A. 16-inch
   B. 12-inch
   C. 8-inch
   D. Cone length is not a factor.

9. Older x-ray machines are AC-based and the newer ones are DC-based; all things being equal, which one is most likely to include the most noise at the ideal exposure time for each one?
   A. The older AC machines
   B. The newer DC machines
   C. Both produce the same amount of noise or lack of it at the ideal exposure factors
   D. Actually the main determining factor is the type of sensor used

10. In terms of radiation safety, which is best?
   A. Standing behind a wall
   B. Using a foot-type exposure switch
   C. Standing behind a barrier with the patient in view
   D. All of the above are equally good safety measures

11. If an intraoral or a pan bitewing is subjected to filters such as *remove noise, de-speckle, sharpen,* and *sharpen edges* it will:
    A. Most likely become less diagnostic for caries
    B. Most likely become more diagnostic for caries
    C. Most likely be unchanged relative to caries diagnosis
    D. None of the above, as caries detection is affected most by other factors such as sensor type

12. Because it is true that an office may have several generations of x-ray machines as well as several different brands of sensors, it is often difficult to get the same excellent results when different combinations of x-ray equipment are used. A practical method of standardizing the sensors and machines is with the use of:
    A. A step wedge
    B. Contrast wells
    C. Line pair resolution measurement tool
    D. All three of these combined in the same quality assurance tool known as the Dental Digital Quality Assurance Phantom (DDQAP)

Chapter (5)

Intraoral Techniques and Errors

Goals

To become familiar with intraoral radiography equipment and supplies
To recognize and correct intraoral technique errors before exposing the radiograph

Learning Objectives

1. Recognize the parts of the x-ray machine
2. Become familiar with the machine controls
3. Understand how to use an exposure chart
4. Know about film and film packets
5. Recognize different film mounts
6. Understand basic patient and operator protection
7. Recognize which patient items can cause artifacts and should be removed
8. Identify errors in setting up the bite block, film, and positioning ring
9. Recognize film-handling errors
10. Identify beam alignment problems

INTRODUCTION

It is probable that almost all training programs now utilize digital sensors to train their dental assisting, dental hygiene, dental students, and most dental graduate program residents. Because of this, we first thought we would focus on digital radiology and eliminate all mention of errors regarding "x-ray film exposure." However, we could not be certain of this fact and could not confirm that everything to do with film is no longer required knowledge for examination purposes for students at all levels. Therefore we provide film-related material in this edition, possibly for the last time. In any case, all of the physical principles as discussed here certainly apply to sensors, although radiation affects film differently than sensors. For example, too much radiation causes a dark image on film while on some sensors, it causes "blooming." Blooming is a dark artifact due to too much radiation interacting with the sensor. The resulting image is partially or fully "blacked out" by this artifact. Also the errors section of this chapter consists of positioning errors in exposing film. Some examples include **elongation, foreshortening,** and **cone cutting**. These and other positioning errors produce the same effects in digital imaging.

Just to review, sensors consist of several types: direct solid state sensors consisting of **charge coupled devices (CCDs)** and **complementary metal oxide sensors (CMOSs)** and indirect type sensors consisting of **photostimulable phosphor plates (PSPs)**; the latter must be scanned into the computer by a laser scanner after the exposure. PSPs must then be erased by a bright light. It must also be recognized that traditionally intraoral imaging has been dominant in most, if not all, dental practices. Some of these practices have adopted intraoral PSPs for intraoral imaging. Dentists are slowly moving away from intraoral imaging as a routine in favor of panoramic imaging that is capable of producing diagnostic bitewing and periapical images as well as normal panoramic images. If desired and equipped, panoramic machines (see Chapter 6) can also be used to make cone beam computed tomography (CBCT; see Chapter 13) images.

SHORT ANSWER QUESTIONS WITH FIGURES
Instructions

Look at each figure and answer the following questions regarding intraoral clinical technique with a short answer. Some questions require you to identify the error, explain how to correct the error, or explain why the error occurred. Compare your answer to the correct answer in the Answer Key at the back of the book.

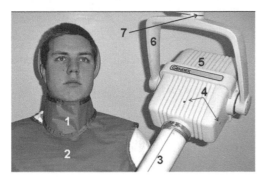

Figure **5-1** Name the labeled items.

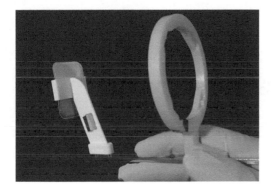

Figure **5-2**
1. Name this instrument.
2. For exactly what purpose is it used?
3. What error has occurred in this setup?

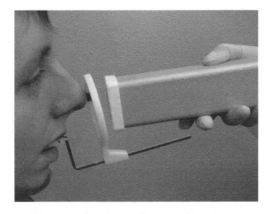

Figure **5-3** Here we see the XCP instrument in use.
1. Which teeth are being radiographed?
2. What type of BID is in use?
3. What error is about to happen?
4. What will this do to the image of the teeth?

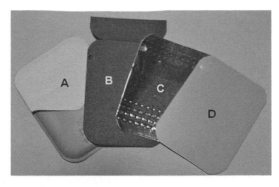

Figure **5-4** This picture demonstrates the contents of an intraoral film packet.
1. Name the labeled items.
2. From front to back, in which order are the items found in the packet?

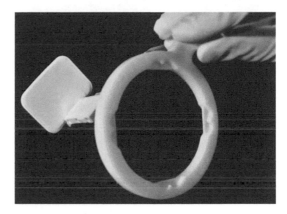

Figure **5-5**
1. What is wrong with this setup?

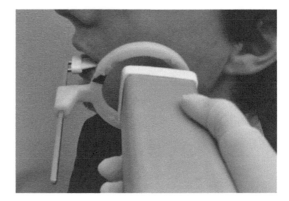

Figure **5-6**
1. What type of intraoral radiograph is being taken?
2. What error is occurring?
3. What will this look like on the radiograph?

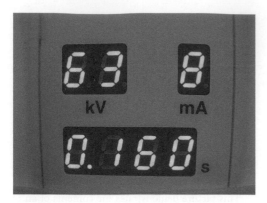

Figure **5-7** This is a part of the control panel of the x-ray machine. List what part(s) or function(s) can be seen in this photo.

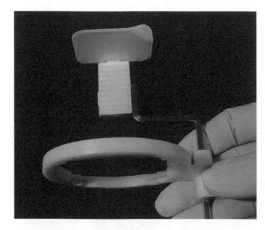

Figure **5-8** This is an XCP setup.
1. For which quadrants is this XCP set up?
2. What size film is being used?
3. What (if any) error has occurred in this setup?
4. How will this appear in the processed image?
5. When using an automatic processor, what can happen to this film?

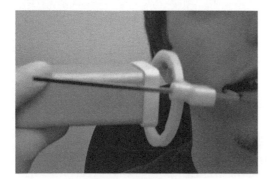

Figure **5-9** A posterior intraoral radiograph is being taken on this patient.
1. Which posterior quadrant is being radiographed?
2. What error is occurring?
3. How will this appear in the processed image?
4. In what situations is it important to avoid this error?
5. In what situations (if ever) is this error desirable?

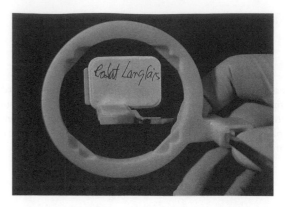

Figure **5-10** Here you can see a setup with a ring-positioning instrument.
1. For what technique (paralleling or bisecting angle) is this setup being used?
2. For what posterior quadrants is the instrument setup?
3. What error(s) do you see here?
4. What will this look like in the processed radiograph?

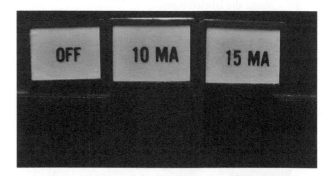

Figure **5-11** Here we see a portion of the control panel of an x-ray machine. List and explain the functions of these controls.

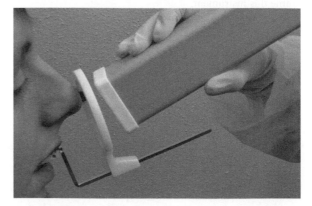

Figure **5-12** Here you can see that the anterior maxillary central incisors are being radiographed.
1. What error is occurring?
2. What will this look like in the processed radiograph?

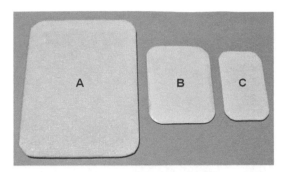

Figure **5-13**   Here we see three commonly used film sizes designed for use primarily in adults.
1. Name the sizes of film depicted in this photograph.
2. Specify what each size is used for.

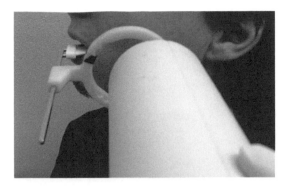

Figure **5-16**
1. Uh-oh! Several errors are in progress! Can you identify the errors?

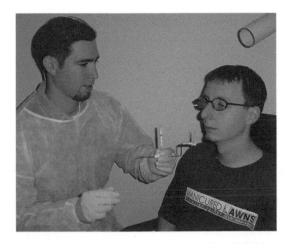

Figure **5-14**   Here we see one or more errors about to happen. Name the error(s).

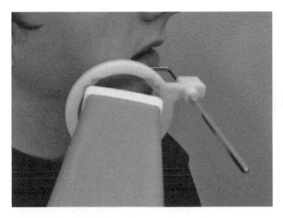

Figure **5-17**   Here we see a lower right posterior periapical radiograph about to be taken.
1. What error has occurred?
2. How will this appear on the processed radiograph?
3. What infection control problem is present?

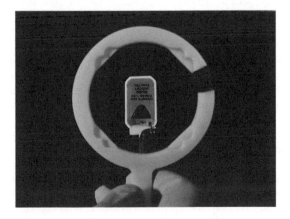

Figure **5-15**   This is a setup for the XCP paralleling instrument.
1. For what teeth is this setup to be used?
2. What error has occurred?
3. How will this look on the processed radiograph?
4. If the image can be seen, should this film be retained or retaken? Explain why.

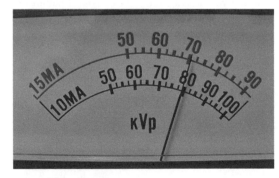

Figure **5-18**   What part of the control panel are we looking at here? Please explain.

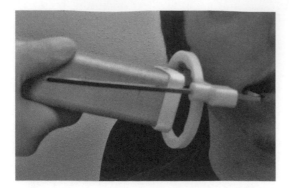

Figure **5-19** Here we see the maxillary right posterior quadrant being set up for an exposure.
1. What error is about to happen?
2. What will it look like in the processed radiograph?
3. What infection control problem is present?

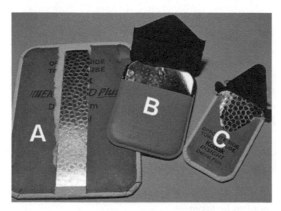

Figure **5-20** Here we are looking at the partially opened film packets of the three most common film sizes used in intraoral radiography.
1. What part of the film packet is immediately behind the back side of the outer envelope?
2. What is the purpose of this item?
3. How would you describe the three embossed patterns seen in the item?

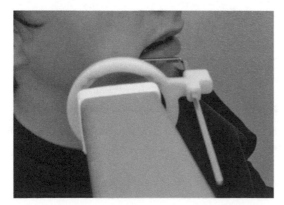

Figure **5-21** Here we see a lower posterior periapical radiograph about to be taken.
1. What error is about to occur?
2. Describe what would be seen on the processed radiograph.

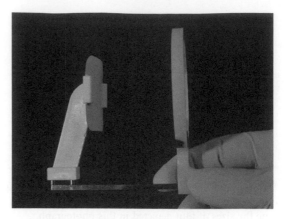

Figure **5-22** This is an incorrect bitewing setup.
1. What is wrong here?
2. What phrase can be used to help remember the correct bitewing setup when viewing the XCP instrument from this angle?

Exposure Chart

Film Type: **Speed Group F**
Kilovoltage = **70 kVp;**   Milliamperage = **15 mA**
BID Length = **LONG** Rectangular or Open
Patient ADULT: **Average** = 120 to 170 lbs.

Max. & Mand.	Adult	Pedo
		(includes erupted 1st perm. Molars only)
Anterior:	18 imp	15 imp
Premolar:	24 imp	18 imp
Molar:	30 imp	

Figure **5-23** This is an actual exposure chart. Use the chart to answer the questions regarding how you will adjust the machine settings (Part 1).
1. What BID length is specified?
2. What is the mA setting?
3. Will the settings be okay for an adult weighing 150 pounds?
4. What speed of intraoral film must we use for these settings?
5. What should we set the kVp at?
6. What will the exposure time be for the maxillary anterior periapicals?

Now you must do a little bit of thinking to answer these more difficult questions about this exposure chart (Part 2). Assume the patient is an average adult unless otherwise specified and that all exposure factors are to remain the same as specified on the chart, except those needing modification, to answer the questions.
1. If you wanted to use a short, 8-inch BID, what would the exposure time be for a premolar periapical radiograph?
2. If the patient weighs 200 pounds, what exposure time would you use for the premolar periapicals? (Select from the settings on the chart.)
3. If you have only "D"-speed film available, what exposure time would you use for a child with erupted 1st permanent molars for a periapical radiograph of the maxillary anterior region? (Select one of the exposure times from the chart.)
4. Let's say you wished to use 10 mA for a molar periapical radiograph. How many impulses would you need to use? Explain.
5. If you are directed to use 85 kVp for a molar periapical view in a 165-pound adult, how many impulses would you have to reset the timer to? Explain. (Select from any of the settings on the chart.)
6. If you wanted to use the fastest available speed of intraoral film, what (if any) modifications would you make to the exposure times on this chart?

7. Say you wanted to switch from a long, 16-inch, round, open-ended cone to a long, 16-inch, rectangular cone, what modifications (if any) would you need to make to this exposure chart?

8. If the patient is a small adult weighing 100 pounds, what exposure time would you use for the molar periapicals? (Select from the settings on the chart.)

9. If one impulse is 1/60 of a second, what fraction of a second is an exposure time of 30 impulses?

10. Someone indicates you must use an exposure time of three fourths of a second (¾ sec), but the timer settings are in impulses; so how many impulses will you set the timer to?

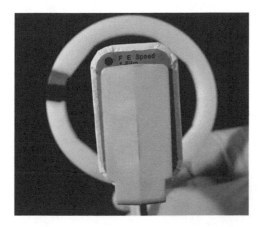

Figure **5-24**   Note this view as the operator studies this XCP setup.
1. What is wrong with this anterior periapical setup?
2. What will it look like in the processed radiograph?

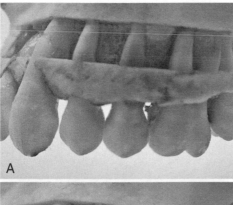

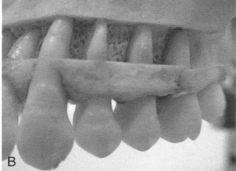

Figure **5-25**   Study carefully images A and B. Answer the following questions:
1. Which periapical region does this represent?
2. Using the chart in Figure 5-23, what would the exposure time be?
3. Which view represents a BID positioning error?
4. What BID positioning error is pictured?

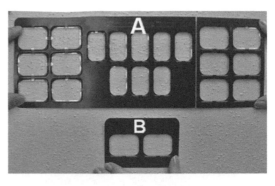

Figure **5-26**   We see two items in this photograph.
1. What is item A called?
2. What is item B called?
3. What film numbers (how many of each) and sizes are used in item A?

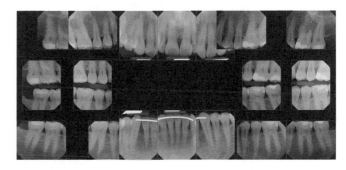

Figure **5-27**   Here we see a full mouth survey.
1. On what type of image capture medium (device) were these images captured?
2. How are these images being viewed? That is, on a view box or a monitor?
3. In either case, the image size is uniform; please explain.
4. Critique the mounting of these images.

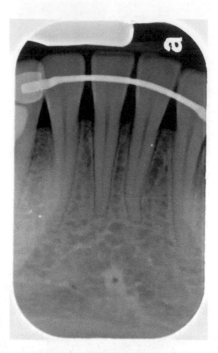

Figure **5-28** Study this image carefully.
1. What type of medium was this image recorded on in the clinic?
2. There are several tiny white spots in the image; what are these?
3. What does the horizontal radiopaque line in the mid-crown areas represent?
4. Is the object in question 3 in the lingual or buccal side of the teeth?
5. What is the little black spot surrounded by a white ring in the lower part of the image? Be as complete as possible.

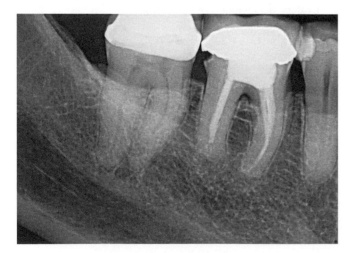

Figure **5-29**
1. This is an electronic sensor image; what technique error has been made here?
2. Comment on the endodontic treatment seen here.

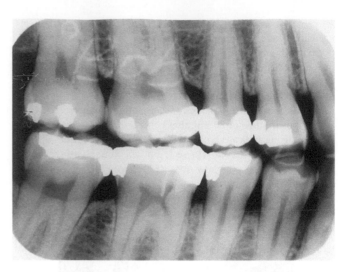

Figure **5-30** It looks like ole Bob had a radiograph taken.
1. What happened here?

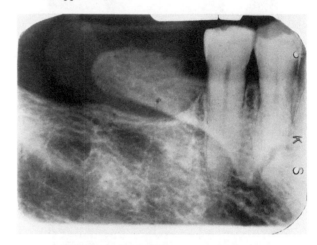

Figure **5-31** Here we see a bone not usually found in intraoral images.
1. What happened here?
2. What term describes this situation?

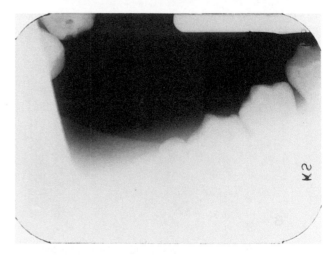

Figure **5-32** Note the partial image of the teeth.
1. What technique error was made here?

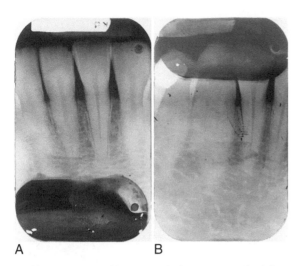

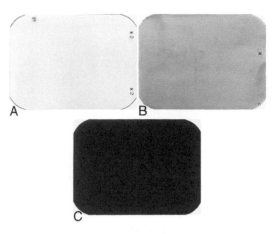

A   B

Figure **5-33** These two films (A and B) were part of a full-mouth survey developed in an automatic processor.
1. What happened to these two films?
2. How can this be corrected?

Figure **5-36** Here we see three "blank" images. You are asked to explain why:
1. Image A is completely clear.
2. Image B is somewhat grayish.
3. Image C is completely black.

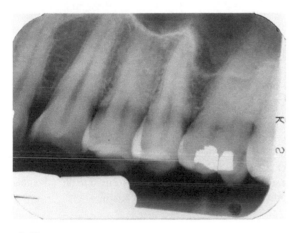

Figure **5-34**
1. Why do the 1st premolar roots appear "fuzzed out"?
2. When may this error be used to our advantage?

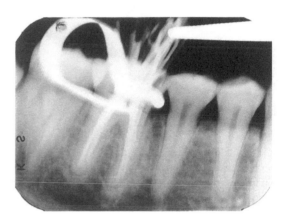

Figure **5-37** There is a certain "fuzziness" to this image.
1. What exposure error(s) was (were) made here? List several possibilities if you are unsure exactly what happened.

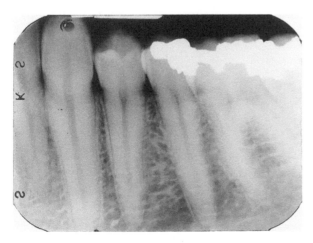

Figure **5-35**
1. Would you call this an acceptable premolar periapical radiograph?
2. In any case, how could you increase the area of periapical coverage?

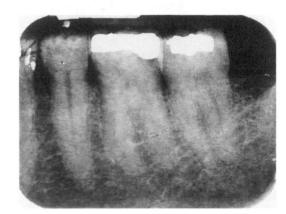

Figure **5-38** This was the student's first opportunity to process a film. She was a little excited and nervous. This film was fed into the automatic processor; the student waited and waited but to no avail. The film just was not coming out. The processor was turned off and opened, and the roller sections were removed. The "lost" film was found in the bottom of the processor.
1. How would you describe the overall appearance of this film?
2. What do you think happened?

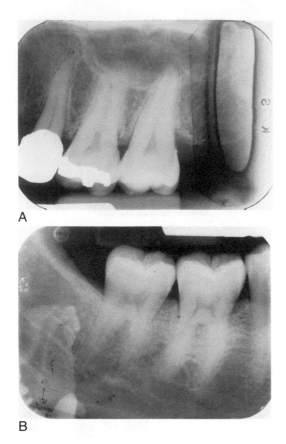

A

B

Figure **5-39**   Radiographs A and B each have a different processing solution stain that can be seen.
1.   What processing solution produced the dark, radiolucent stain?
2.   What processing solution caused the whitish, radiopaque stain?

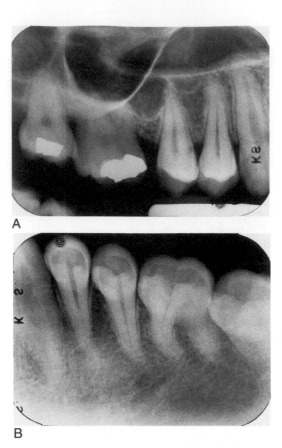

A

B

Figure **5-41**   In images A and B, the same exposure error was made. Part A represents the maxillary posterior region and B the mandibular posterior area.
1.   State what error was made.
2.   What features in A and B allow you to identify the error?
3.   In some situations, could this error be used to our advantage, or performed on purpose by the clinician?

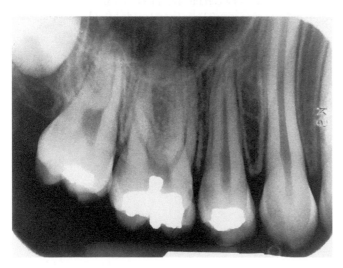

Figure **5-40**
1.   What film-handling error was made here?

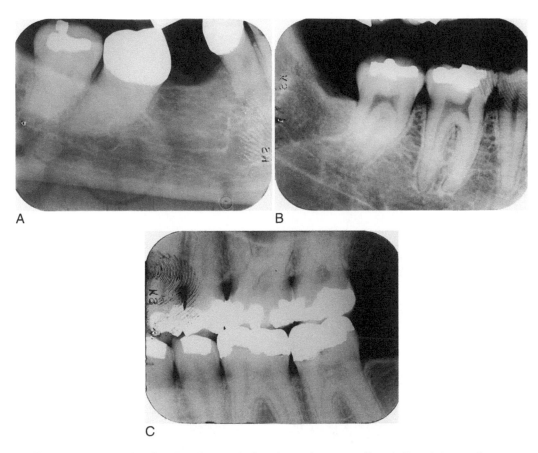

A   B

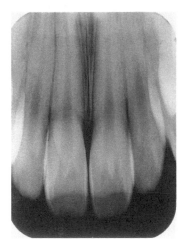

C

Figure **5-42**   Sloppy film handling has resulted in chemical stains on films A, B, and C. In each case, contaminated fingers marred the films.
1.   Which one of three different chemicals produced each of the errors?

Figure **5-43**
1.   What term best describes what has happened to these teeth?
2.   Explain how this occurred.

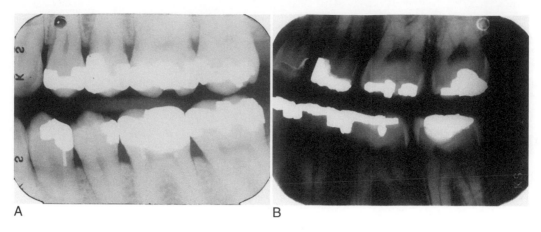

Figure **5-44**   These are two bitewing radiographs. Example A is too light, and B is too dark.
1.   List some reasons film A is too light.
2.   List some reasons film B is too dark.

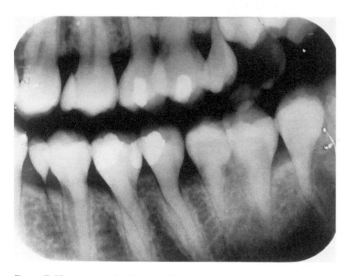

Figure **5-45**   Strange looking teeth...
1.   What exposure error was made here?

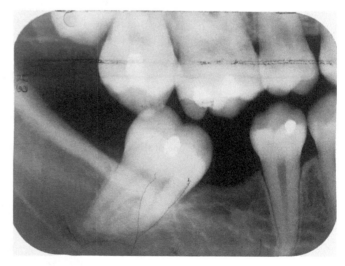

Figure **5-46**   This radiograph was processed in an automatic processor in Alaska during the coldest part of winter.
1.   List two processing errors seen here.
2.   Explain how each can be corrected.

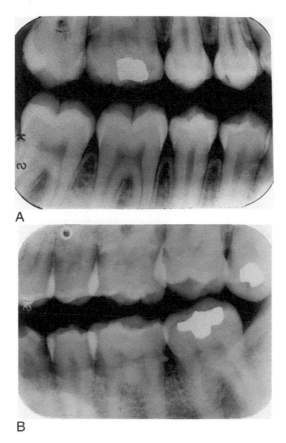

A

B

Figure **5-47** Here are two bitewings: A (premolar) and B (molar).

1. What is wrong with bitewing A?
2. What is wrong with bitewing B?
3. Which (if any) need(s) to be retaken?

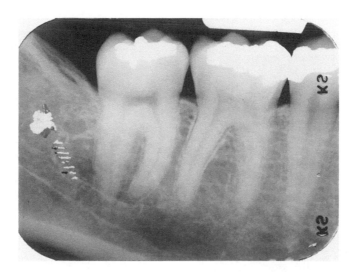

Figure **5-48**

1. What film-handling error produced this radiopaque artifact distal to the 2nd molar?

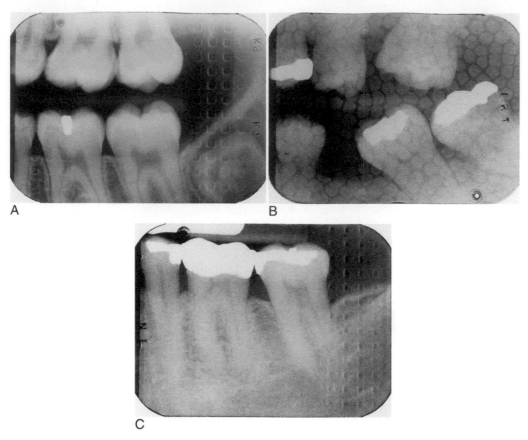

Figure **5-49**   Examples A, B, and C have all occurred as a result of the same error.
1. What error has occurred here?
2. Example C (and possibly the others) seems quite readable. Why is it better to retake all three of these radiographs?
3. Notice the patterns are a bit different from each other. Could this have to do with film type?

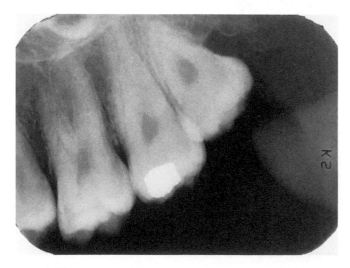

Figure **5-50**
1. Why were the apical regions of the 2nd and 3rd maxillary molars missed?
2. What is the radiopaque object with the embossed KS mark superimposed?

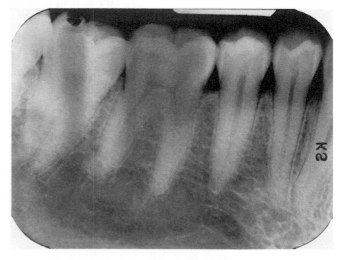

Figure **5-51**   Clinically this radiograph looked a little greenish and lacked translucency.
1. What processing error was made?

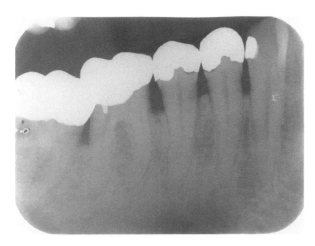

Figure **5-52**   This is a fogged film.
1.   List possible reasons for this problem.

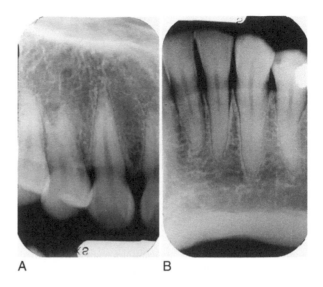

A   B

Figure **5-54**   Examples A (maxillary canine) and B (mandibular canine) both illustrate the same two errors.
1.   Name the two errors.

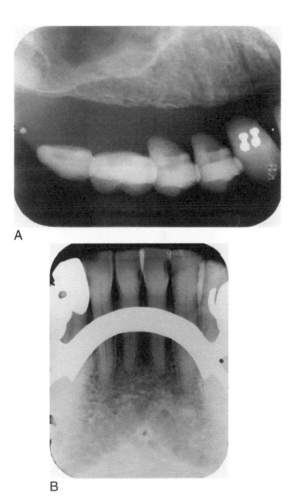

A

B

Figure **5-53**   This is from the "stuff left in or on" department.
1.   What happened here?
2.   Do both examples A and B represent technique errors?

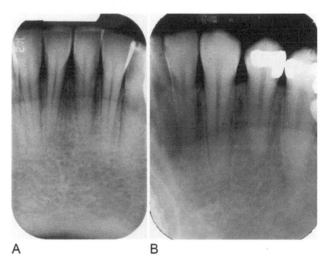

A   B

Figure **5-55**   This patient was really cooperative though the bite block was uncomfortable when she bit down.
1.   What error occurred in both examples A and B?
2.   What further error occurred in example B?

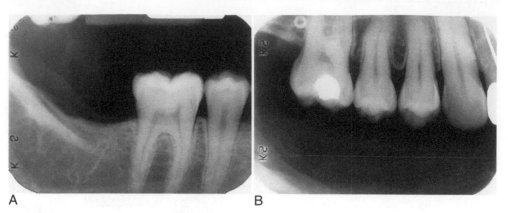

A   B

Figure **5-56**   In examples A and B we see inadequate periapical coverage because of the exact same error.
1.   What error occurred here?

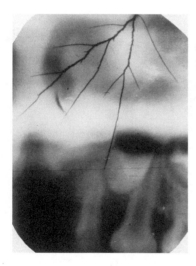

Figure **5-57**   Okay. You asked for it, and here it is…but look closely because there may be more than one problem!
1.   What problems do you see? Ignore the background image quality.

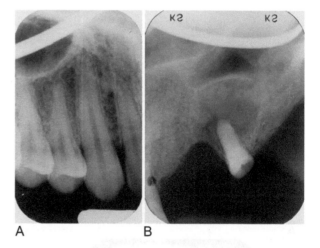

A   B

Figure **5-58**   In examples A and B, one error is common to both images and involves some sort of foreign body or material. Both A and B are views of just about the same anatomic region, though the film size is different.
1.   State what error has occurred.
2.   From what material(s) is the foreign object made?
3.   What film sizes do we see here?

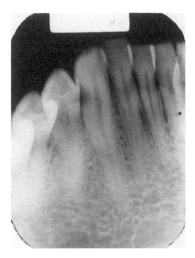

Figure **5-59**   Notice the distal portion of the mandibular canine.
1.   What error does the radiolucent area represent?
2.   Why would you not think it is caries?
3.   Would you repeat this view?

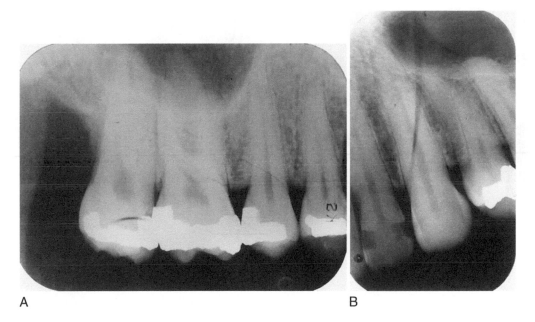

A   B

Figure **5-60**   Examples A and B have a similar but not identical error. Both are the result of mishandling the film.
1.   State what errors you are being asked to identify.

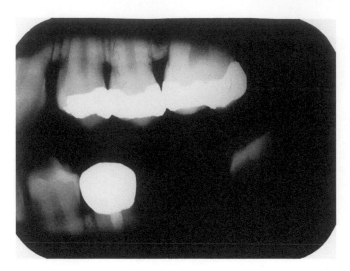

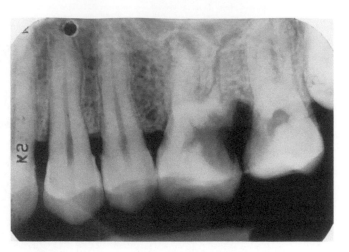

Figure **5-61**
1.   What happened to this radiograph?

Figure **5-62**   This film involves inadequate apical coverage in general and specifically at the apex of the 1st premolar.
1.   In general, how could you increase the apical coverage?
2.   What happened at the apex of the 1st premolar?

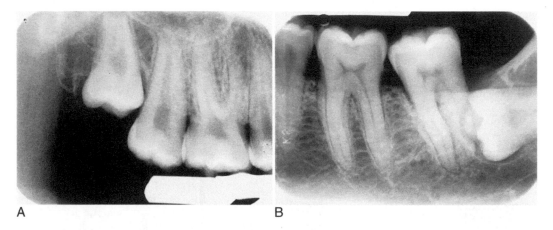

A   B

Figure **5-63**   Both of these 3rd molars lack apical coverage.
1.   In examples A and B, what could you do to correct this?

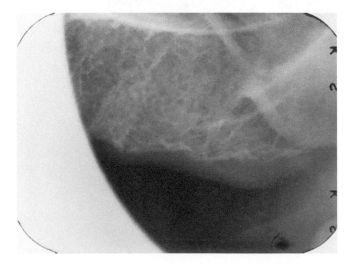

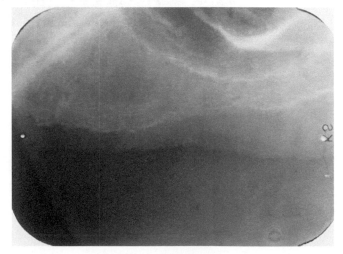

Figure **5-64**   What error(s) occurred here?

Figure **5-65**   What error(s) occurred here?

Figure **5-66**   What error(s) occurred here?

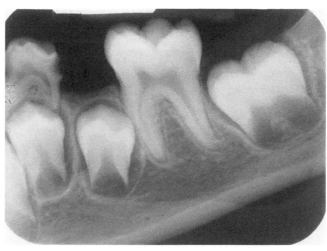

Figure **5-69**   What error(s) occurred here?

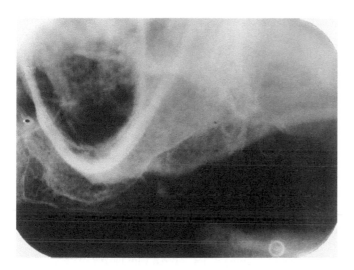

Figure **5-67**   What error(s) occurred here?

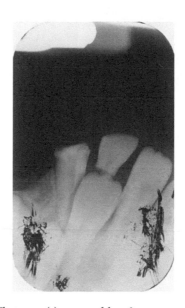

Figure **5-70**   What error(s) occurred here?

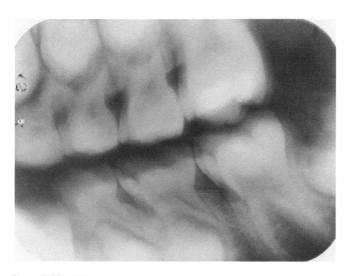

Figure **5-68**   What error(s) occurred here?

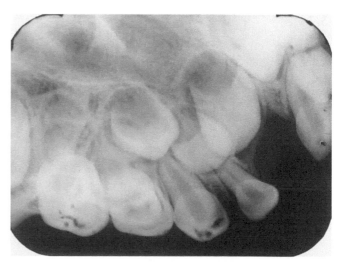

Figure **5-71**   What error(s) occurred here?

MULTIPLE CHOICE QUESTIONS WITH FIGURES

Instructions

Please select the best answer and check your selection with the correct answers in the Answer Key at the back of the book.

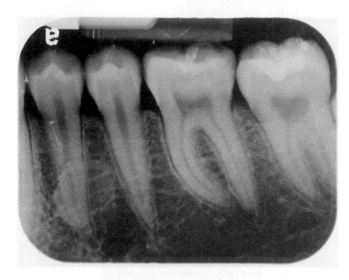

Figure **5-72**

1. What type of image is this?
   A. PSP with minor scratches
   B. Dark film
   C. Unacceptable dark and scratched film
   D. Electronic sensor-generated image

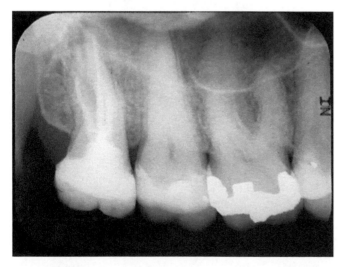

Figure **5-73**

1. What type of image is this?
   A. It is a film image as indicated by the speed letters "IN"
   B. It is an underexposed image
   C. The roots of the first molar indicate poor technique
   D. All of the above are true
   E. None of the above are true...this is a PSP image

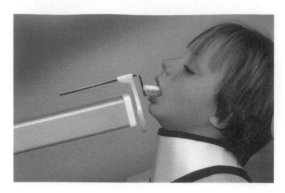

Figure **5-74**

1. What error is seen here?
   A. The child's chin is too high
   B. The thyroid collar is no longer needed
   C. There is an infection control issue
   D. None of the above

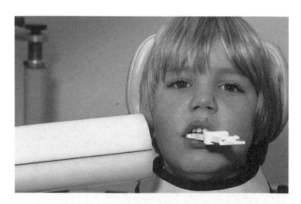

Figure **5-75**

1. Here we see an image about to be taken. The problem is:
   A. The BID (cone) is not covered with barrier material
   B. The lips are open
   C. The head is turned slightly
   D. The film/sensor holder is in upside down
   E. All of the above

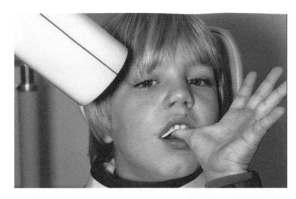

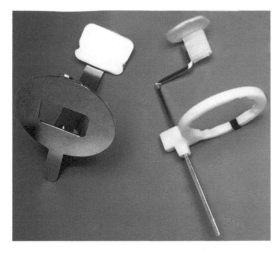

Figure **5-76**

1. This is Mark and this image was taken 30 + years ago. Given that both infection control measures, such as covering the cone with barrier material, were not in effect, and panoramic imaging was much less available and of poorer quality, what is the one most important technique error in this photo?
   A. The vertical angulation of the cone appears to be too high
   B. The film could be bent with the finger pressure causing image distortion
   C. The tip of the cone appears to be too far back for this anatomic region
   D. Today, the thyroid collar would not be needed

Figure **5-78**

1. We are getting ready to take a posterior periapical image in a 5-year-old child. Which setup would you recommend?
   A. The one on the left
   B. The one on the right
   C. Each one has advantages
   D. None of the above

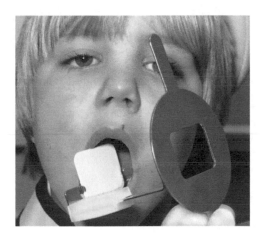

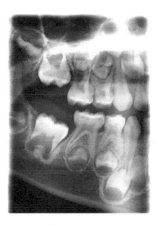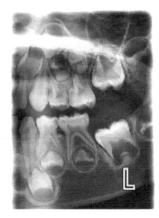

Figure **5-77**

1. In the day, this was a highly touted technique because, before rectangular BID or cone development, this device blocked out all of the unneeded radiation. What error is present?
   A. The technique as illustrated is contraindicated in this circumstance
   B. Child-size film and film holder-localizer should have been used
   C. A #2 film (as seen here), placed occlusally, may have been an option
   D. All of the above
   E. None of the above

Figure **5-79**

1. This is an example of a panoramic bitewing. Which of the following statements is *not* true?
   A. Panoramic bitewings are recommended in children
   B. Pan bitewings (BWs) are not as diagnostic for incipient caries as intra BWs
   C. Pan BWs involve less radiation than a full-mouth survey
   D. Pan BWs deliver a similar radiation dose as four collimated intra BWs

2. Looking at the pan BW in Figure 5-79, in the interproximal space of all of the primary molars there is caries. On the right side as well as the upper left, the interproximal contacts seem to overlap. This is because this represents:
   A. Visible loss of space because of contact destruction
   B. Poor patient positioning technique by the operator
   C. Good positioning but with the wrong jaw size setting
   D. An eruption anomaly in the primary dentition

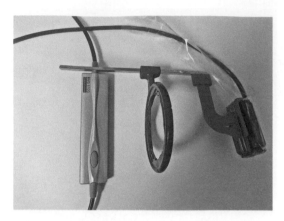

Figure **5-80**   Here we have a setup to take a digital image.

1. What type of image is this setup for?
   - A. Posterior periapical
   - B. Anterior periapical
   - C. Bitewing
   - D. All of the above

2. Looking at the above illustration, the gray rectangular device is connected to the power cord of the sensor. This device is a:
   - A. Powered USB router (connected to the treatment room laptop computer)
   - B. Network junction box connector serving the treatment room
   - C. Filter which removes noise because the x-ray machines are AC types
   - D. Step-down transformer to prevent sensor burn out

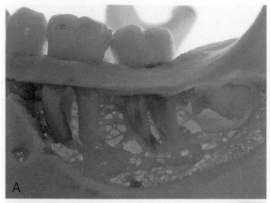

A

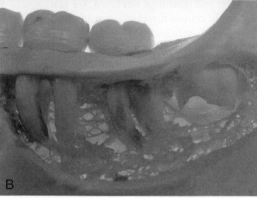

B

Figure **5-81**   Here we have a simulation of two periapical images. Looking carefully at images A and B to answer the following questions:

1. If the cone of the x-ray machine was aimed at images A and B, which periapical image would this be equivalent to?
   - A. The lower left molar region
   - B. The lower right molar region
   - C. A distalized view of the third molar
   - D. None of the above
   - E. Any one of the above

2. Technique-wise, which image would produce the most accurate periapical x-ray image?
   - A. Image A
   - B. Image B
   - C. Either image A or B
   - D. Neither image A nor B

3. If you feel that one of the images represents the most accurate image, then what error (if any) would the second image produce in the radiograph?
   - A. Either image is equally acceptable
   - B. Neither image is perfectly acceptable
   - C. Image B represents an example of foreshortening
   - D. Image A represents an example of elongation

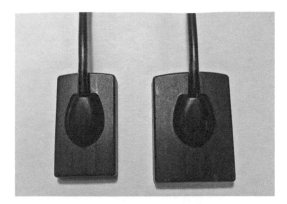

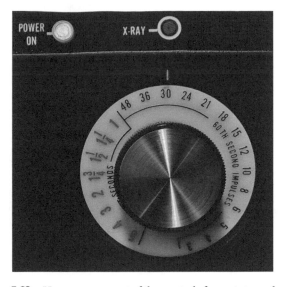

Figure **5-82** Here you are looking at a couple of x-ray imaging devices.

1. What type of imaging devices are these:
   A. PSP sensor
   B. CMOS sensor
   C. CCD sensor
   D. Any of the above
   E. Either B or C

2. What size are these two imaging devices?
   A. Size 0 on the left; size 1 on the right
   B. Size 0 on the left; size 2 on the right
   C. Size 1 on the left; size 2 on the right
   D. Either B or C could be correct

3. Infection control-wise what protection would you place on each of these sensors while in use?
   A. Vinyl sleeve only for the sensor and about 1 foot of the wire
   B. Finger cot only to protect the sensor from saliva leakage
   C. Either A or B is acceptable
   D. Both A and B are recommended

Figure **5-83** Here we see a part of the controls for an intraoral x-ray machine.

1. What type of x-ray machine was this control used for?
   A. Handheld portable
   B. Wall-mounted AC type
   C. Wall-mounted DC type
   D. Either B or C would be correct

2. Note the orange light indicating the power is on. There is also a red light that was not on at the time the photograph was taken. This light will go on when:
   A. The machine is turned off
   B. Excess exposure time is selected according to the selected kVp
   C. Excess kVp is selected according to the selected exposure time
   D. The exposure switch is depressed, indicating radiation emission

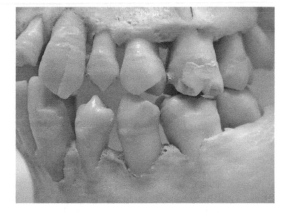

Figure **5-84** Here we see a photo that simulates the clinical view of the teeth when lining up the x-ray machine to take a bitewing image.

1. What routine bitewing (BW) view is closest to what we see here?
   A. The anterior BW
   B. The posterior BW
   C. The BW using #3 film
   D. None of the above

2. Characterize the bitewing that used #3-size film.
   A. This method exists only in Dr. Miller's mind
   B. This is a special method invented by Dr. Langlais
   C. There is no and never was such a thing as a #3 bitewing
   D. A single #3 film covered the whole quadrant

Chapter 6

Panoramic Radiology: Principles and Error Identification

Goals

To understand correct clinical techniques in panoramic radiology
To know how to recognize and correct errors seen in panoramic radiographs

Learning Objectives

1. Recognize the parts of the panoramic machine
2. Know how to use a panoramic machine and its components
3. Identify errors in taking the panoramic radiograph
4. Know how to correct errors in taking the panoramic radiograph
5. Recognize panoramic concepts that contribute to clinical decision-making

INSTRUCTIONS

Carefully read the introductory information on panoramic principles and error identification presented here. The machines illustrated represent several different brands. Whether the machine is an older film-based panoramic machine or a newer digital machine, all of them can be operated in basically the same way. Slight differences in technique exist from one brand or model to another; however, the errors remain the same. The principles for the recognition and correction of errors are relatively universal. Having said that, some brands or models may be more prone to certain errors or artifacts and some may even produce unique errors. The information here is the basis for understanding, recognizing, and correcting problems for most machines, models, and situations. Once this basic information is mastered, unique problems can be identified and corrected; and by the way, we often forget to refer to the owner's operating manual where most of the answers to common problems can be found.

BASIC CONCEPTS

The simple goal of this chapter is for users of panoramic radiology to perfect their panoramic technique and get the most diagnostic panoramic images possible with the equipment in use. Luckily most of the errors are not machine brand–specific. We have placed several really nice panoramic images in this chapter so the reader can appreciate the full potential of modern digital panoramic machines. For this edition we removed many film-based panoramic error images and replaced them with digital radiographs. We have also redrawn the diagrams illustrating in color the salient features of each of the positioning errors.

One great advantage of digital technology is that there are no film-based errors such as scratches or cloudy, outdated film. Also, there are no problems with cassettes such as the development of light leaks or scratches on the screens. However, photostimulable

phosphor plates (PSPs) use cassettes, and these are subject to scratches and light leaks, although PSPs are less sensitive to light than film; but remember, bright light is used to erase PSPs. Also there are no darkroom-associated problems such as fog resulting from light leaks or an unsafe darkroom light or from old, used-up solutions, and there are no automatic processor problems such as faulty rollers or solution-heating mechanisms. Most of the digital panoramic problems are limited to faulty patient positioning in the machine and are therefore highly advantageous. Additionally, the image quality or certain details within the image can be improved after the image has been taken with the digital software. Therefore there are fewer problems with digital panoramic radiography. In this edition, we used color images that are more demonstrative, in that the positioning lights standout more in color. Therefore in this edition, we have combined the clinical positioning photos, color diagrams of the errors, and the image troubleshooting into one comprehensive chapter. Finally, the protective lead apron is no longer required for panoramic imaging (see Chapter 2). Having said this, some patients, especially pregnant patients may prefer to have the (unneeded) protection of the lead apron, and so if an apron is available, it is best to use it for the patient's peace of mind.

INTRODUCTION

Panoramic (pan) radiology has evolved in a significant way over the past dozen years. This evolutionary process has moved the technology from film-based systems capable of a standard panoramic image with or without a cephalometric (ceph) attachment to machines capable of bitewings and cone beam computed tomography (CBCT) plus other functions. These functions, such as panoramic bitewings and panoramic periapical images, are now included in this edition. Historically, this development included a phase where standard pan or pan-ceph images could be converted to indirect digital images with the use of PSPs, which require scanning into a special laser scanner, instead of the regular film-based cassette system. The most recent technology includes a single digital direct capture system usually consisting of the complementary metal oxide sensor (CMOS) type, which can capture standard pans, pan bitewings (pan BWs), pan periapicals (pan PAs), CBCT, and digital ceph functions. A new type of sensor designated as a cadmium telluride photon counting (CdTePC) sensor has been introduced on some panoramic machines in Japan and Finland. At present this sensor is available on one or more pan-CBCT machines in the U.S. market. This new sensor will reduce the current low digital pan and CBCT doses by up to three- to fivefold, be capable of sharper images, and allow for an improved technology known as tomosynthesis whereby overlapping interproximal tooth contacts on the pan BWs can be opened after the exposure. The new pan-CBCT machines will be capable of capturing the whole head for cephalometric and other applications and at doses as low as or lower than current ceph technology with the use of the standard digital CMOS sensors. In addition, the practitioner will be able to choose dose levels, such as standard, low, and ultra-low dose levels for all volume sizes as recommended in Publication 129 of the International Commission on Radiological Protection (ICRP 129). The highest of these CBCT doses offered by manufacturers are presently less than or similar to a digital full-mouth intraoral survey using the long, round cone.

THE PARTS (ANATOMY) OF THE PAN-CEPH MACHINE

Although not all pan-ceph machines are exactly the same as the one portrayed here, this is one example of such a device. Some parts of this machine are unique to this model; however, the goal of all brands and models of such machines is to properly position the patient in the device so as to obtain the best image quality possible. In the end, all machines produce various types of panoramic images such as the traditional panoramic as well as the newer pan BW and both lateral and posteroanterior (PA) images.

Instructions

Study Figures 6-1 to 6-5 and identify the labeled parts of the machine. Compare your answer to each question to the correct answer in the Answer Key at the back of the book.

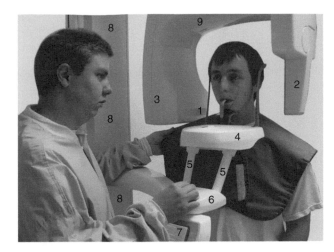

Figure **6-1** Name or identify the numbered parts.

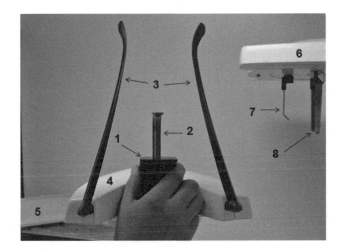

Figure **6-2** Name or identify the numbered parts.

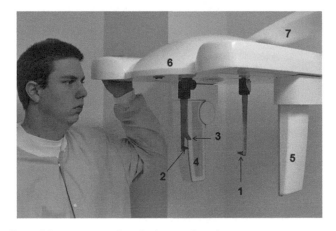

Figure **6-3** Name or identify the numbered parts.

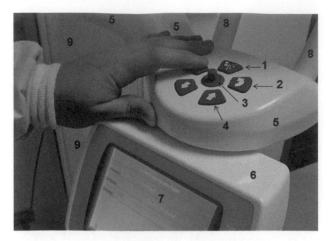

Figure **6-4**   Name or identify the numbered parts.

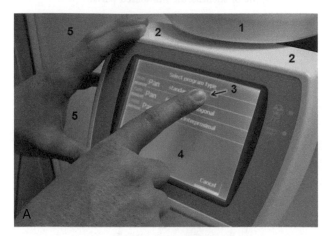

Figure **6-5A**   Name or identify the numbered parts.

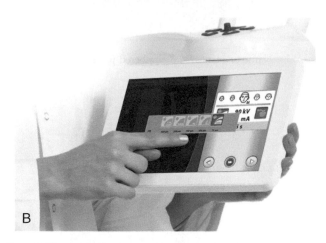

Figure **6-5B**   Study this figure carefully. Look at the icons and compare to Figure 6-5A. What does this illustration represent? (Figure courtesy of Planmeca USA, Roselle, IL.)

PANORAMIC PROJECTION GEOMETRY: A CONCEPTUAL APPROACH

To understand technique errors and both the advantages and limitations of panoramic imaging, it is important to know how the pan projection geometry affects the image. All manufacturers design their machines slightly differently; however, in spite of the resulting variables, there is a commonality to all of the brands of machines in terms of analyzing the image for technique errors. As such we have developed five concepts that will help you to learn why certain things happen to the image and why some aspects relating to the interpretation of the image are subject to limitations, which may be significant with respect to applications such as implant measurements or space analysis for orthodontic applications. Because the following information may not be well articulated in standard textbooks, we have elected to place it here. Part of the reason for this is that panoramic error troubleshooting is often poorly understood and poorly executed in many practices. We hope to help with this aspect of panoramic radiology. For this first section on the concepts, there is text only; there are no questions or answers.

Concept #1: Pan "Tomographic" Layer and Focal Trough

Panoramic machines have an axis of rotation whereby the x-ray tube head and the film or PSP cassette or sensor assembly rotates. Because the rotation point moves during the exposure, this axis is termed the *rotation center*. The *path of the rotation center* places the layer in focus (**focal trough**) within the structures to be imaged. As such a layer of tissues in focus usually consists of the entirety of the jaws, including the teeth, as well as the lower parts of the nose and sinuses and the upper parts of the neck including parts of the cervical spine, airway, and hyoid bone (Figure 6-6).

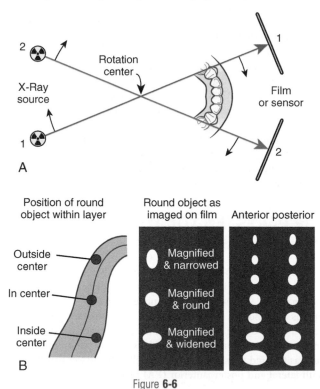

Figure **6-6**

In Figure 6-6A, the x-ray tube head and capture device (film, PSP, or sensor) rotate around an axis of rotation to form a layer in focus (focal trough) such that the structures of the jaws appear in the image. The focal trough is consistent with the shape of the jaws, but it is narrower in the anterior region and wider in the posterior area of the jaws. The layer is such that objects in the middle of the layer have their correct shape and proportions. However, objects buccal to the center of the layer are narrowed and objects lingual to the center are widened.

Figure 6-6B demonstrates that buccal objects outside the center but within the layer are narrowed and lingual objects outside the center are widened. This distortion is greatest in the narrow parts of the layer, which is the anterior region in the patient.

This first concept is the basis for troubleshooting the following patient positioning errors: patient too far forward (teeth are narrowed); patient too far back (teeth are widened); and patient turned in the machine (teeth narrowed on one side and widened on the other). These errors will be further illustrated in this chapter with diagrams, clinical photos, and radiographs. This concept is also the basis for inaccurate horizontal measurements, such as space analysis when a pan film is used in orthodontic planning, and for replacement of teeth by implants or other prosthetic appliances, such as a fixed bridge.

Concept #2: Projection Angle of the Pan Beam is Upward

Pan machines *do not* normally project the x-ray beam perpendicular to the teeth and jaws. Instead, the projection of the beam is in an upward direction as it passes through the anatomy, such as the jaws, and then exposes the film, PSP, or sensor. The reason for this design feature is to allow the x-ray beam to pass under the thick occipital part of the skull in the back of the head.

In Figure 6-7, the pan beam is directed from the focal spot in the tube head, through the patient, and to the sensor at an upward angle, to pass under the thick occipital part of the skull in the back of the patient's head.

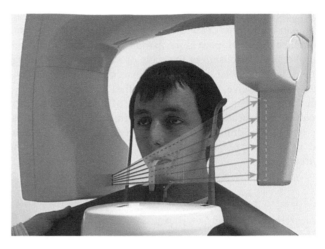

Figure **6-7**

This *negative vertical angulation* of the beam keeps the radiation dose lower but does cause an inaccurate vertical relationship of objects in the image. This beam projection geometry causes *all objects* to be higher up in the image, and buccal objects will be lower than lingual objects when objects are actually on the same horizontal plane in the patient.

In Figure 6-8, the negative projection angle of the pan beam causes lingual objects on the same plane to be projected higher and buccal objects in the same plane to be projected lower in the pan image. The lingual objects are labeled 1; those in the middle of the layer are labeled 2; and the buccal objects are labeled 3. This causes inaccurate structural relationships in the vertical dimension.

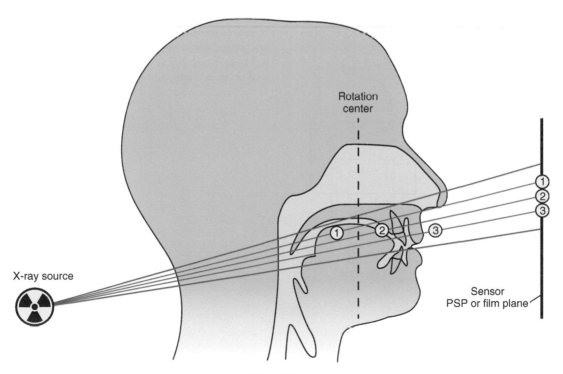

Figure **6-8**

This concept is the basis for inaccurate vertical measurements when panoramic images are used for implant planning regarding the available vertical space in the mandible or maxilla. In another example, the relationship of the roots of an impacted 3rd molar to the inferior alveolar canal may be inaccurate. This canal contains a major nerve, artery, and vein that may be intertwined with the roots of an impacted 3rd molar. Misjudging the inferior alveolar canal's location could result in unintended trauma, excessive bleeding, and/or a temporary or permanent loss of sensation in certain structures such as the tongue and lips on the injured side.

Concept #3: Vertical Relationships in the Mandible and Maxilla

The vertical relationship of objects within the layer in focus (focal trough) is different in the mandible than in the maxilla. That is to say, the vertical separation of buccal and lingual objects on the same horizontal plane in the patient is more severely affected in the maxilla than in the mandible.

In Figure 6-9A, note how the pan beam spreads out more in the maxilla than the mandible. As the pan beam is projected in an upward direction, it spreads out more in the maxilla than in the mandible due to the negative projection angle of the beam.

This concept explains why there is a greater vertical separation of objects in the maxilla than the mandible in pan images. This is an additional factor that contributes to the inaccuracy of vertical measurements between buccal and lingual objects on the same horizontal plane that are in the mandible vs. the maxilla.

In Figure 6-9B, note the difference in the vertical relationship of buccal and lingual objects in the lower jaw (mandible) vs. the upper jaw (maxilla). The buccal objects are narrowed in both jaws, and the lingual objects are widened in both jaws compared with those in the middle of the layer, which represents the true shape of the object. The difference is that the vertical separation of these objects is much greater in the maxilla. These latter two concepts are the reasons why making vertical measurements using pan images for treatment planning for implants, endodontics, or surgery may be inaccurate and may contribute to less than desirable or unpredictable clinical outcomes.

THE BOTTOM LINE (CONCEPTS 1-3): These three simple panoramic concepts that apply to all panoramic machines help to identify pan technique errors, which if appreciated, will lead to the correction of those errors and better pan images. Second, pan imaging has some significant limitations with regard to making both horizontal and vertical measurements as they apply to various treatment planning procedures. What is the solution? While good technique is helpful, the above limitations are inherent and thus unavoidable in this technology, and this is true for all brands of panoramic machines. The solution to this problem is the acquisition of a pan machine capable of standard panoramic functions as well as CBCT with which all measurements and structural relationships are accurate including cephalometric measurements (see Chapter 13 on CBCT).

Concept # 4: Formation of Double Images

In panoramic radiology, images may be classified as follows: **real images** and **ghost images**. Real images can be divided into single real images and double real images. The first three concepts deal with single real images.

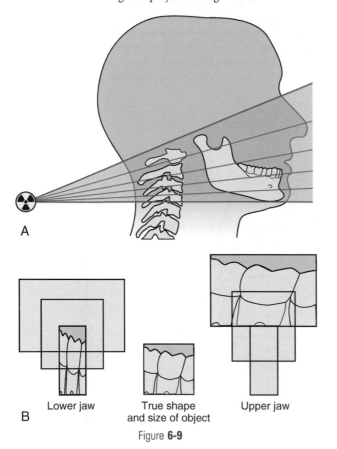

A

B   Lower jaw   True shape   Upper jaw
                   and size of object

Figure **6-9**

As illustrated in Figure 6-12, the result of the exposure of the left and right sides of the patient produces a central diamond-shaped area illustrated in green, which is exposed twice. This area forms an additional layer within which structures appear in the image. Anatomic structures in this area are seen as **double images**.

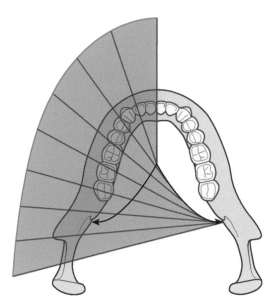

Figure **6-10**

In Figure 6-10 the thick, curved black line represents the path of the rotation center of the pan beam. The beam emerges at a tangent to the path of the rotation center and exposes the *left side of the patient* as viewed from above.

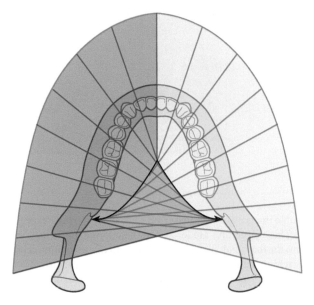

Figure **6-12**

When both sides of the scan are combined, the formation of real double images occurs in anatomic structures situated within the green diamond-shaped central area in Figure 6-12. The anatomic structures that fall into this diamond-shaped area consist primarily of the hard palate, the cervical spine, and the hyoid bone as well as the airway.

Figure 6-13 shows real double images of objects in the diamond-shaped area. The white arrows point to the *vertebrae of the cervical spine;* the yellow arrows point to the *body of the hyoid bone;* and the orange arrows point to the *hard palate;* the airway is just anterior to the cervical spine bilaterally and extends into the nasal area. Note there are two more images of the hard palate above each of the real images; the upper palate images each represent the ghost image of the real hard palate image on the opposite side. Ghost image formation will be explained in the next concept.

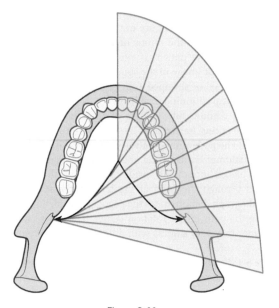

Figure **6-11**

In Figure 6-11, here once again, the thick, curved black line represents the path of the pan rotation center of the beam as the opposite side is being imaged. Also on this side, the beam emerges at a tangent to the path of the rotation center and exposes the *right side of the patient* as viewed from above.

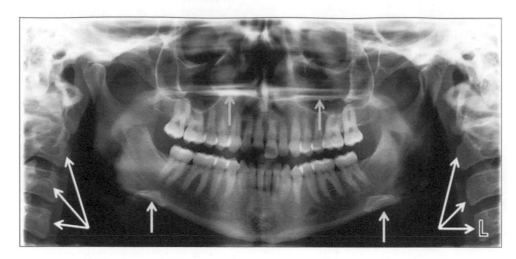

Figure **6-13**

Double images are seen twice and each is the mirror image of the other. These structures are located in the midline of the patient and fall into the diamond-shaped area of the path of the rotation center of the machine, and within which, single midline structures are seen twice, one on each side of the image. More anterior structures within the diamond-shaped area, such as the posterior part of the hard palate, are seen bilaterally toward the middle of the pan image, and the more posterior structures, such as the spine, are portrayed toward the edges of the image bilaterally. In addition, though these structures are located in the patient's midline, they are not always located in the midline of the pan image. Also, the farther toward the right and left edges of the pan image (posterior in the patient), the more posterior they are anatomically within the diamond-shaped area. If these structures are not exactly in the same place on opposite sides of the pan image, then the patient's head was turned to one side when positioned in the machine. Thus this concept also helps us to address patient positioning problems.

In summary, single real images are located in front of the path of the rotation center but not within the diamond-shaped area. In the diamond-shaped area, real double images are formed, and each of these produces a ghost image on the opposite side and slightly above its real counterpart. The hard palate (orange arrows) is an example where this effect is seen, whereby the real image is the lower structure, and the ghost image of the hard palate on the opposite side is the upper, more blurry structure. Ghost images are the next topic.

Concept # 5: Formation of Ghost Images

First, some structures that fall behind the path of the rotation center may also produce **ghost images**. Second, because the diamond-shaped area is behind the path of the rotation, real double images of some structures are formed, and these structures may also produce ghost images; an example of this is the hard palate. Other structures not within the diamond-shaped area but behind (posterior to) the rotation center, such as the **ramus** and spine, may also form ghost images.

This concept allows us to figure out other positioning problems. Some structures, such as the ramus of the mandible, may produce ghost images when the patient is positioned too far back in the machine, or the ghost image of the spine appears in the image when the patient is stooped or slumped. Once again, this concept helps us to address patient positioning problems.

Figure 6-14A demonstrates a zone of ghost image formation in blue. Notice the ramus, hard palate, hyoid bone, and spine are in this ghosting zone. The path of the rotation center is the black line, which defines the anatomic limits of the ghosting zone. Figure 6-14B is a film that was placed horizontally inside a phantom with multiple horizontal slices through the head at the level of the mandible. The resulting radiograph demonstrates the pagoda-shaped, thin black line representing the path of the rotation center. The exact path of the rotation center may vary slightly with different brands of panoramic machines.

In Figure 6-14C, a blurry ghost image of the spine is seen in the midline. Ghosting of the ramus bilaterally is seen as blurry white shadows medial to and on the opposite ramus. Thus the patient was too far back and slumped. (These errors will be illustrated clinically.).

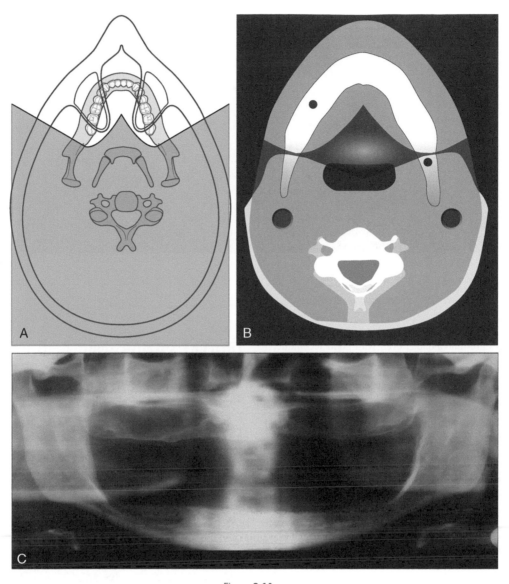

Figure **6-14**

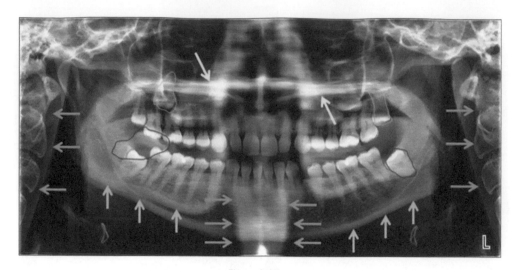

Figure **6-15**

Some ghost images are unavoidable, even with good technique, and tend to be those located within the diamond-shaped area such as the hard palate. Avoidable ghost images, such as the ghost images of the ramus and spine, are almost always an indication of a technique error. Once we learn and understand this information, it leads to the recognition of errors and their cause and ultimately good technique through the correction of these positioning errors.

In Figure 6-15, the patient was positioned too far back and "slumped" in the machine. First, the yellow arrows point to the real image of the hard palate on the left side and its ghost image on the right side of the image; this occurs in a normally positioned patient. The right side of the hard palate also produced real and ghost images but they are not indicated by arrows. Second, the ghost image of the left mandibular body and ramus (green arrows) as well as the real and ghost images of the right mandibular body and ramus not indicated by arrows indicate the patient was too far back in the machine; this also caused all four 3rd molars to be positioned behind the rotation center in the ghosting zone and resulted in ghost images and real images of the upper and lower third molars as outlined in red and orange for the left side. Third, the real images of the spine are illustrated by the blue arrows at the right and left edges of the image and the ghost image is the blurred vertical radiopacity in the center of the image. The ghosting of the spine occurred because the patient was "slumped" in the machine, that is to say the neck was not vertically positioned when the image was taken. In summary, this analysis of the image indicates the patient was positioned incorrectly in the machine. The patient was too far back and was "slumped" when the image was taken.

DIGITAL PANORAMIC AND CEPHALOMETRIC IMAGING

The development of panoramic and cephalometric imaging has gone through several phases since the advent of digital radiographic imaging in dental offices. One of the first digital panoramic images was taken in a laboratory at the University of Texas Health Science Center Dental School using a prototype digital panoramic machine. The volunteer patient was Dr. Langlais, and you can see him in Figure 6-16 and the resultant image in Figure 6-17.

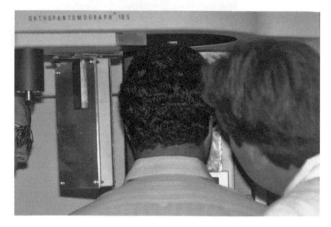

Figure **6-16**

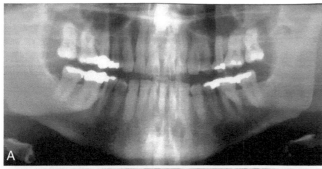

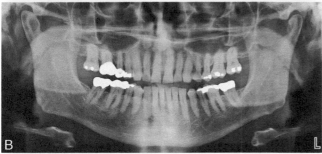

Figure **6-17**

In Figure 6-16, Dr. Langlais is being positioned in possibly the first digital panoramic machine. The sensor was from an early airport baggage scanner.

Figure 6-17A may possibly represent the first digital panoramic image taken in the 1980s and Figure 6-17B was taken in 2015. You can see that, in both cases, Dr. Langlais was positioned too far back (ghosting of the ramus bilaterally) and slumped in the machine, which produced ghosting of the spine vertically in the midline of the image.

This section, which explains the basis for troubleshooting panoramic positioning errors, is really important to understand. You should refer to this information as you go through the remaining sections of this chapter. This will help you identify positioning errors before taking an image, as well as after the image is taken, so corrective action can be taken to improve your technique. We have developed new diagrams illustrating the salient features of each positioning error. It is not uncommon to find several errors in a single panoramic image. All errors can be identified by their unique characteristics in the pan image. These features, though slightly variable, are essentially the same for all brands of panoramic machines.

QUESTIONS PART 1: IDENTIFICATION OF ERRORS IN CLINICAL TECHNIQUE

Figures 6-18 to 6-30 are examples of most of the possible errors in the positioning of the patient in the machine. The student may feel the errors are obvious. However, when the reader gets to the second part of this chapter consisting of the errors in the images, it becomes obvious that these errors happen and many of them continue to occur because neither the dentist nor the staff member is able or desires to recognize the problem(s) in the images themselves. Therefore the easier step in the learning process, and part of a good quality assurance program, is to identify positioning errors and correct them before the image is taken. Note that most operators of the machine tend to make the same error over and over again, until someone corrects the error, and different operators tend to make different errors. Thus when there are several operators in the office, each unique operator can be identified by the errors they tend to make. In this next section, it is our goal to show you virtually all of the positioning errors so that you can prevent them. Most of the pictures are of Dr. Langlais (the older one), Dr. Miller (the younger one) and Dr. Langlais' two sons Mark and Paul who "volunteered" for the pictures.

Instructions

Identify the errors illustrated in the following clinical photos (Figures 6-18 to 6-30) then check your answers with the Answer Key. Students may refer to the diagrams for a review of what effect these malpositioning problems have on the image. The next section will feature the images, and in the last section, we will ask you to match the clinical photo with the corresponding erroneous image. Our emphasis is to identify the error before taking the image because errors make images less diagnostic and can require a retake that doubles the radiation dose to the patient.

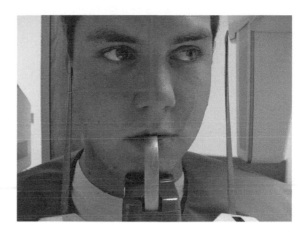

Figure **6-18**   Only one technique error has occurred or is the most obvious in this figure. Name the error, and state how the error can be corrected.

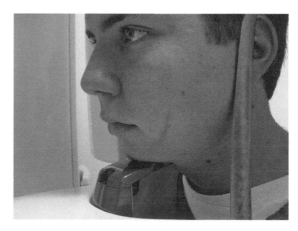

Figure **6-19**   Only one technique error has occurred or is the most obvious in this figure. Name the error, and state how the error can be corrected.

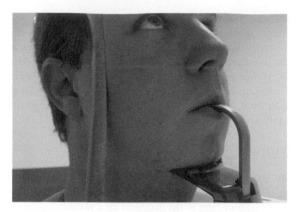

Figure **6-20**   Only one technique error has occurred or is the most obvious in this figure. Name the error, and state how the error can be corrected.

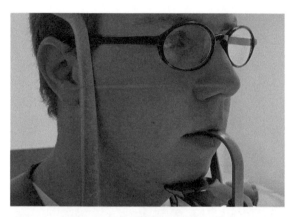

Figure **6-21**   Identify the technique error and state how the errors can be corrected.

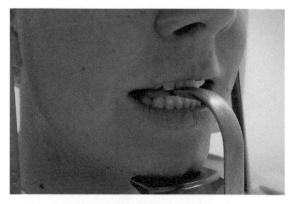

Figure **6-22**   Identify the technique errors and state how the errors can be corrected.

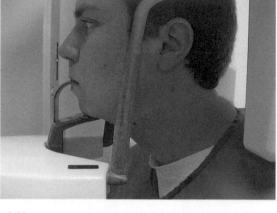

Figure **6-23**   Only one technique error has occurred or is the most obvious in this figure. Name the error, and state how the error can be corrected.

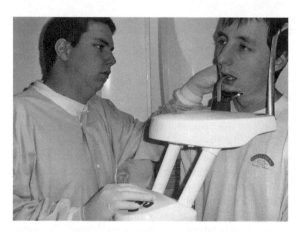

Figure **6-24**   Several errors have occurred in this picture. Name the errors, and state how the errors can be corrected.

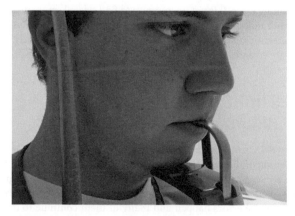

Figure **6-25**   Only one technique error has occurred or is the most obvious in this figure. Name the error, and state how the error can be corrected.

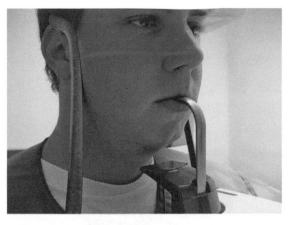

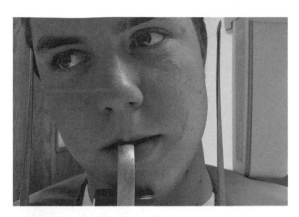

Figure **6-26** Only one technique error has occurred or is the most obvious in this figure. Name the error, and state how the error can be corrected.

Figure **6-27** Only one technique error has occurred or is the most obvious in this figure. Name the error, and state how the error can be corrected.

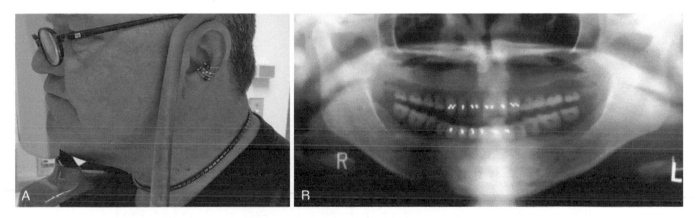

Figure **6-28** A and B: First the dad, who represents an edentulous older patient (father and son like to dress alike). Study the picture and radiograph carefully and see how many errors you can find.

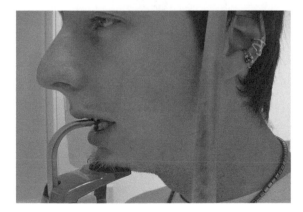

Figure **6-29** Identify the technique errors in this image.

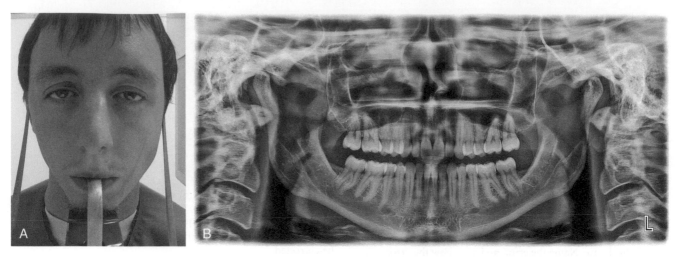

Figure **6-30**   This is the son. See how many errors you can find here.

A VISUAL REFERENCE FOR PANORAMIC TECHNIQUE TROUBLESHOOTING

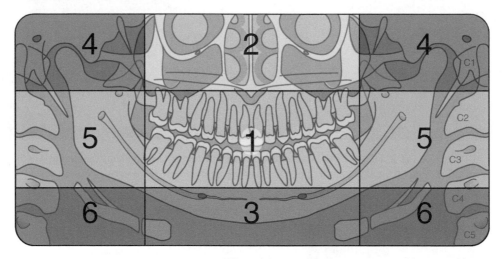

Figure **6-31**

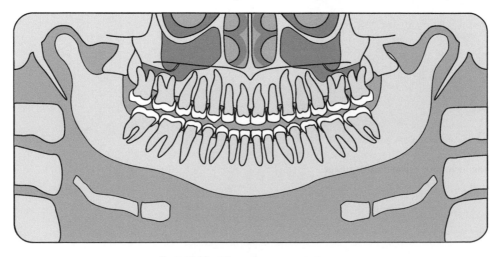

Figure **6-32**   Normal panoramic image.

Zones for the Analysis of Panoramic Errors

See Figure 6-31. Panoramic images should be reviewed for technical quality by zone. There are three zones in the midline and three bilateral zones.

ZONE 1: The dentition. There should be a gentle curve at the occlusal plane, not flat or overly curved; the occlusal plane should be symmetric and not higher up or lower down on one side or the other. The teeth, especially the anteriors, should not be excessively narrowed or widened and the posterior teeth should not be wider or narrower on one side or the other. The contacts should be slightly overlapped on both sides; not open on one side and excessively overlapped on the other side. The root tips of the anterior teeth should not be cut off.

ZONE 2: The nose-sinus. The turbinates, especially the lower turbinates, should be within the nose and not spread out across the maxillary sinus. Within the sinus, there are usually the real and ghost images of the hard palate equally on both sides. Also the malar process of the maxilla (root of the zygomatic arch) and a portion of the maxillary process of the zygomatic arch may be present.

ZONE 3: The inferior mandible midline. The inferior border should be slightly curved downward vertically and not flat or excessively curved. The ghost image of the spine should not be seen here at the midline. The inferior cortex should not be wiggly or have jagged discontinuities.

ZONE 4: The temporomandibular joints (TMJs). The condyles should be in the middle of this area bilaterally, not higher up toward the top of the images or to the sides. The condyles should both be at the same level, not one higher or lower than the other.

ZONE 5: The ramus-spine. There should be separation between the ramus and the spine. The spine should not be superimposed on the ramus bilaterally or on one side only. The spine should be vertical. If the spine is not seen, this may also be normal. The ramus itself should not be wider on one side than the other and should be clear of the ghost image of the opposite ramus.

ZONE 6: The hyoid bone. There is usually a double image of the hyoid bone because it falls in the diamond-shaped area created by the rotation center; but it should not extend more than a few centimeters into zone 3. It should be equal and symmetric on both sides.

Panoramic Error Identification Reference Diagrams

The following diagrams may be used as a reference for the identification of the positioning errors on panoramic images. Look carefully at the radiographs and see if you can find the same features in the diagrams. Remember there may be more than one error in the radiograph.

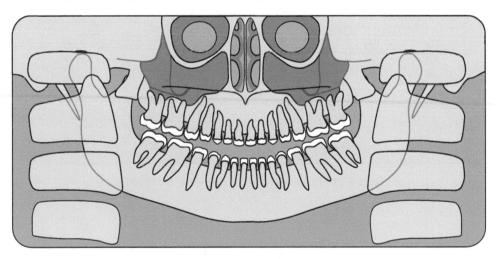

Figure **6-33** Patient too far forward.

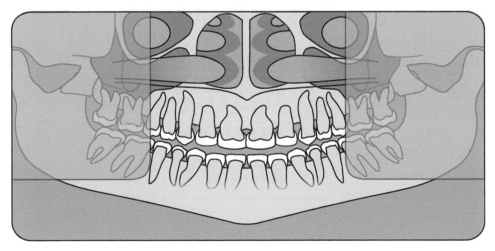

Figure **6-34** Patient too far back.

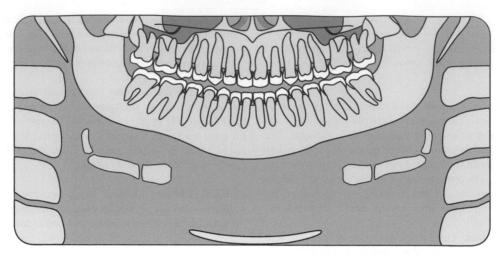

Figure **6-35**   Patient's chin not on the chin rest.

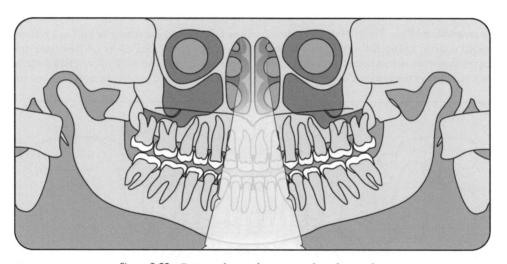

Figure **6-36**   Patient slumped or stooped in the machine.

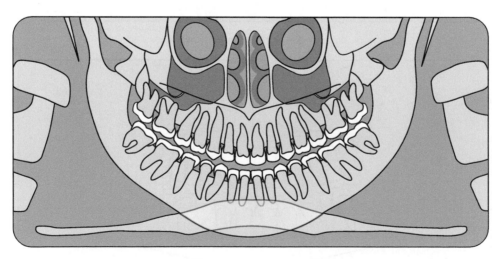

Figure **6-37**   Patient's chin tilted too low.

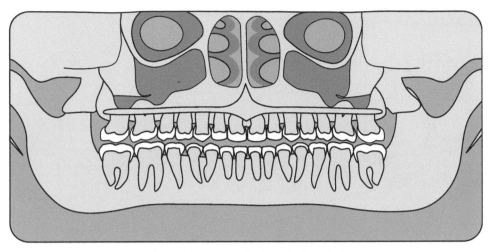

Figure **6-38** Patient's chin tilted too high.

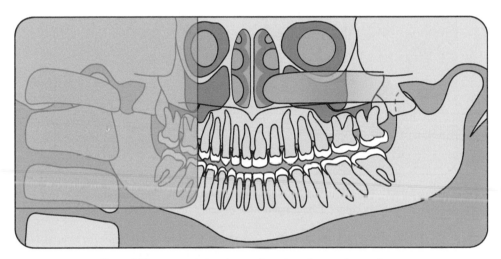

Figure **6-39** Patient's head turned to the side; not facing front.

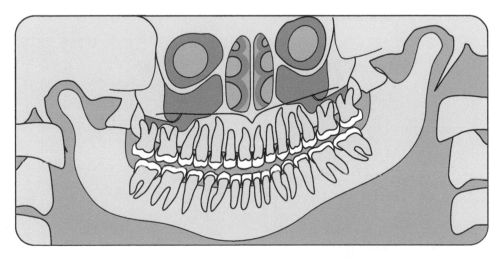

Figure **6-40** Patient's head tilted or canted to one side.

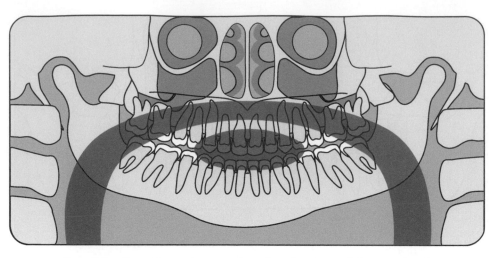

Figure **6-41**   Patient's tongue not against the palate; patient's lips not closed.

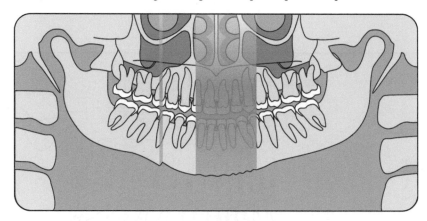

Figure **6-42**   Patient movement during the exposure, often because of the machine rubbing against the patient's neck or upper back.

QUESTIONS PART 2: IDENTIFICATION OF ERRORS IN RADIOGRAPHS
Instructions

Identify the errors in the following radiographs and answer any included questions. When asked to identify errors in a radiograph, give a three-part answer: (1) Name the error(s), (2) when possible, list one characteristic feature of the error as seen in the teeth and one anatomic feature, and (3) explain how to correct each error. Compare your answers to the correct answers in the Answer Key at the back of the book.

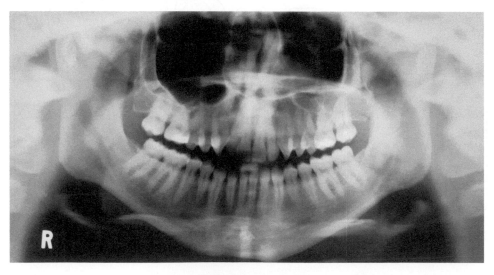

Figure **6-43**   Identify one error.

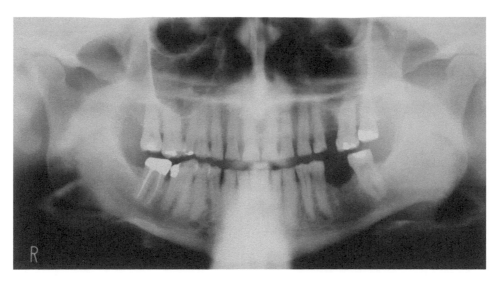

Figure **6-44**   Identify one error.

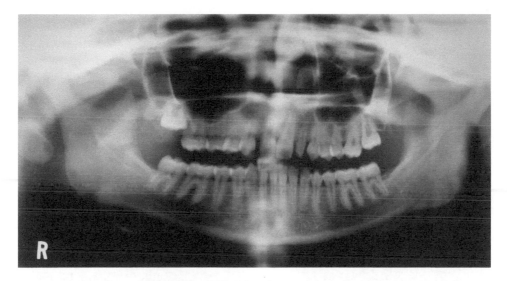

Figure **6-45**   Identify two errors.

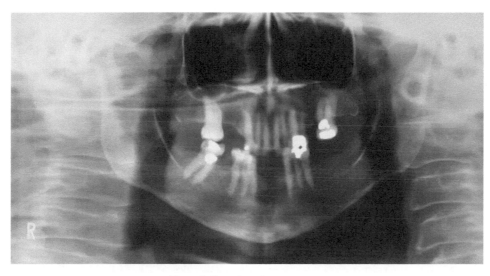

Figure **6-46**   Identify two errors.

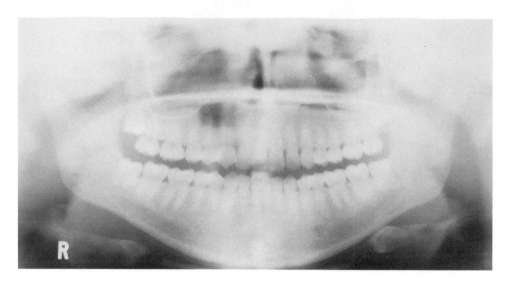

Figure **6-47**   Identify one error.

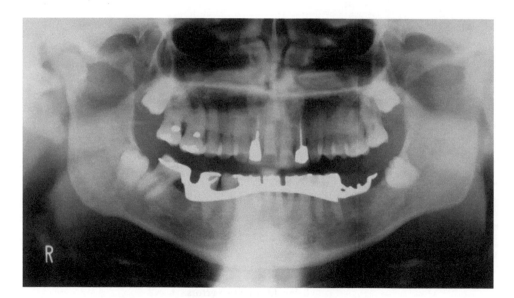

Figure **6-48**   Identify two errors.

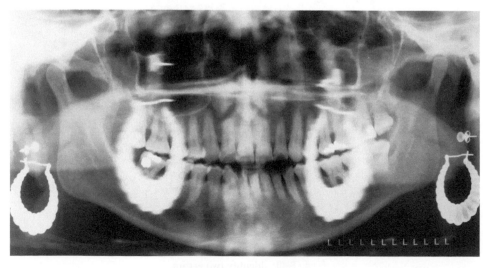

Figure **6-49**   Identify one error.

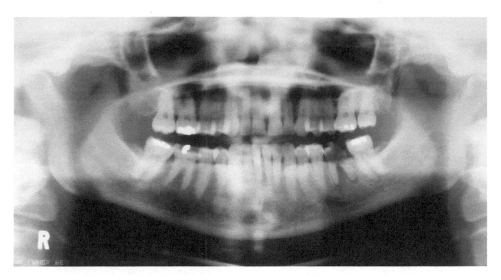

Figure **6-50**   Identify two errors.

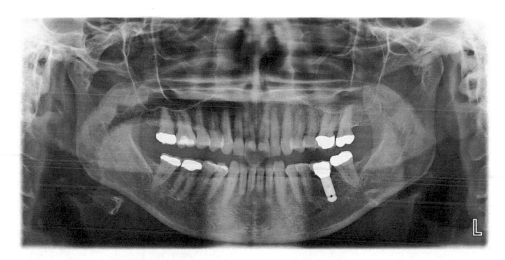

Figure **6-51**   Identify one error.

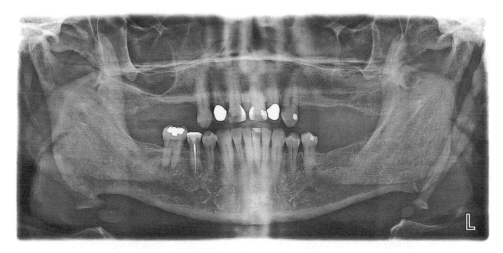

Figure **6-52**   Identify two errors.

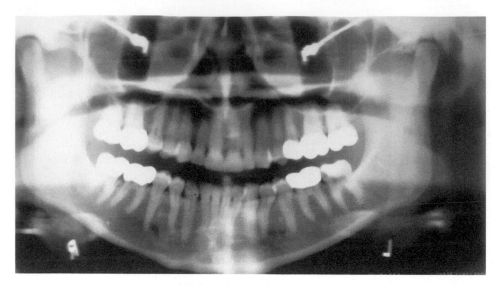

Figure **6-53**   Identify three errors.

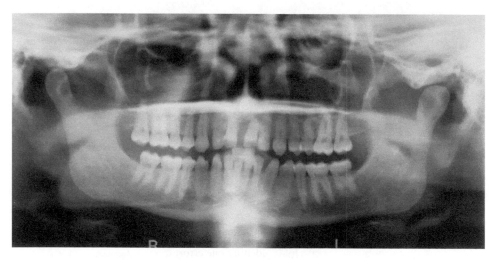

Figure **6-54**   Identify four errors.

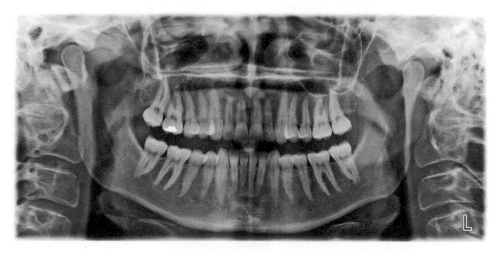

Figure **6-55**   Identify two errors.

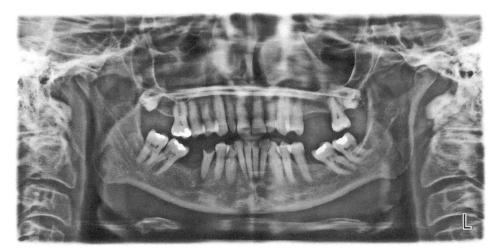

Figure **6-56**   Identify three errors.

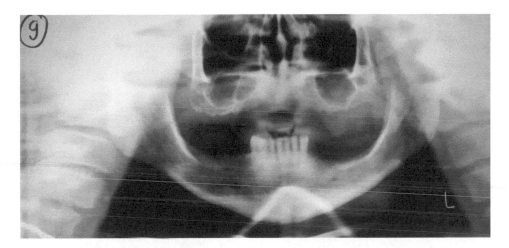

Figure **6-57**   Identify two errors.

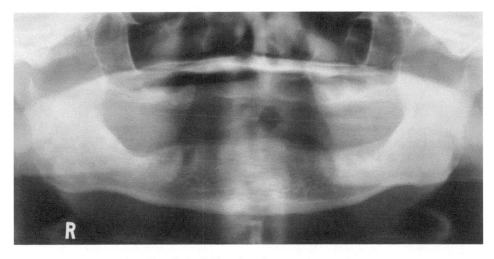

Figure **6-58**   Identify two errors.

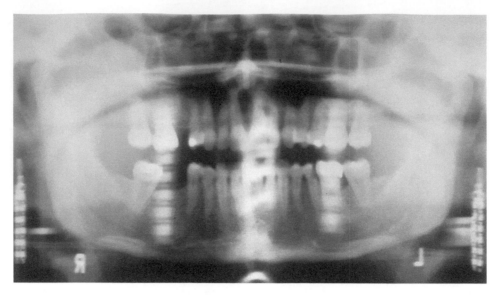

Figure **6-59**   Identify five errors.

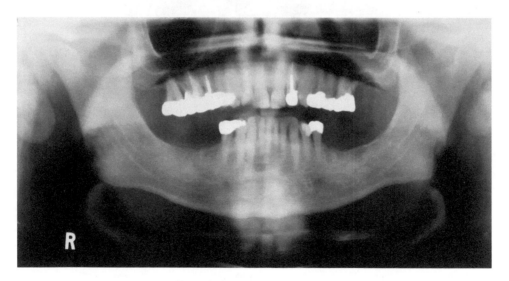

Figure **6-60**   Identify two errors.

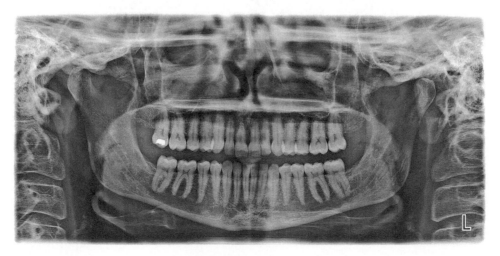

Figure **6-61**   Identify three errors.

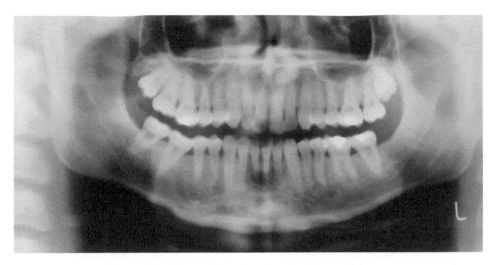

Figure **6-62** Identify one error.

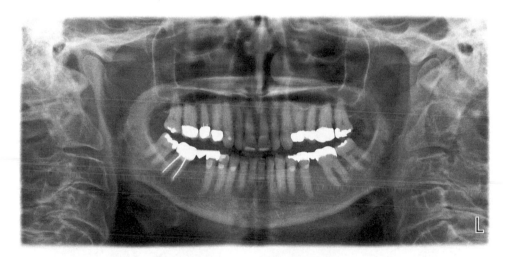

Figure **6-63** Identify two errors.

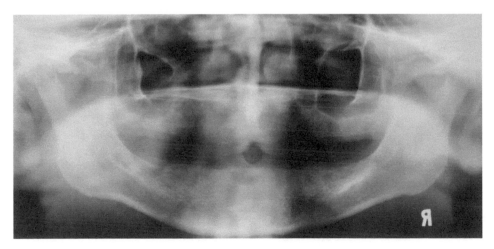

Figure **6-64** Identify one error.

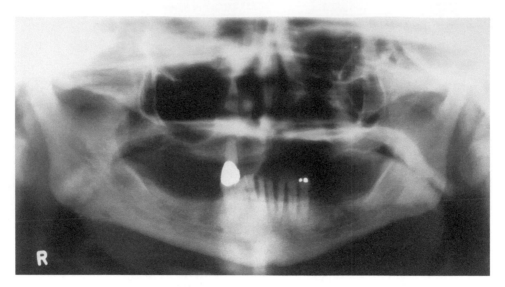

Figure **6-65**   Identify one error.

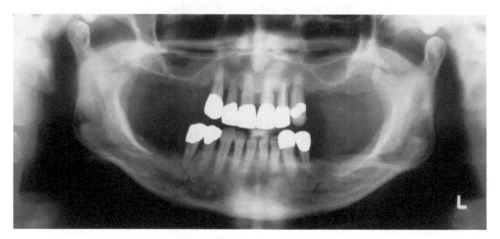

Figure **6-66**   Identify one error.

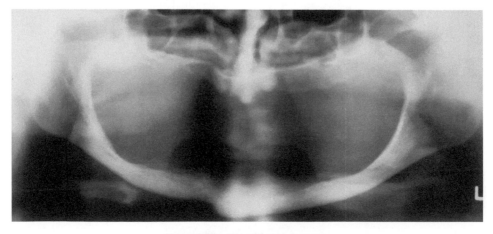

Figure **6-67**   Identify three errors.

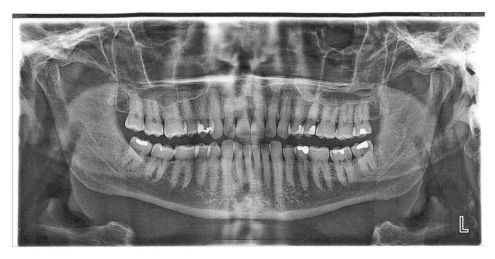

Figure **6-68**   Identify four errors.

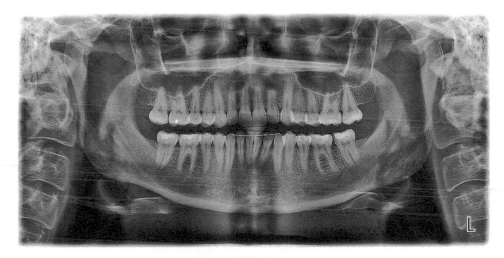

Figure **6-69**   Identify two errors.

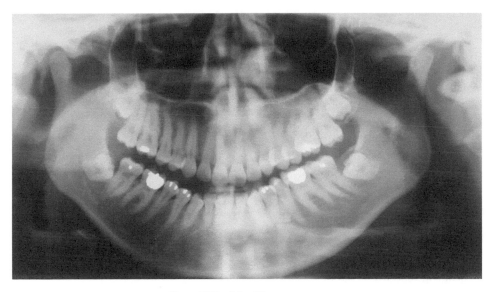

Figure **6-70**   Identify two errors.

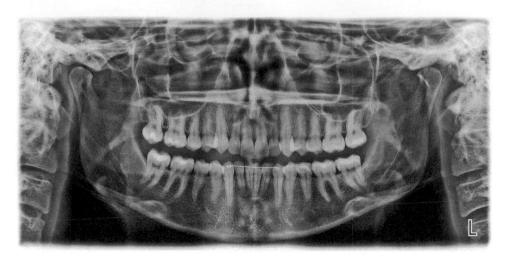

Figure **6-71**   Identify one error.

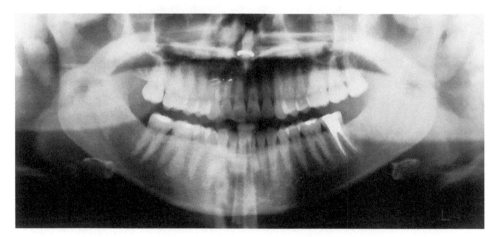

Figure **6-72**   Identify four errors.

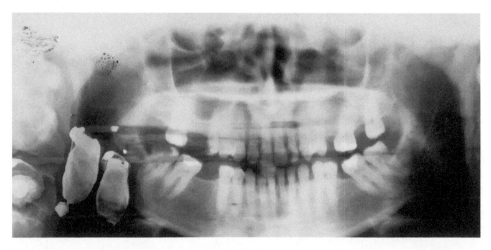

Figure **6-73**   This film is marred by chemical stains.
1.   State what chemical(s) has (have) affected this image.

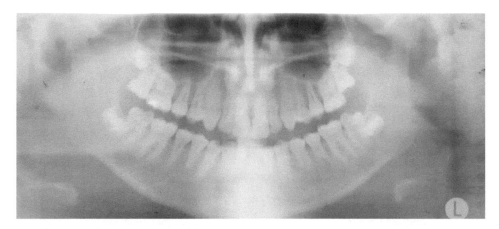

Figure **6-74** Though it is hard to see here, this film has an overall grayish look to it.
1. State what problem caused this.

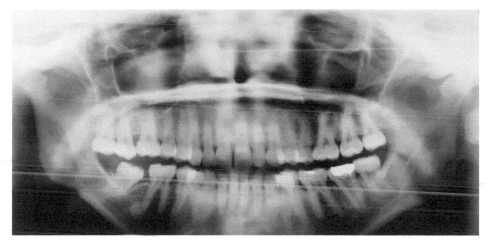

Figure **6-75** This film has an undesirable horizontal white line on it, and every film taken with the same cassette had the same mark.
1. State what the problem is.

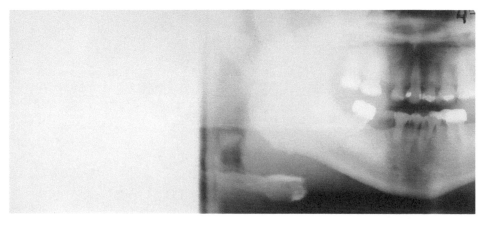

Figure **6-76** Only half of this film was exposed, but the exposure was not aborted.
1. What happened here?

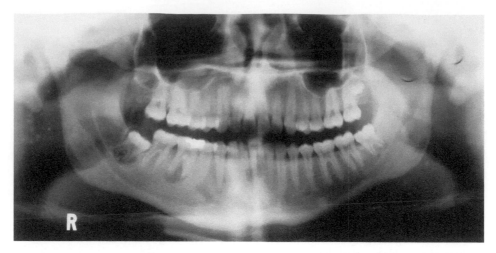

Figure **6-77**   There are two different problems here:
1.   What are the black, crescent-shaped marks from?
2.   What are the little whitish spots at the right- and left-hand edges of the film?

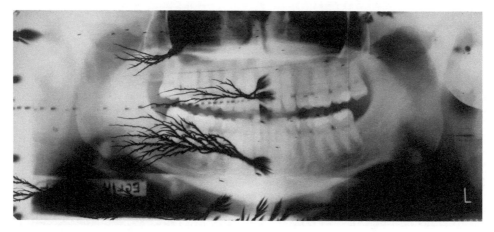

Figure **6-78**   Observe the black spots and lightninglike marks.
1.   What happened here?
2.   How can this be prevented?

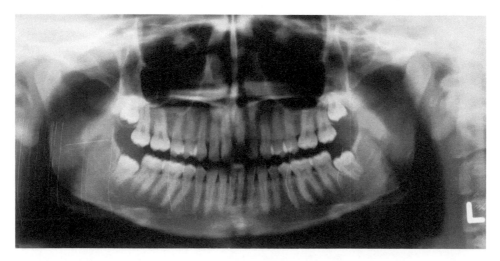

Figure **6-79**   Observe the radiopaque vertical lines in this image.
1.   What could these be?

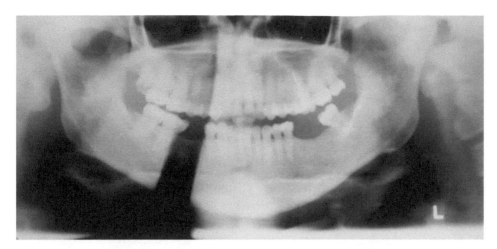

Figure **6-80** Here's a clue regarding the nature of this problem. The cassette is an old plastic one that is wrapped around a drum.
1. What is the undesirable black mark on the film?

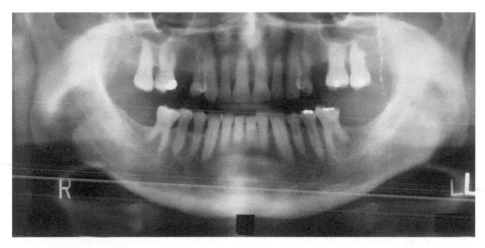

Figure **6-81** Look at the squiggly, thin, white vertical line on the patient's left. Every film taken with this cassette had this mark.
1. What is the problem?

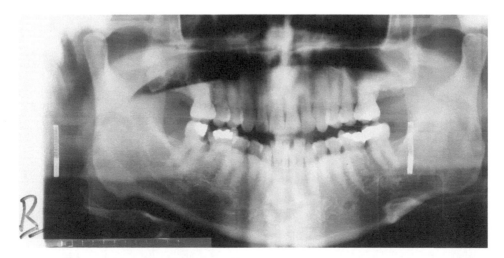

Figure **6-82** Notice the "Ls" at the bottom left of the figure and an "R" written in. There are also a couple of springs and darker square or rectangular areas.
1. Can you state what happened?
2. Would you keep this film?

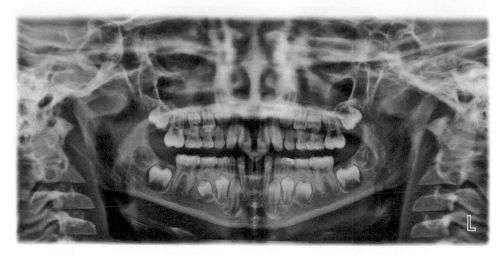

Figure **6-83** Identify two errors.

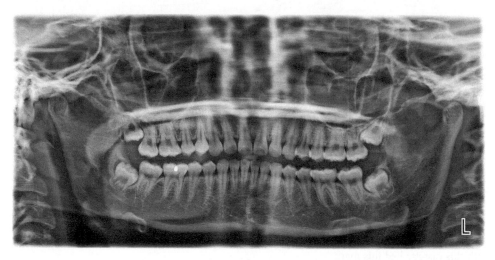

Figure **6-84** Identify two errors.

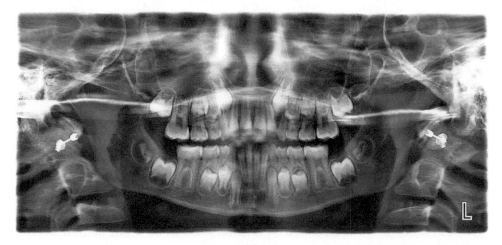

Figure **6-85** Identify three errors.

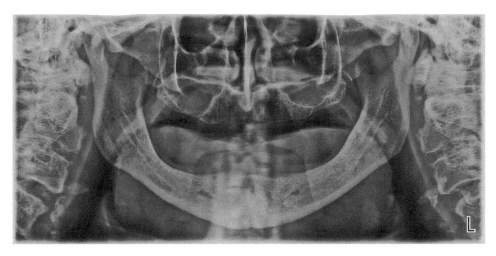

Figure **6-86** Identify two errors.

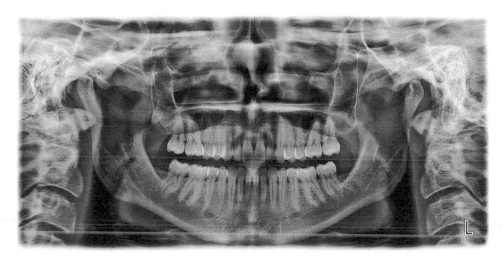

Figure **6-87** Identify three errors.

QUESTIONS PART 3: MATCHING THE CLINICAL ERROR WITH THE RADIOGRAPH

Instructions

We finally get to see both a clinical picture and a selection of radiographs, one of which will most closely match the clinical picture. To do this in the best way, try to identify the one or two major positioning errors in the clinical image and then look for the closest match in the series of radiographs. Most of the pictures including Dr. Miller, Dr. Langlais, and his son Paul Langlais are seen erroneously positioned in a variety of panoramic machine models. The error(s) should be identified clinically first, but if you cannot, then look at the radiographs and try to find that error in the clinical photo. Remember that the object is to first recognize and correct the error before taking the radiograph. However, if the pan image has been taken, then recognition of the error(s) in the image can still lead to improved technique. There is one picture of a darkroom safelight, and there is a corresponding pan image as well. Also, there is a patient with a barbell in his tongue, and it is unrelated to any of the other photographs anywhere in this book. Look carefully at these examples to improve your radiographic techniques.

Match the clinical pictures numbered 6-88 through 6-97 with the radiographs numbered 6-98 to 6-107. Check the correct answers in the Answer Key at the back of the book.

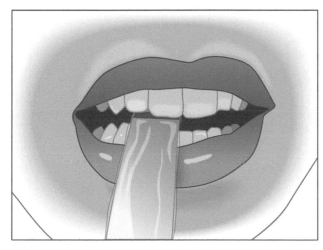

Figure **6-88**

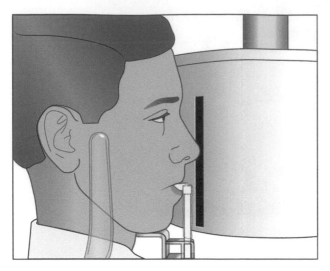

Figure **6-89**

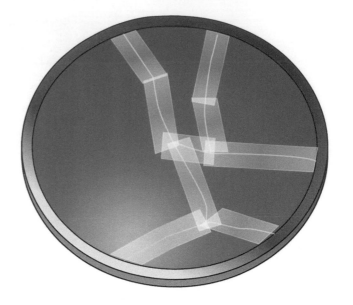

Figure **6-91**

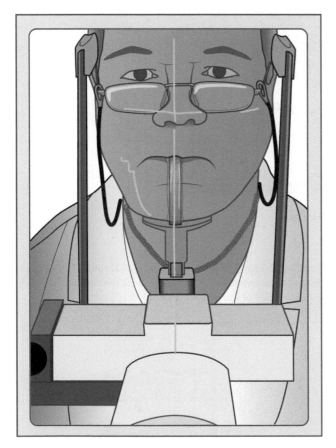

Figure **6-90**

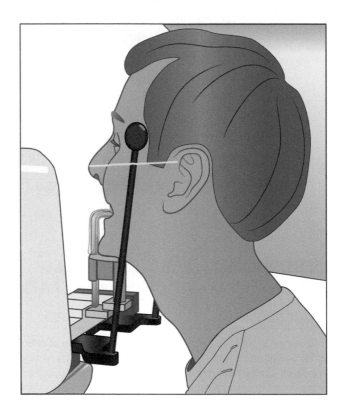

Figure **6-92**

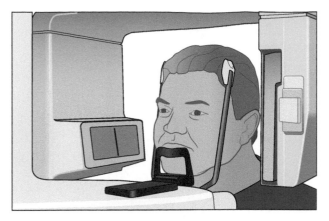

Figure **6-93**

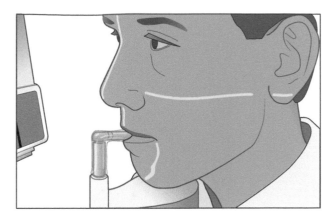

Figure **6-96**

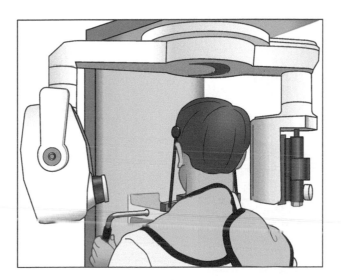

Figure **6-94**

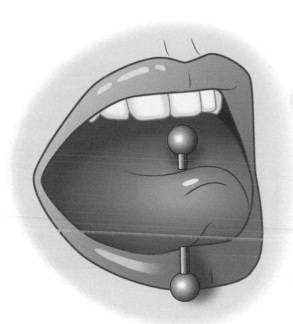

Figure **6-97**

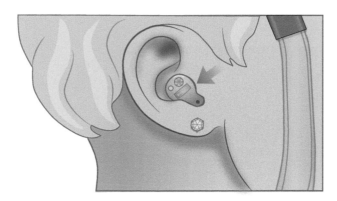

Figure **6-95**

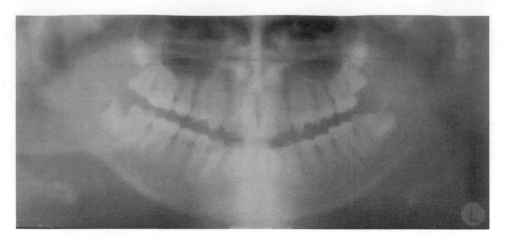

Figure **6-98**

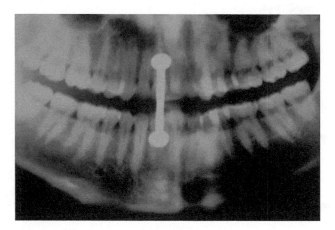

Figure **6-99**

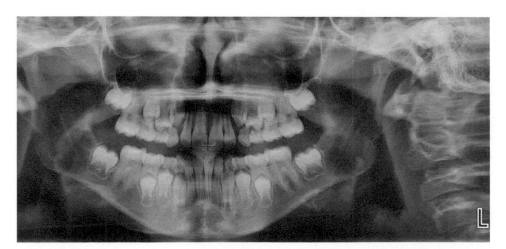

Figure **6-100**

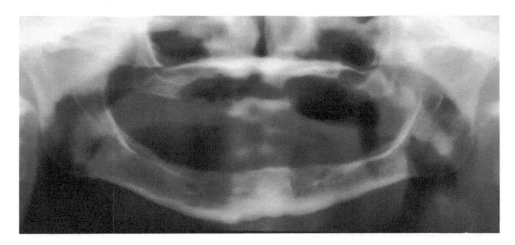

Figure **6-101**

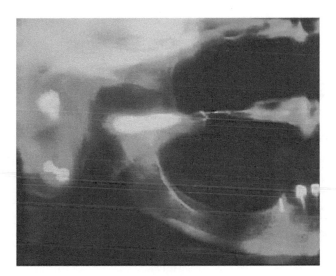

Figure **6-102**

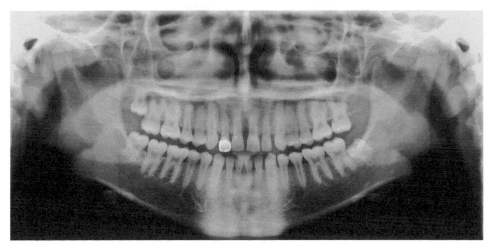

Figure **6-103**

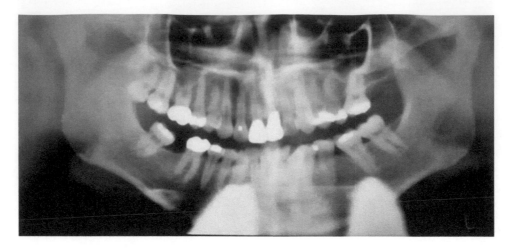

Figure **6-104**

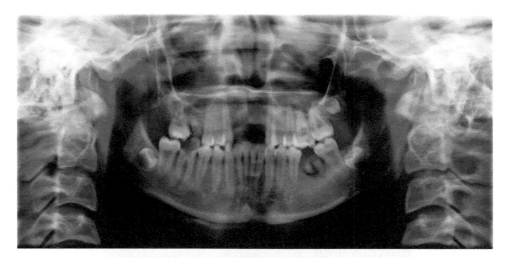

Figure **6-105**

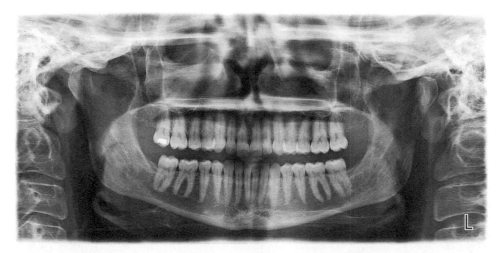

Figure **6-106**

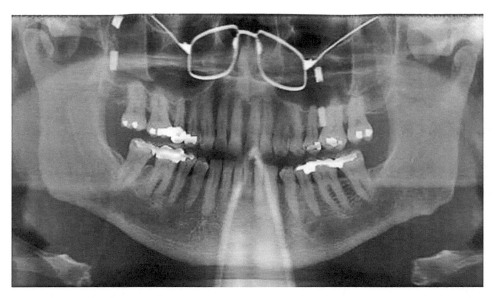

Figure **6-107**

QUESTIONS PART 4: MULTIPLE CHOICE QUESTIONS WITHOUT FIGURES

Instructions

Please select the best answer and check your selection with the correct answer in the Answer Key at the back of the book.

1. In panoramic radiology, it is possible to capture the image on:
   A. Film
   B. Photostimulable phosphor plates
   C. Electronic sensors
   D. All of the above

2. In a properly positioned patient, the projection angle of the beam causes buccal objects to be projected _____ in the image.
   A. Upward
   B. Downward
   C. On the same horizontal plane
   D. Upward or downward, depending on the anatomic location

3. The projection angle of the panoramic beam is:
   A. Perpendicular to the jaws
   B. Upward relative to the jaws
   C. Downward relative to the jaws
   D. Is a horizontal fan beam with an angle of 230 degrees

4. In a properly positioned patient, and in terms of the horizontal magnification of objects within the panoramic layer:
   A. Buccal objects are narrowed
   B. Buccal objects are widened
   C. Buccal objects are unaffected in terms of horizontal magnification
   D. Buccal objects may be widened or narrowed, depending on patient size

5. In a properly positioned patient, buccal and lingual objects are subject to more vertical displacement:
   A. In the maxilla
   B. In the mandible
   C. In the center of the layer
   D. There is no difference between buccal and lingual objects

6. In standard panoramic projection geometry, the beam is said to:
   A. Emanate from the path of the center of rotation
   B. Be perpendicular to the path of the center of rotation
   C. Be perpendicular to the contact points of the posterior teeth
   D. Be a tangent to the path of the rotation center

7. The so called diamond-shaped anatomic area is where _____ images are generated.
   A. Ghost
   B. Double-ghost
   C. Double-real
   D. Double-real and ghost

8. If an anatomic structure is located behind the rotation center, it may produce:
   A. Double-real images
   B. Ghost images
   C. Single-real images
   D. All of the above

9. If we are looking at a lower 1st molar edentulous space and we can clearly see the alveolar canal and the crest of the mandibular ridge, we may:
   A. Make vertical measurements using a 25% magnification factor
   B. Make vertical measurements using a 33% magnification factor
   C. Make vertical measurements using a magnification factor as determined by the measurement of a fiduciary object, such as a BB, in the region of interest
   D. Not reliably make vertical measurements

10. A ghost image is _____ in the radiographic image:
    A. Always above the real image
    B. Always on the opposite side of the real image
    C. A and B
    D. Neither A nor B as real images superimpose ghost images on the same side

11. If the upper 3rd molars are impacted and you see an additional molar in the maxillary sinus on the same side:
    A. It may be an ectopically erupted supernumerary molar
    B. It may be an oval-shaped osteoma in the maxillary sinus
    C. It may represent the ghost image of the opposite maxillary 3rd molar
    D. It may represent an object in the diamond-shaped area as there is a similar ghost image in the opposite maxillary sinus, the two representing a double image of a single object

12. In panoramic radiology, there is more widening and narrowing of the teeth in the:
    A. Anterior region
    B. Posterior region
    C. Both the anterior and posterior regions
    D. Middle of the layer

13. In a panoramic image, the hard palate produces:
    A. Double-real images
    B. Double-ghost images
    C. Double-real and ghost images
    D. Thin and hard-to-see images

14. If a patient's chin is positioned too high up during the exposure, the hard palate:
    A. Real and double images may be superimposed on each other
    B. Real and double images may be superimposed on the apices of the upper teeth
    C. May have a radiolucent band of air below it due to air because the tongue was not against the hard palate
    D. All of the above

15. If a patient is positioned too far forward in the pan machine, features of this error in the image consist of which of the following?
    A. The anterior teeth appear narrow and the spine is superimposed on the ramus
    B. The anterior teeth are too wide and the spine is not in the image
    C. The hard palate shadow is superimposed on the apices of the upper teeth and the occlusal plane is flat
    D. This error is difficult to identify in the image

Chapter 7

Normal Anatomy

Goal

To learn to recognize normal anatomic structures as they appear in various radiographs

Learning Objectives

1. Learn to identify anatomic structures on labeled photographs and diagrams
2. Recognize anatomic structures as labeled on cone beam computed tomography (CBCT) three-dimensional (3D) reconstructions in coronal, sagittal, and axial views
3. Learn by correlating diagrammatic and 3D anatomic diagrams and images with the structures as projected on the radiographic image
4. Identify anatomic structures in intraoral radiographs
5. Recognize anatomic structures in panoramic radiographs
6. Begin to correlate anatomic distortions and panoramic technique errors

---

NOTE TO STUDENTS

Some of the structures identified in this chapter may not seem relevant. However, anatomic identification is key to diagnosing abnormalities. Remember, we will be looking at not only intraoral and panoramic images, but also CBCT images, which will sometimes involve more extensive anatomic coverage, depending on the volume.

INTRODUCTION

Learning normal anatomy as displayed on radiographs has always been important. Up until recently, dental offices were limited to the use of two-dimensional radiographic imaging consisting mainly of intraoral, panoramic, and cephalometric machines. In intraoral imaging, undesirable distortions of certain anatomic structures can signal a technique error, which can be corrected by retaking the radiograph. Distortion can be defined as unequal magnification in different parts of the image. This can result in inaccurate structural relationships and measurements that are needed for endodontic, implant, surgical, and orthodontic applications, just to name a few. Furthermore, some digital intraoral sensors are bulky and have a smaller image area than film or photostimulable phosphor plates (PSPs), which have been discussed in Chapter 1 and Chapter 4. In some cases, there is a limitation in the size of the intraoral beam such as with rectangular collimation or cone-cutting errors. The aforementioned developments in digital intraoral imaging may result in missing the apical regions and inadequate bitewing coverage, especially in the canine or first premolar areas due to discomfort caused by office personnel who are inexperienced in the use of some bulky electronic sensors.

Since the previous edition of this book, there has been much progress in panoramic imaging. While electronic digital panoramic images have coverage equal to that of film and PSP-based digital panoramic images, they are also subject to the same distortions of anatomic structures. Some of these anatomic distortions may be due to a technique error in patient positioning. Advances in panoramic imaging now make it possible to collimate the beam to a specific region resembling a periapical image but without the loss of apical coverage and/or discomfort of digital electronic sensors. In addition, panoramic bitewings are now available and will be discussed in Chapter 9. Panoramic bitewings provide visualization of the interproximal contacts and periapical regions. However, like intraoral bitewings, panoramic bitewings may have overlapped interproximal contacts due to specific errors related to panoramic bitewing techniques that can be recognized, analyzed, and corrected.

Another new technology that is now becoming much more commonplace is cone beam computed tomography (CBCT). CBCT is less subject to technique errors, although the structures of interest must be included in the volume. On occasion, structures may be missed due to malpositioning or the selection of too small a volume. CBCT has not been recommended for bitewing techniques and the present authors do not recommend CBCT for the diagnosis of interproximal caries. The great advantages of CBCT include an absence of distortions in anatomic structures, accurate linear and angular anatomic measurements, and the ability to view any anatomic structure, area, or lesion in all three dimensions. In addition, the user can scroll through the entire volume in any one of the three selected planes or view the entire volume as a three-dimensional image just as we have illustrated in this chapter.

One item of note is that CBCT, unlike medical CT, can be utilized with radiation doses no greater than a series of intraoral images, a panoramic radiograph, or cephalometric image. In intraoral imaging, significant increases in dosage can occur when utilizing a short, 8-inch or 12-inch or even a round, 16-inch cone vs. a rectangular round cone and also "D" speed film vs. digital sensors. While most dental assisting, hygiene, and dentist training is with rectangular collimation, in the experience of the authors, it is not commonly used in dental practices.

The above short narrative has been included to explain why the authors have revised this chapter to not only include intraoral and panoramic anatomy, but also an added introduction to CBCT anatomy. Furthermore, color pictures of the bony structures have been substituted for some of the diagrams, and 3D-colorized CBCT images have been used instead of skull photographs. This is because CBCT displays the bony anatomy as never seen before, and CBCT cases will be included in this edition. Also several cuts from each of the three anatomic viewing planes in CBCT consisting of axial, coronal, and sagittal views have been included with the anatomic structures identified.

In short, our knowledge of anatomy as displayed in dental radiographic images has always been important. However, this knowledge has never been as important as it is now because of the tremendous advances in dental radiography in recent years.

SHORT ANSWER QUESTIONS WITH FIGURES
Instructions

For each question please answer the following:

Part 1: Identify the overall anatomic structure(s) in the illustration (example: mandible).
Part 2: State whether this is a view from the buccal or lingual.
Part 3: Identify anatomic landmarks as indicated by the numbered arrows.

Compare your answer to the correct answer in the Answer Key at the back of the book

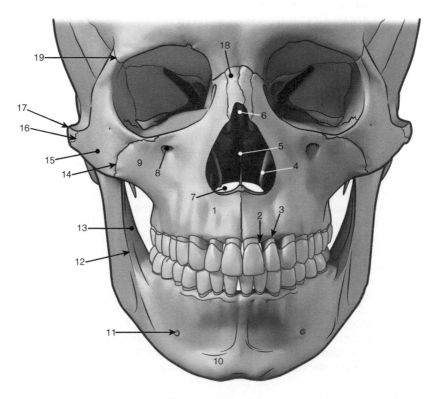

Figure **7-1** Identify the overall structure, view, and indicated bony landmarks.

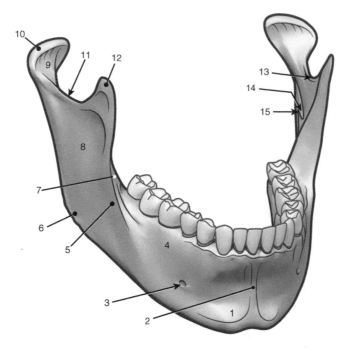

Figure **7-2** Identify the overall structure, view, and indicated bony landmarks.

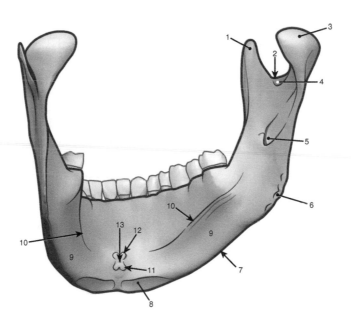

Figure **7-3** Identify the overall structure, view, and indicated bony landmarks.

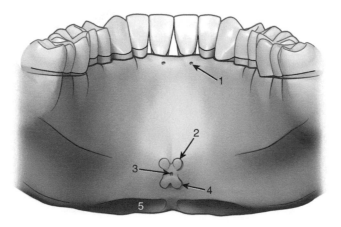

Figure **7-4** Identify the overall structure, view, and indicated bony landmarks.

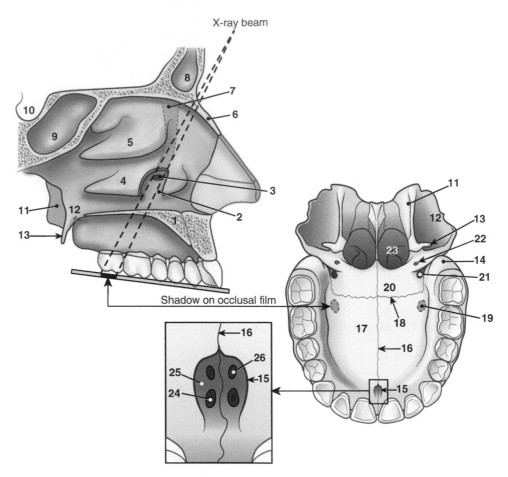

Figure **7-5** Identify the overall structure, view, and indicated bony landmarks.

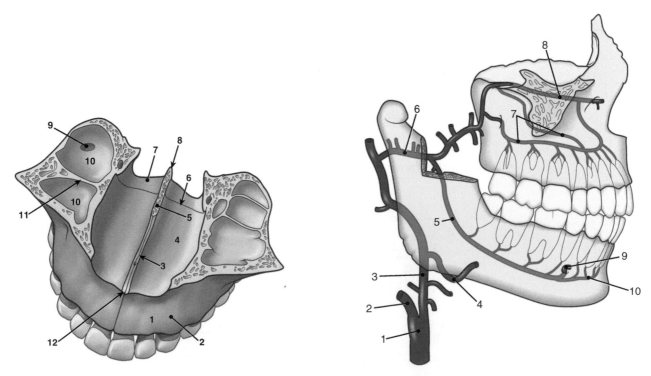

Figure **7-6** Identify the overall structure, view, and indicated bony landmarks.

Figure **7-7** Identify the overall structure, view, and indicated anatomic structures.

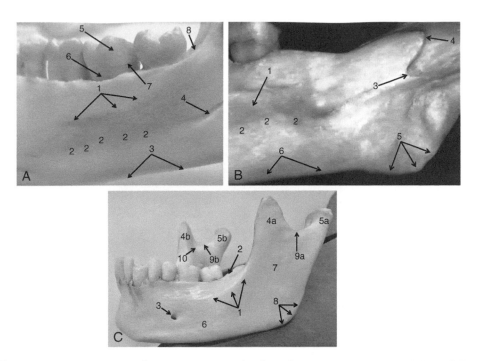

Figure **7-8** Identify the overall structure, view, and indicated anatomic structures in A, B, and C.

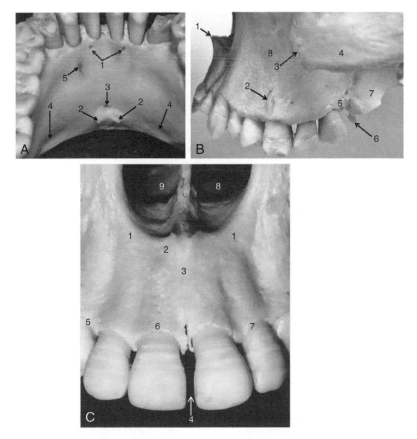

Figure **7-9** Identify the overall structure, view, and indicated bony landmarks in A, B, and C.

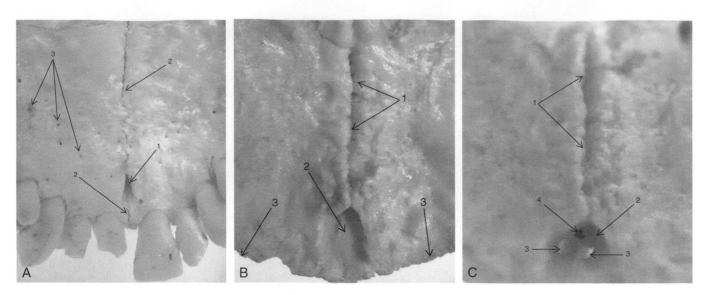

Figure **7-10**   Identify the overall structure, view, and indicated bony landmarks in A, B, and C.

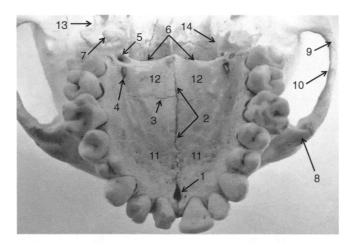

Figure **7-11**   Identify the overall structure, view, and indicated bony landmarks.

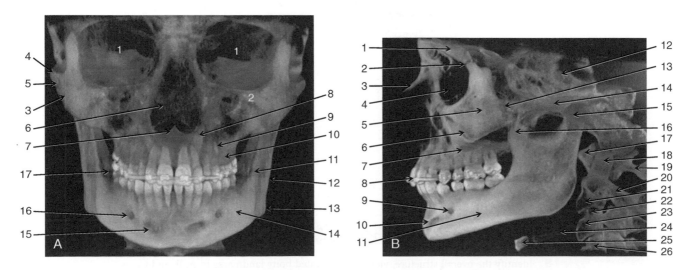

Figure **7-12**   Identify the overall structure, view, and indicated bony landmarks in A and B.

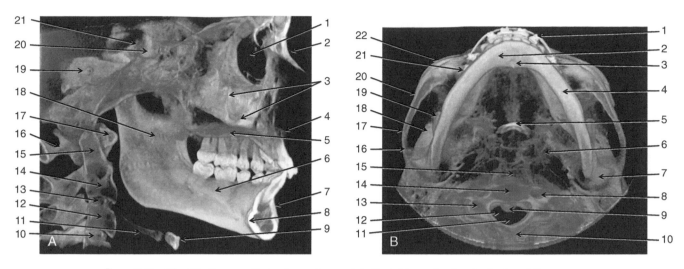

Figure **7-13** Identify the overall structure, view, and indicated bony landmarks in A and B.

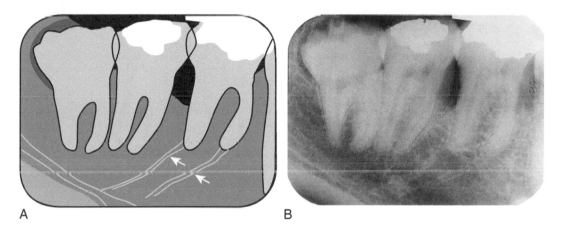

Figure **7-14** Identify the indicated structures.

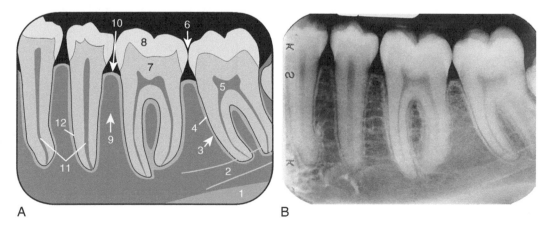

Figure **7-15** Identify the indicated structures.

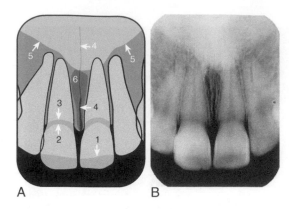

Figure **7-16** Identify the indicated structures.

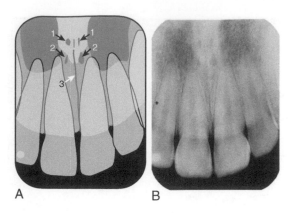

Figure **7-19** Identify the indicated structures.

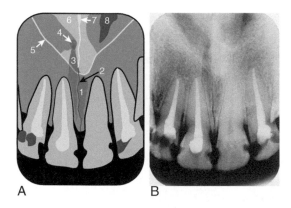

Figure **7-17** Identify the indicated structures.

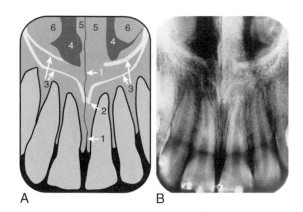

Figure **7-20** Identify the indicated structures.

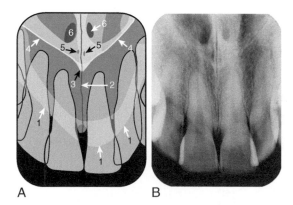

Figure **7-18** Identify the indicated structures.

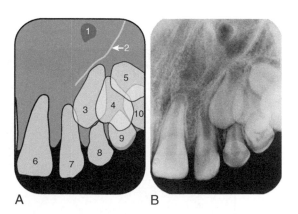

Figure **7-21** Identify the indicated structures.

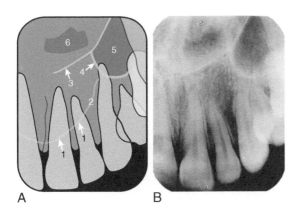

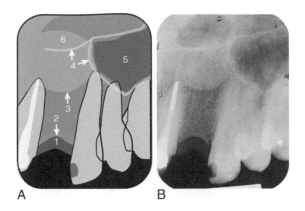

Figure **7-22** Identify the indicated structures.

Figure **7-23** Identify the indicated structures.

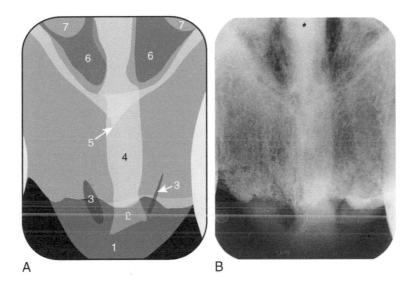

Figure **7-24** Identify the indicated structures.

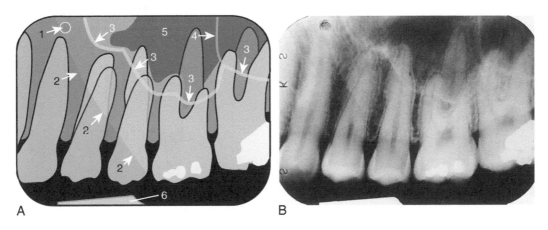

Figure **7-25** Identify the indicated structures.

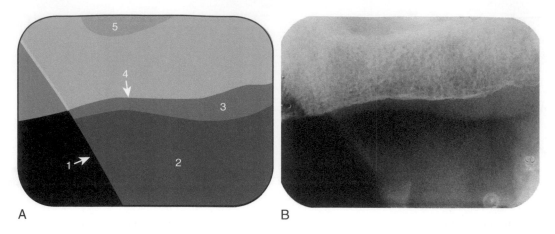

Figure **7-26** Identify the indicated structures.

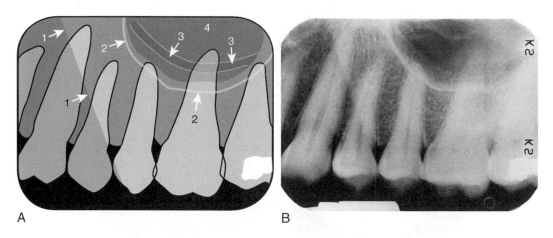

Figure **7-27** Identify the indicated structures.

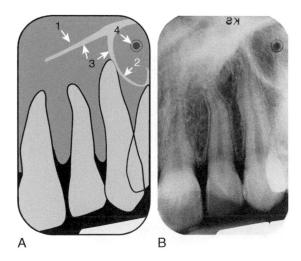

Figure **7-28** Identify the indicated structures.

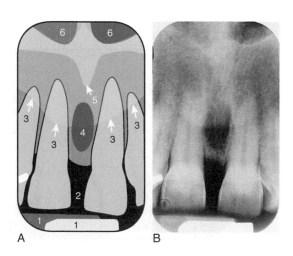

Figure **7-29** Identify the indicated structures.

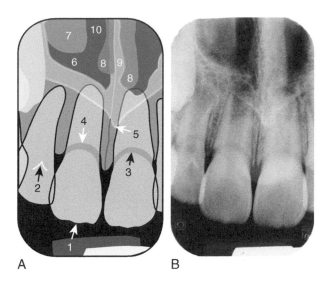

Figure **7-30**   Identify the indicated structures.

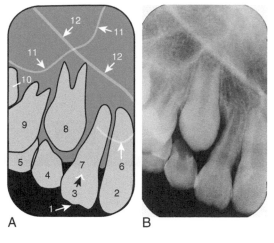

Figure **7-32**   Identify the indicated structures.

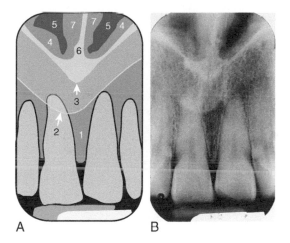

Figure **7-31**   Identify the indicated structures.

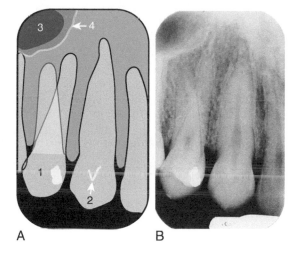

Figure **7-33**   Identify the indicated structures.

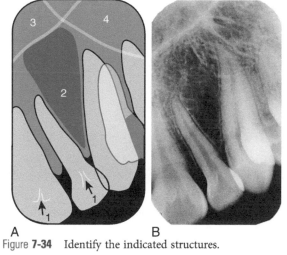

Figure **7-34**   Identify the indicated structures.

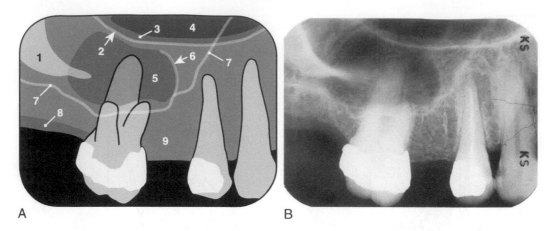

Figure **7-35**   Identify the indicated structures.

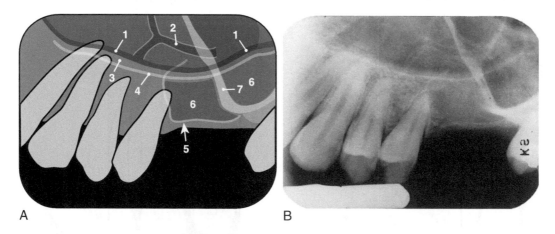

Figure **7-36**   Identify the indicated structures.

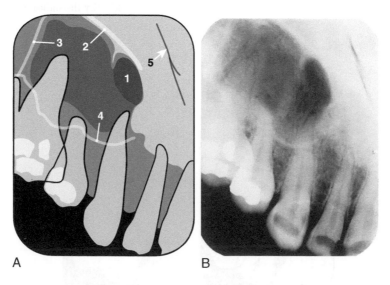

Figure **7-37**   Identify the indicated structures.

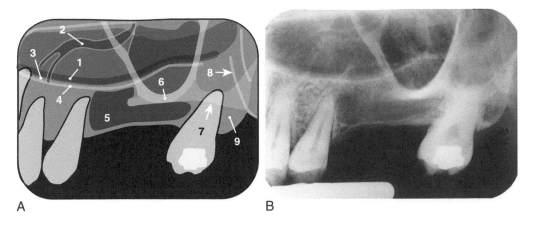

Figure **7-38**   Identify the indicated structures.

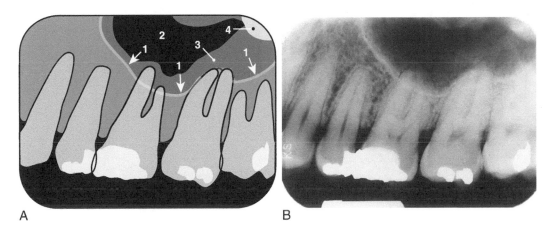

Figure **7-39**   Identify the indicated structures.

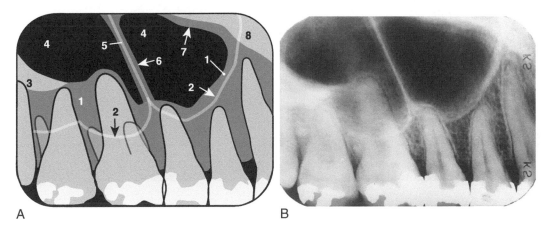

Figure **7-40**   Identify the indicated structures.

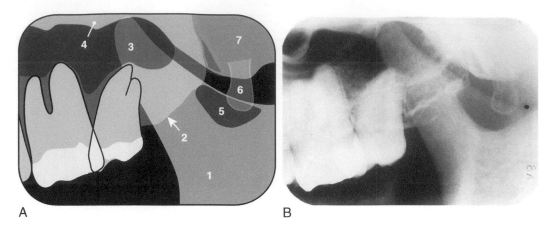

Figure **7-41**   Identify the indicated structures.

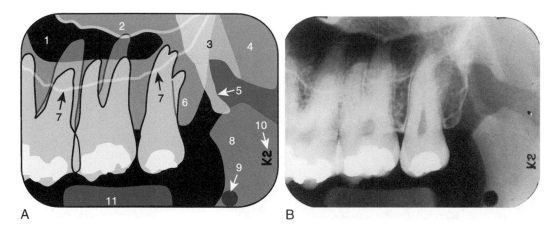

Figure **7-42**   Identify the indicated structures.

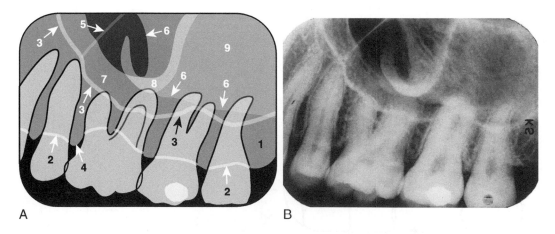

Figure **7-43**   Identify the indicated structures.

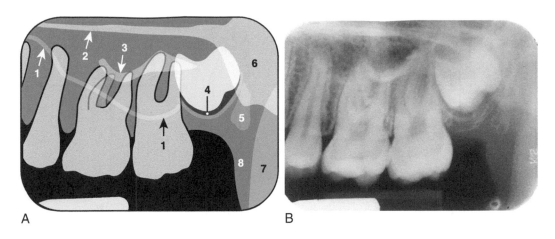

Figure **7-44** Identify the indicated structures.

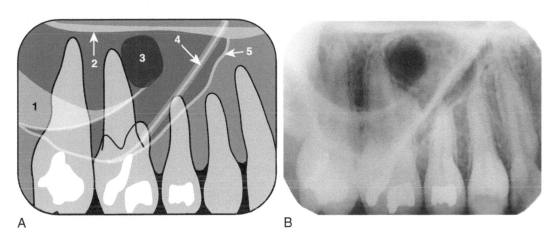

Figure **7-45** Identify the indicated structures.

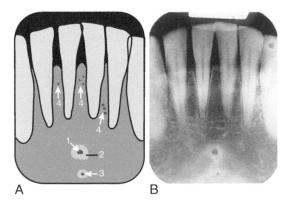

Figure **7-46** Identify the indicated structures.

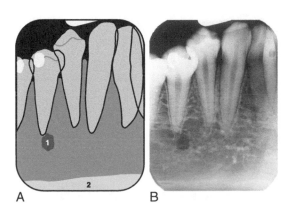

Figure **7-47** Identify the indicated structures.

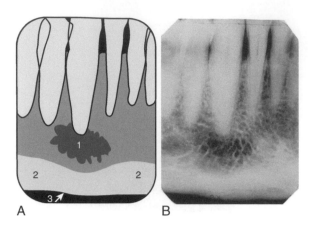

Figure **7-48**   Identify the indicated structures.

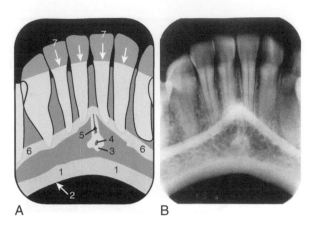

Figure **7-51**   Identify the indicated structures.

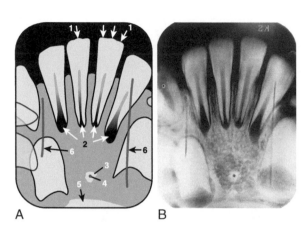

Figure **7-49**   Identify the indicated structures.

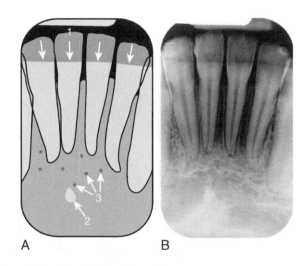

Figure **7-52**   Identify the indicated structures.

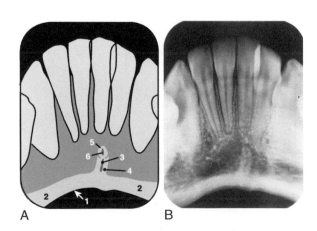

Figure **7-50**   Identify the indicated structures.

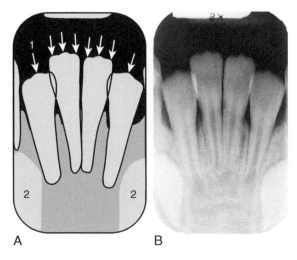

Figure **7-53**   Identify the indicated structures.

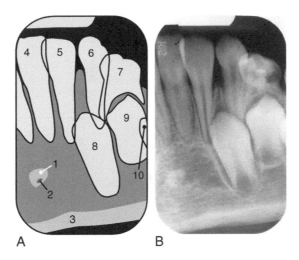

A   B

Figure **7-54**   Identify the indicated structures.

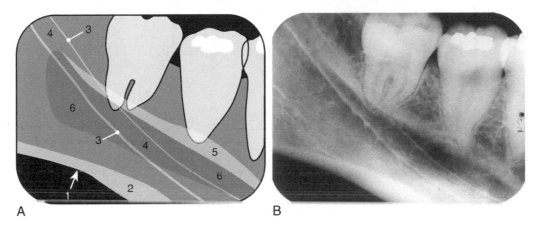

A   B

Figure **7-55**   Identify the indicated structures.

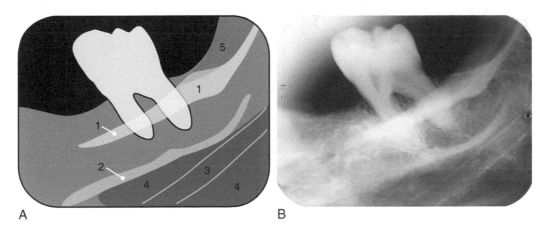

A   B

Figure **7-56**   Identify the indicated structures.

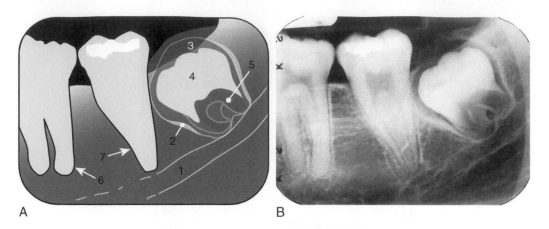

Figure **7-57**   Identify the indicated structures.

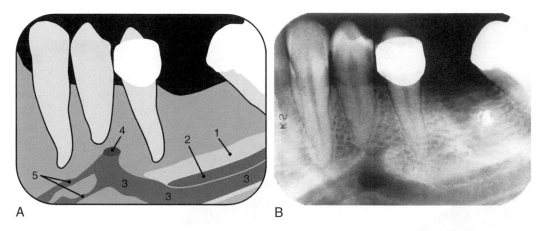

Figure **7-58**   Identify the indicated structures.

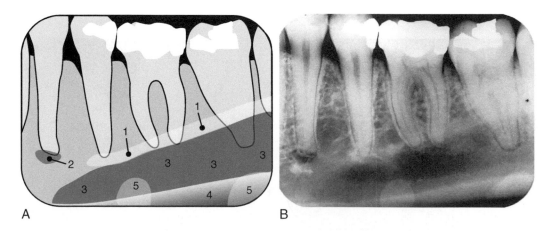

Figure **7-59**   Identify the indicated structures.

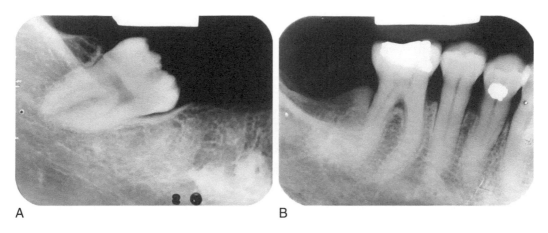

A   B

Figure **7-60**   Parts A and B are variants of the same anatomic structure (crest of ridge distal to molar).
1.   Name the structure.
2.   Can you explain the difference between situations A and B?

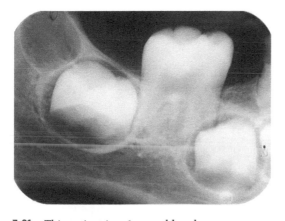

Figure **7-61**   This patient is a 6-year-old male.
1.   Identify the radiolucent area distal to the developing 2nd molar.

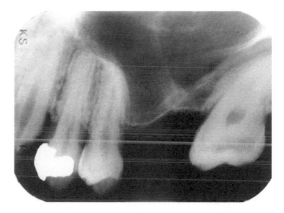

Figure **7-62**   Here we see that several molars have been extracted. As a result, the sinus has enlarged to where the floor of the sinus is at the crest of the alveolar ridge.
1.   What term is used to describe the sinus enlargement?

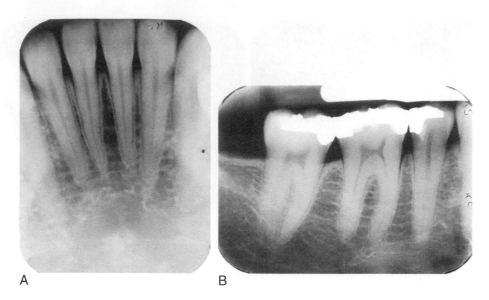

A   B

Figure **7-63**   This question is about a specific trabecular pattern seen in parts A and B. In part A, it is between the central incisors, and in part B, it is between the 1st molar roots.
1.   What term best describes this trabecular pattern?
2.   Is this of any significance?

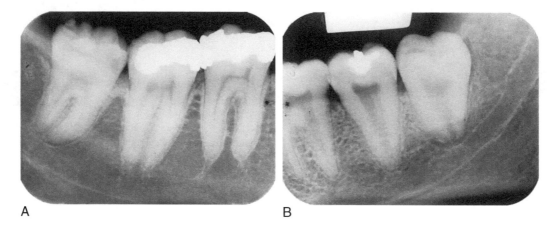

A   B

Figure **7-64**   This question is about trabecular patterns in general as seen in parts A and B.
1.   What term best describes the trabecular pattern in part A?
2.   What term best describes the trabecular pattern in part B?
3.   In which part of the alveolar bone is the trabecular pattern? (Cortex vs. spongiosum or marrow space.)

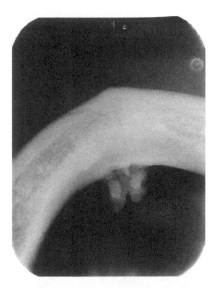

Figure **7-65** Here you see a #2 film oriented like an occlusal view.
1. What structures do we see at the lingual midline?
2. Of what significance (if any) are these?

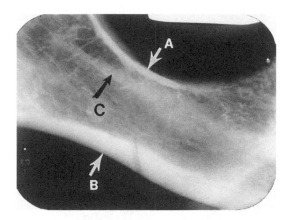

Figure **7-66** Here you see an edentulous mandible.
1. To what structures are arrows A, B, and C pointing?

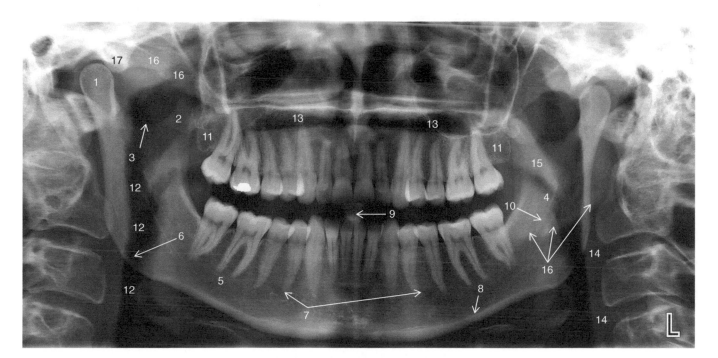

Figure **7-67** Identify the indicated structures.

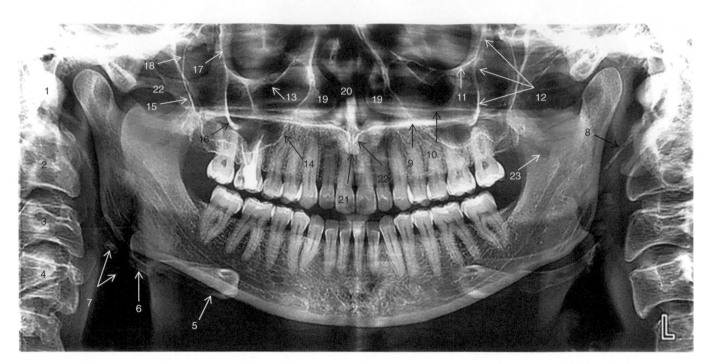

Figure **7-68** Identify the indicated structures.

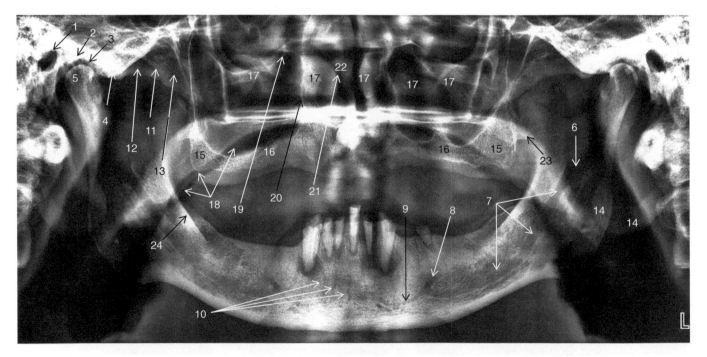

Figure **7-69** Identify the indicated structures.

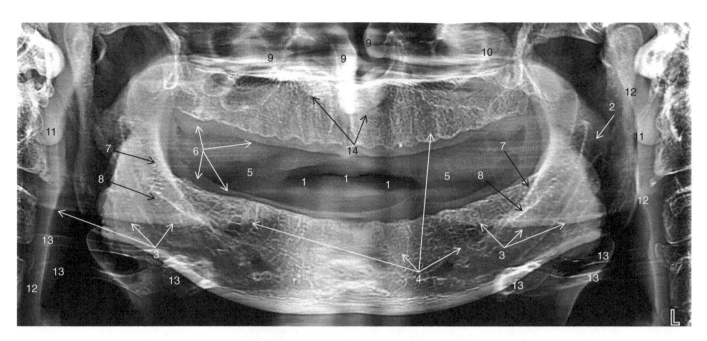

Figure **7-70** Identify the indicated structures.

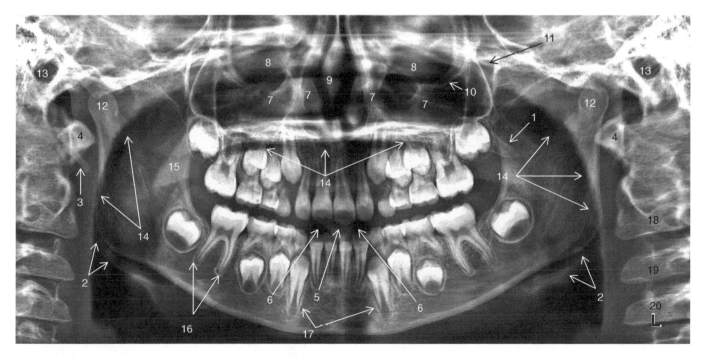

Figure **7-71** Identify the indicated structures.

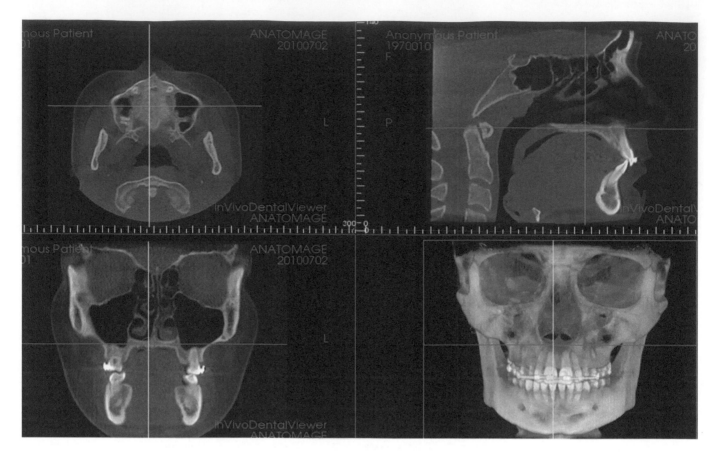

Figure **7-72**

1. What type of radiographic image is seen on this computer screen?
2. Identify the views from upper left to lower right.

Instructions

In Figures 7-73 through 7-78, identify:
1. The view and anatomic level
2. The labeled anatomic structures

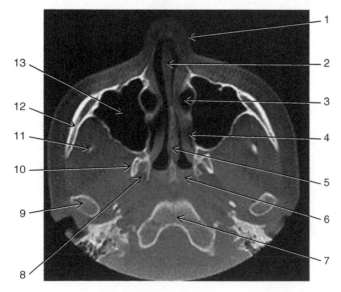

Figure **7-73**

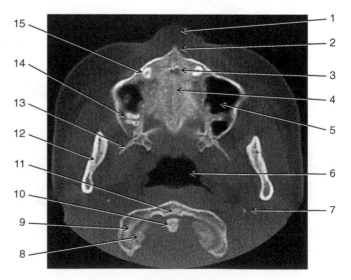

Figure **7-74**

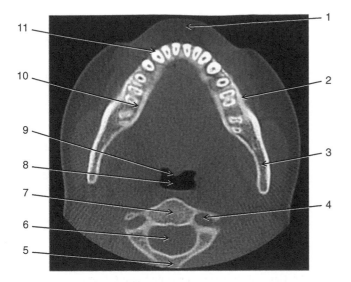

Figure **7-75**

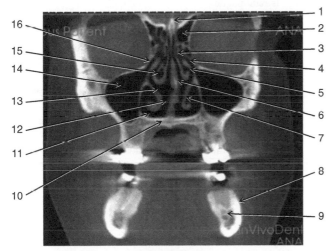

Figure **7-76**

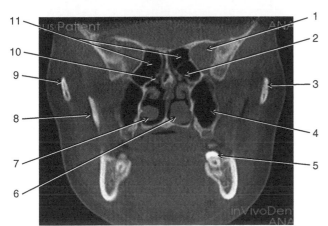

Figure **7-77**

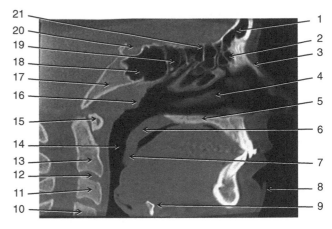

Figure **7-78**

MULTIPLE CHOICE QUESTIONS WITHOUT FIGURES

Instructions

Please select the best answer and check your selection with the correct answer in the Answer Key at the back of the book.

1. Which anatomic structure attaches to the internal oblique ridge of the mandible?
   A. The fascia of the submandibular gland
   B. The internal oblique muscle
   C. The mylohyoid muscle
   D. The glossopharyngeal muscle

2. Which anatomic structure is associated with the mylohyoid groove?
   A. The mylohyoid artery
   B. The mylohyoid muscle
   C. The inferior alveolar artery and nerve
   D. The submandibular salivary gland duct

3. Where is the medial sigmoid depression?
   A. In the medial aspect of the anterior mandible
   B. Just inferior to the sigmoid notch on the buccal side
   C. Just inferior to the sigmoid notch on the medial side
   D. On the lingual aspect of the posterior mandible

4. The mental foramen:
   A. Is on the buccal aspect of the body of the mandible
   B. Contains the mental branch of the inferior alveolar vessels and nerve
   C. Is a source of pain under some dentures
   D. All of the above

5. The lingual artery:
   A. Passes through a foramen centered between the genial tubercles
   B. Can be found on the surface of the posterior mandible
   C. Passes in a notch in the mandible parallel to the tongue
   D. Is entirely within the tongue and is its main blood supply

6. The genial tubercles:
   A. Are normally four in number and are located in the anterior maxilla
   B. Are normally four in number on the buccal aspect of the anterior mandible
   C. Serve as the attachments of the genioglossus and geniohyoid muscles
   D. Are protrusions of the genial bone

7. The hamular process attaches to:
   A. The maxilla
   B. The medial pterygoid plate
   C. Lateral pterygoid plate
   D. Hamulus of the mandible

8. Which of the following is centered on the anterior maxilla?
   A. Foramen of Scarpa
   B. Foramen of Stenson
   C. Foramen ovale
   D. Incisive foramen

9. Which foramen is the most lateral?
   A. Foramen of Scarpa
   B. Foramen of Stenson
   C. Foramen ovale
   D. Mandibular foramen

10. On a panoramic image, the location of the bifurcation of the carotid artery is most frequently:
    A. Between C3 and C4 on the pan image
    B. Level with C3
    C. Level with C4 and the hyoid bone
    D. On the medial aspect of the mandible, near the lingula

11. The body of each cervical vertebra is:
    A. Posterior to the spinal canal
    B. Anterior to the spinal canal
    C. Just posterior to the pedicle
    D. A bilateral structure just lateral to the spinal canal

12. The inferior turbinate is located anatomically:
    A. Above the inferior meatus
    B. On the mandibular condyle
    C. On the lingual side of the mandible, below the external oblique ridge
    D. As a depression in the orbit for the lacrimal gland

13. The panoramic innominate line:
    A. Is a continuous horizontal radiopaque line consisting of the lateral wall of the orbit and the malar process of the maxilla
    B. Is a panoramic landmark with no name
    C. Can only be seen on a cone beam CT scan
    D. None of the above

14. When air is seen in a panoramic radiograph it:
    A. Is radiopaque
    B. Is radiolucent
    C. Always indicates a technique error
    D. Means the patient moved during the exposure

15. The odontoid process is:
    A. The part of the zygomatic arch that has its root apical to the upper molars
    B. A supernumerary cusp on the palatal side of the maxillary incisors
    C. A bony toothlike process located on the hyoid bone
    D. A part of the second cervical vertebra

Chapter (8)

Materials and Foreign Objects

Goal

To recognize materials and foreign objects in intraoral and extraoral radiographs

Learning Objectives

1. Recognize the appearance of dental materials in the radiographs
2. Identify foreign objects in the radiographs
3. Describe the features of materials and foreign objects as seen in intraoral radiographs
4. Describe the features of materials and foreign objects as seen in panoramic radiographs

INTRODUCTION

The identification of materials and foreign objects can be important. First, a foreign object may be the cause of a patient's symptom(s) or of an abnormal clinical finding. For example, a metal fragment from a long-forgotten injury may suddenly become infected and cause pain or swelling. In another instance, an amalgam tattoo in the gingiva may resemble a bluish pigmented macule called a nevus; however the radiograph will demonstrate a metallic density fragment at the site of the gingival abnormality. In other instances, fixed appliances such as bridges, removable cast metal partial denture frameworks, implants, or orthodontic materials can be identified and examined for any defects. Restorative materials can be seen as well. Some of these may include retentive pins, gutta percha root canal fillings, composite, amalgam, porcelain, gold foil, or cast metal restorations. In older restorations, liners, composite, silicate and acrylic restorations were radiolucent, although most of these will have been replaced in patients being seen nowadays as these older esthetic restorative materials often fail over time.

The identification of restorative materials may also be useful for insurance claims or even legal procedures whereby lost or destroyed dental appliances or restorations represent a claim being made by an injured party. The written dental record may or may not include a full description of lost or destroyed dental restorations or appliances, and in the absence of clinical photographs, the radiographs may serve as unquestionable proof of the validity of the patient's claim.

An additional application of this aspect of dental radiology is in the area of forensic science. An unknown victim can be identified with certainty based on a comparison of the antemortem and postmortem dental radiographs. Most persons serving in the U.S. military have a copy of their panoramic radiograph on file in the central forensics facility in Hawaii. In military situations, a victim of severe injury may be ultimately identified by radiographic examination of the jaws, although nowadays DNA is becoming the method of choice for such forensic identifications. Finally, apart from the above applications, the identification of a restorative material may be a part of the process to determine whether the restoration is failing. For example, a radiolucent area under a radiopaque restoration could represent redecay, "pull back" of a composite, or a radiolucent liner beneath the restoration. An amalgam overhang may be associated with periodontal disease characterized by gingival bleeding and/or bone loss or a patient's complaint of the shredding of floss. Some cast or other restorations have a leaky margin, which is suspected if more radiopaque secondary dentin can be identified beneath the restoration, even in the absence of x-ray evidence of the defective margin.

As a parting thought, it should be remembered that anything in a radiograph that may be related to a patient's complaint should obviously be looked for by the hygienist or dentist. Sometimes it is the patient's complaint that causes us to take a closer look for any subtle radiographic evidence of the problem, and this evidence may relate to materials or foreign objects seen in the radiographs.

SHORT ANSWER QUESTIONS WITH FIGURES

Instructions

Look at the figures and identify the materials, foreign objects, or case-related information in the following questions. Compare your answer to the correct answer in the Answer Key at the back of the book.

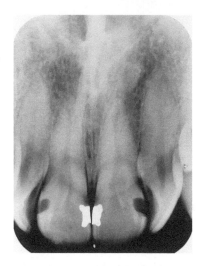

Figure **8-1**   What materials could have been used to restore the:
1. Mesial portion of the central incisors?
2. Distal portion of the central incisors?

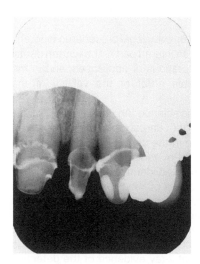

Figure **8-2**
1. With what metals might this patient's prosthesis have been made?
2. With what materials are the crowns of the anterior teeth restored?
3. What are the radiopaque lines seen in the cervical areas of these teeth?

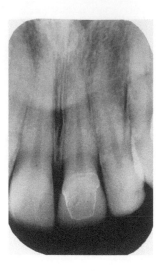

Figure **8-3**
1. What type of crown has been placed on the left central incisor?
2. What is the radiopaque line within the crown area?

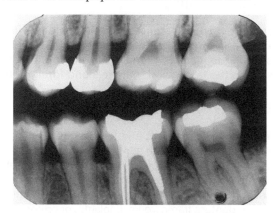

Figure **8-4**
1. What materials can we see in the lower 1st molar?
2. What is the radiolucent area on the distal cervical area of the lower 1st molar?

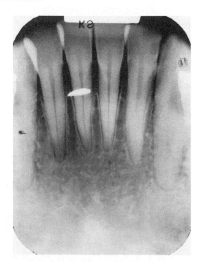

Figure **8-5**   This is a 23-year-old. The radiograph revealed a radiopaque area on the right central incisor. There was no restoration on this tooth, but she had been in an auto accident several months previously.
1. What do you think this radiopacity might represent?
2. What else could look like this?

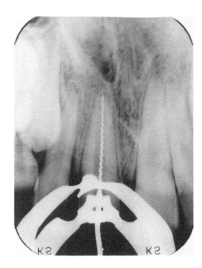

Figure **8-6**
1.   Name two metallic objects seen in this radiograph.

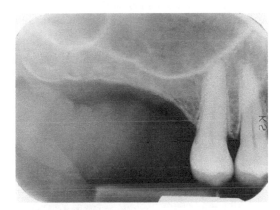

Figure **8-7**   Here we can see three different materials associated with taking this radiograph.
1.   Can you enumerate them?

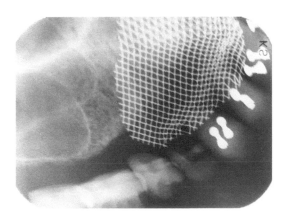

Figure **8-8**   This patient wears a complete upper denture against his natural lowers and keeps breaking the denture while masticating food.
1.   What materials can you see here?
2.   What material can you not see?

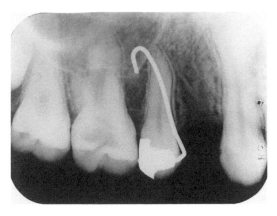

Figure **8-9**   This patient is 13 years old and needs several carious lesions restored. She is also missing both central incisors, which were extracted for caries.
1.   What do you think this radiopaque object superimposed on the premolar represents?

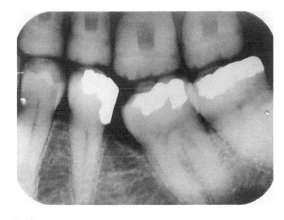

Figure **8-10**
1.   Can you account for the strange appearance of the maxillary teeth?

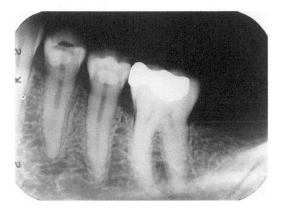

Figure **8-11**
1.   What restorative material is observed in the premolars?
2.   What restorative material is observed in the molar?

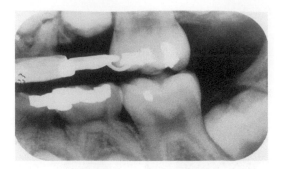

Figure **8-12**
1. What type of appliance do we see in the maxilla of this 10-year-old boy?

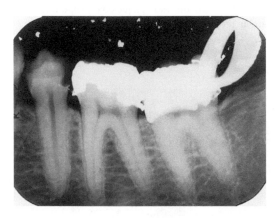

Figure **8-13**
1. What materials do you see in this radiograph?
2. What dental materials are present but not seen in this radiograph?

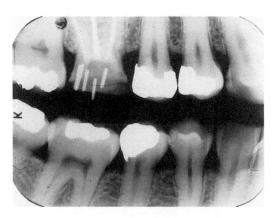

Figure **8-14**
1. What materials do we see in the upper 1st molar?

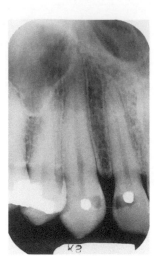

Figure **8-15**   Look at the lateral incisor and canine teeth. Each tooth has a radiopaque and a radiolucent restoration in proximity to each other. Ignore the restoration on the distal of the canine.
1. What materials were used, and where on the teeth are they?

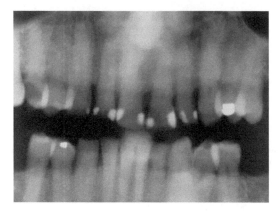

Figure **8-16**
1. What restorative material do we see in these anterior teeth?

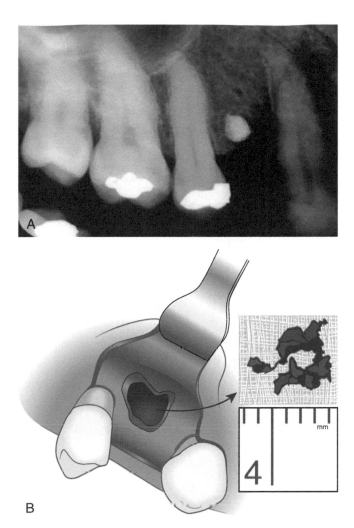

Figure **8-17**   This patient presented with gingival redness in the upper right canine/1st premolar region and a draining fistula in the area of the 1st premolar. There was severe bone loss associated with the canine and a radiopacity which resembled a fragment of tooth material. Based on the radiographs and illustration of the surgical specimen, what do you think the problem was?

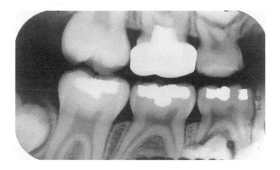

Figure **8-18**

1. Compare and contrast the treatment and materials in the upper and lower primary 2nd molars.

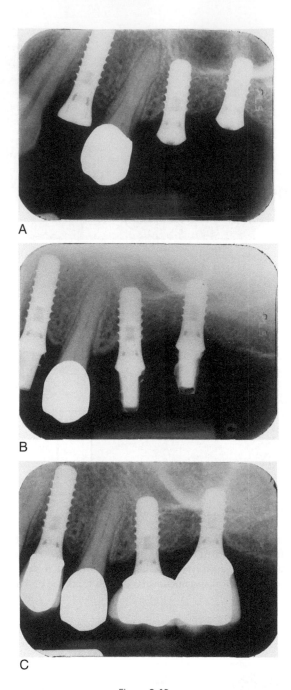

Figure **8-19**

1. This case illustrates three different phases in the treatment of this patient. Apart from the crown on the 2nd premolar, which appears to be all gold, what materials do we see in parts A, B, and C?

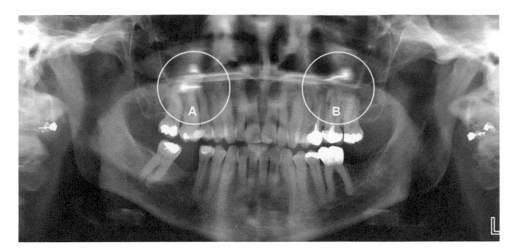

Figure **8-20**
1. How many earrings is this patient wearing?
2. Circle A: What do the two blurry radiopacities represent?
3. Circle B: What does the blurry radiopacity represent?

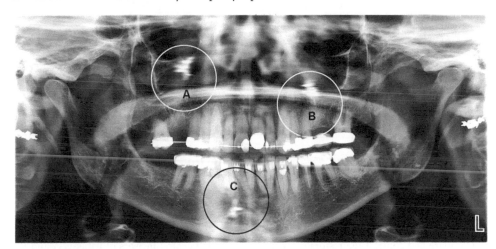

Figure **8-21**
1. Why is the ghost image in circle A higher than the one in circle B?
2. What does the fuzzy radiopacity in circle C probably represent?
3. Where is the object in circle C located?
4. What type of active treatment does the patient appear to be undergoing?

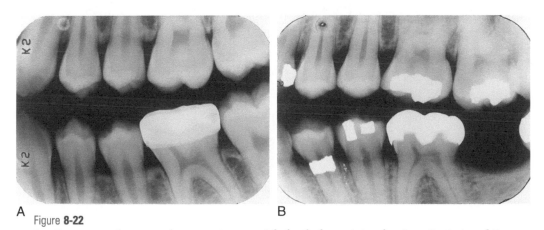

A   B

Figure **8-22**
1. Compare and contrast the restorative materials for the lower 1st molars in patients A and B.
2. Which one has the amalgam tattoo?

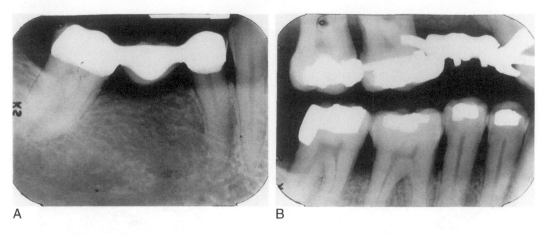

A   B

Figure **8-23**

1. Compare and contrast the two prostheses seen in patients A and B.

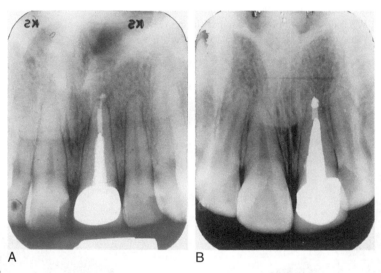

A   B

Figure **8-24**

1. Compare and contrast the restorative materials in the left central incisors of patients A and B.

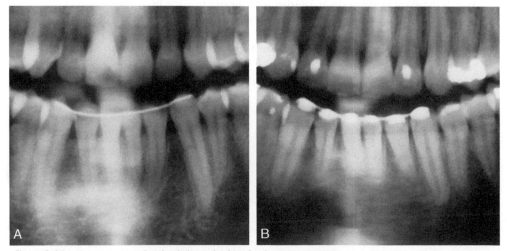

A   B

Figure **8-25**   Patients A and B both have had orthodontic treatment.

1. What orthodontic appliance does each have?
2. Compare and contrast the two appliances.

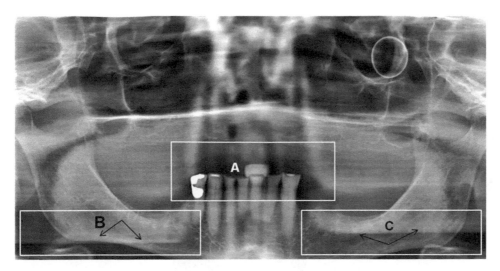

Figure **8-26**

1. Anatomically, where is the radiopaque circle in the upper left (patient's left) part of the image?
2. What does this object represent?
3. In rectangle A, are the patient's lips sealed as they should be for proper panoramic technique?
4. Can you explain what the horizontal white shadows are in the two rectangles labeled B & C?

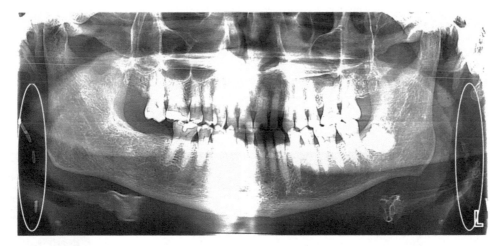

Figure **8-27**

1. Compare and contrast the radiopaque objects in the two ovals.

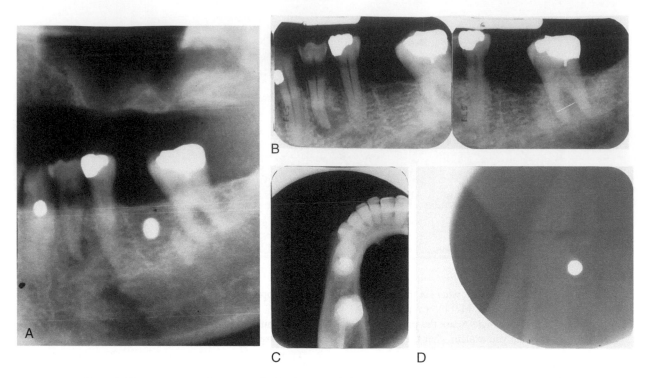

Figure **8-28**   A mystery object. Here's the history of this case: Part A, the panoramic radiograph (cropped), was taken first. On the same day image B, the periapicals from the full-mouth survey, were taken. To investigate the unusual radiopaque object further, image C, the occlusal, was taken. However, no solution to the mystery was obtained. So, image D was taken, and the mystery was solved. Now you will also have a chance to solve the mystery.
1. Part D is a radiograph of what area? How was this taken?
2. What is the solution to the mystery, and what and where is the foreign object seen in A and D?

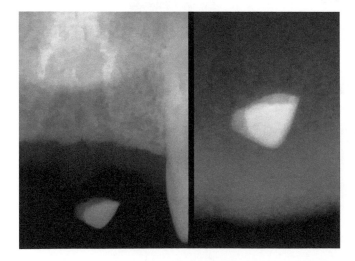

Figure **8-29**
1. What types of radiographs do you see in the left and right images?
2. What most likely is the radiopacity seen in these images?

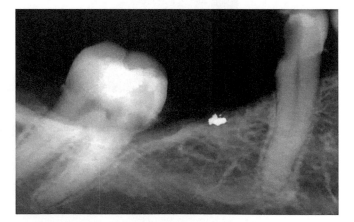

Figure **8-30**
1. On clinical examination this patient demonstrated a bluish-black macule on the lower right edentulous ridge. Clinically, the surrounding tissue appeared healthy. What is the cause of the macule?
2. Is any treatment needed?

MULTIPLE CHOICE QUESTIONS WITHOUT FIGURES

Instructions

Please select the best answer and check your selection with the correct answer in the Answer Key at the back of the book.

1. In panoramic radiography, earrings can appear as both "real" and "ghost" images when:
   A. More than one earring is worn on the same ear
   B. The earring is located behind the path of the center of rotation
   C. The earring is located in front of the path of the center of rotation
   D. The patient is malpositioned too far forward in the machine

2. With regard to dental restorations, which of the following is *not true?*
   A. Most current restorative materials can be seen and are radiopaque
   B. Radiographs can usually detect redecay under a restoration when it cannot be seen clinically
   C. Over-processing of a digital radiograph with software can create an artifact beneath restorations that resembles redecay
   D. Overhangs cannot be detected in composite restorations

3. In panoramic radiographs, foreign objects:
   A. May produce ghost images
   B. Even if present or suspected clinically, may not be seen in the pan radiograph
   C. May produce both real and ghost images in pan images
   D. All of the above

4. In a panoramic radiograph, which of the following *may* not be seen?
   A. Evidence of coronary artery surgery consisting of clips
   B. Implants made of ceramic material
   C. Newer composite restorations
   D. Nose jewelry

5. Which of the following is *not* true?
   A. A foreign metallic object may look like a retained root tip
   B. A subcutaneous amalgam fragment may only be suspected after taking a radiograph
   C. In a pan radiograph, a foreign object may actually be higher up or lower down in the patient than in the radiograph
   D. A panoramic radiograph cannot always rule out the presence of a metallic foreign object.

6. When using software filters such as "sharpen," "sharpen edges," and "remove noise" in a patient with metallic restorations in the panoramic radiograph:
   A. A radiopaque artifact may appear under the restoration
   B. A radiolucent artifact may appear under the restoration
   C. Such artifacts only occur with composite restorations
   D. The artifact is called "beam hardening"

7. You have an upper molar periapical radiograph with an implant in the image. The apical portion of the implant appears to have perforated into the maxillary sinus. In this type of image:
   A. Perforation of the sinus may have occurred
   B. The implant may actually be buccal to the sinus floor
   C. The implant may be lingual to the sinus floor
   D. All of the above are possible

8. You have a panoramic radiograph of a patient with two implants replacing a lower left 2nd premolar and a lower left 1st molar. According to the patient's chart, both implants were identical in length and width. However, one implant appears to be narrower than the other in the radiograph. The reason for this is:
   A. One implant is higher than the other in the bone
   B. One implant is located more to the buccal than the other
   C. One implant is located more to the lingual than the other
   D. Only B is correct
   E. Either B or C is correct

9. You have a panoramic radiograph of a patient with two implants replacing a lower left 2nd premolar and a lower left 1st molar. According to the patient's chart, both implants were drilled to the same depth in the bone. However, one implant appears to be higher than the other in the radiograph. The reason for this is:
   A. One implant was placed more to the lingual than the other
   B. One implant was placed more to the buccal than the other
   C. The difference is due to the curvature of the mandible in this location
   D. Either A or B is correct

10. In a panoramic radiograph you see the patient has an oval metallic object about 3 mm in height and about 2.5 mm in width in the position of the missing lower left 1st molar of the mandible. The periapical image of the area shows no evidence of a metallic object in the bone. The patient admits to having been shot as a child with a BB gun. The most likely location of this BB is:
    A. In the buccal mucosa or cheek
    B. In the tongue
    C. Within the alveolar bone
    D. Not a BB but an ovoid amalgam restoration that fell into the extraction socket
    E. Either C or D

Chapter 9

Caries Detection and Panoramic Bitewings

Goal

To know the advantages of and be able to interpret panoramic bitewings

Learning Objectives

1. Know the radiographic methods of identifying interproximal caries
2. Understand the differences between classic intraoral bitewings and panoramic bitewings
3. Discover the unique advantages of panoramic bitewings
4. Learn how to identify and correct pan bitewing technique errors

RADIOGRAPHIC CARIES DETECTION

Many types of carious lesions can be detected clinically, without a radiograph. Some of these include occlusal (class I) caries, buccal and lingual caries, root (class V) caries as well as caries that develop on cusp tips (class VI). Interproximal caries involving the anterior teeth can be easily detected with transillumination and are classified as class III. If class III caries involve or extend to the incisal surface, they are referred to as class IV. Bitewing radiographs have an important role in detecting interproximal caries in the posterior teeth. These caries are classified as class II, and the goal is to detect them when they are very small lesions, before they progress. The smallest lesions are called "*incipient,*" and these are less than halfway through the enamel. The role of traditional bitewings is to detect these small interproximal caries lesions before they can generate symptoms, such as sensitivity to sweets or to hot or cold temperatures, and before they get larger. Radiographic detection of caries is accepted practice in dentistry. There are guidelines from the U.S. Food and Drug Administration (FDA) and the American Dental Association as to how frequently bitewings should be taken depending on the age and caries susceptibility of the patient (see *J Am Dent Assoc 2006;137;1304-1312*).

Traditional intraoral machines have used alternating current (AC) and required higher mAs (milliamp second) settings to properly expose x-ray film. This has been largely replaced by digital sensors and lower mA (milliamperage) direct current (DC) machines, which are also lighter. Another development has been the handheld intraoral x-ray machine (Figure 9-1). This device has the advantage of portability for public health and military applications outside of the dental office as well as within any dental practice. Through FDA testing and research at the University of Texas Dental School in San Antonio, the handheld intraoral machine has been found to be safe for intraoral imaging in dental offices.

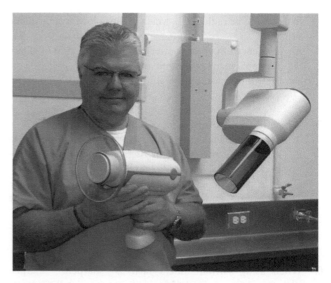

Figure **9-1**

Figure 9-1 shows Dr. Langlais with the available handheld intraoral x-ray machine, which has been shown to be safe to use.

The big problem in 2016 is that, even though **panoramic bitewings** (pan BWs) are available and have advantages, many in the profession don't know about this technique or do not have the equipment. Thus one of the goals of this chapter is to show that pan BWs are at least as diagnostic as intraoral bitewings (intra BWs), and in fact, may be slightly more diagnostic, especially for incipient interproximal lesions in the posterior teeth.

PANORAMIC BITEWINGS

The accuracy of detecting and interpreting interproximal caries in posterior teeth on panoramic radiographs compared with intraoral bitewing images appears to have been first reported by Dr. Robert Langlais and colleagues in 1985. The project was presented orally at the Congress of the International Association of Dentomaxillofacial Radiology in London, England, and subsequently published as a supplement to the journal, *Dentomaxillofacial Radiology (Dentomaxillofac Radiol Supp. 1985; 7:40).*

This classic study involved 659 interproximal surfaces that were read in a double-blind manner by eight raters on both standard panoramic x-rays (pans) and intraoral bitewings (intra BWs). Only individual posterior interproximal contacts that were open on both the pan and corresponding intra BWs were included for study. The Kappa statistic was used to measure the agreement between the two imaging modalities. Interestingly, there were no significant differences in the detection of small (incipient), medium (limited to enamel), and larger (into dentin) caries between the two modalities. A limitation of this study was that panoramic machines of that era were not specifically designed to open the posterior interproximal contacts. Additionally, the perception that incipient caries could be detected in panoramic radiographs was a hard sell in the mid-1980s because pan image quality was much lower 30 years ago when the study was done.

Some years later Dr. Langlais sent a panoramic image with the posterior contacts open to the Planmeca Company in Finland. The manner in which this could be accomplished was described. As a result of this impetus, panoramic machines with a posterior bitewing function became available from several manufacturers. These devices are now designed and programmed to open the posterior contacts when in bitewing mode. Also most parts of the ramus, including the parotid gland, are not exposed to x-radiation in the pan BW exposure, and these structures are not imaged in the pan BW image. Thus pan BWs reduce dosage to sensitive tissues and provide a targeted view of the interproximal surfaces.

Presently (2016) a study has been completed at the University of Minnesota, and one has been completed at the University of Texas in San Antonio. Using receiver operating characteristic (ROC) curves, the San Antonio investigators found no statistical difference between pan BWs and intra BWs for the detection of interproximal caries at all depths including incipient caries.

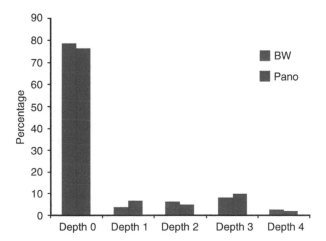

Figure **9-2** Percentages of surfaces read by both modalities demonstrating the absence of caries (depth 0) or presence of caries at different depths. Depth 1 is caries less than ½ way through the enamel; depth 2 is enamel caries to the dentino enamel junction (DEJ); depth 3 is caries into dentin less than ½ way to the pulp; depth 4 is caries into dentin more than ½ way to the pulp.

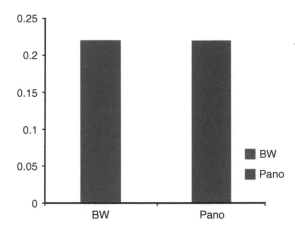

Figure **9-3** Mean number of overlaps per contact for each modality.

Also, Dr. Langlais has completed another pilot project in which the detection of interproximal caries at four different depths, including incipient caries as well as the incidence of overlapped contacts for both methods, was recorded. The salient findings in this pilot study were that pan BWs detected caries similar to conventional intraoral BWs, regardless of the depth of the caries, and there was no difference in the incidence of overlapping posterior contacts between the two methods, as shown in Figures 9-2 and 9-3.

Figure 9-2 shows the percentages of surfaces read in both modalities, demonstrating the absence of caries (depth 0) or presence of caries at different depths (depths 1-4). Incipient caries are annotated by depth 1.

Figure 9-3 shows the mean overlaps per contact (in millimeters) for each modality indicating no difference between the intra BWs and pan BWs.

Suffice it to state that, at this moment, the available evidence indicates the pan BWs are at least as diagnostic as intra BWs for all sizes of posterior interproximal caries, and pan BWs offer some significant advantages over intra BWs. The advantages of pan BWs are listed below in no particular order of importance.

1. **Time:** It involves fewer steps and takes much less time to expose a pan BW than to acquire four intra BWs. This means less cost in terms of labor for the doctor and a shorter appointment for the patient.
2. **Comfort:** Intraoral electronic sensors are bulky and may cause patient discomfort, especially in the anterior floor of the mouth and sometimes the hard palate or when infection or lesions such as oral ulcers are present. Some discomfort may be especially associated with the proper positioning of the sensor for the anterior BW. There is no intraoral discomfort associated with the pan BW.
3. **Ease of use:** Panoramic BWs are as easy to take as a standard pan. In contrast, intra BWs may involve the use of bulky sensors that are more difficult to manage. Intra BWs also require positioning devices to ensure proper alignment of the x-ray beam.
4. **Versatility:** The pan machine with a BW function is often manufactured to include traditional pan imaging, cropped partial pan images, and cone beam computed tomography (CBCT) imaging as well as cephalometric functions. Intraoral machines can not capture a CBCT image.
5. **Low radiation dose:** The panoramic BW dose is less than all intraoral BW techniques, except when the long, rectangular cone (or rectangular collimation) with "F"-speed film or a digital sensor is used, in which case the doses are similar. In the experience of the authors, most educational programs teach

the long, rectangular-cone technique; however, most dental practices are equipped with round cones of varying lengths, and in these instances, the intraoral BW doses will be higher than the pan BW doses (*Ludlow, J JADA. 139: Sept 2008*).

6. **Parotid salivary gland cancer risk:** Malignant disease of the parotid gland has been shown to be significantly related to previous exposure to dental radiation in combination with additional sources of medical radiation. Both the anterior and posterior intra BWs involve some direct as well as exit radiation to the parotid gland on the opposite side, whereas the pan BW involves a highly collimated thin vertical slit beam, which exposes very little, and in some cases, involves no exposure to the parotid gland (*Preston-Martin S, Thomas DC, White SC, Cohen D. Prior exposure to medical and dental x-rays related to tumors of the parotid gland. J Natl Cancer Inst 80:943-949; 1988.*)

7. **Children:** The pan BW is really fantastic for the examination of children. The interproximal contacts of the primary teeth open very easily and consistently with the pan BW function on children, and there is no need for bulky objects such as film or sensors, sensor holders, and aiming devices. All of the developing teeth are also seen in the pan BW image.

8. **Image quality:** Visually, the pan BWs often look as sharp as some film-based images and some sensor images. It must be remembered that even if the pan BW images are less sharp, it does not imply, and there is no proof, that they are less diagnostic for the detection of interproximal caries.

9. **Diagnostic quality:** In a pilot study as described in this chapter, pan BWs have been shown to be equivalent to intra BWs for the detection of interproximal caries in general, including incipient caries, and the rate of overlapped contacts for the pan BWs is the same as for the intra BWs. Further studies confirming these pilot data will soon be published.

10. **Diagnostic coverage:** Because bulky electronic digital sensors cover approximately 25% to 33% less area than film or digital photostimulable phosphor plates (PSPs), periapical visualization may be difficult. Pan BWs include regions well beyond the apices of all the teeth, except the central and lateral incisors. The pan BW covers nearly all of the teeth in a full-mouth survey and there is much more periapical coverage.

11. **Diagnostic sensitivity:** The detection of periapical pathology of pulpal origin and other lesions may on occasion be visible on the pan BW, completely absent on the intraoral *periapical* images, and impossible to visualize in the intra BWs because intra BWs do not cover the periapical regions.

12. **Evidence-based:** There is a growing body of evidence supporting the pan BW for the efficient, effective, and accurate detection of interproximal carious lesions of all sizes including incipient caries. This evidence is currently being prepared for publication.

13. **Affordable:** The BW function is supplied as a normal feature on many newer pan machines. The savings in infection control products and procedures needed for intraoral imaging vs. a simple bite sleeve over the pan bite block as well as the labor cost of the excess time needed for intraoral techniques, which may include the need for some periapical images and disinfection and sterilization are ample justification for the purchase of a new machine. This new machine may now include cone beam computed tomography (CBCT) for which the normal pan and pan BW functions can be major financial affordability factors when considering the adoption of the extra CBCT technology.

Why Pan BWs May Be Better: The Role of Saturation

In all probability, the biggest hindrance to the more rapid adoption of pan BW technology is the inherent belief of many, if not most doctors, hygienists, and dental assistants, that there is no way any pan image can be as good diagnostically for interproximal caries detection as an intraoral bitewing image. Many clinicians inaccurately believe that, in terms of sharpness and detail, the pans will just not compete. Many may also believe the pan dose is greater than the dose of a set of intra BWs. But what if the diagnostic efficacy of the pan BW has nothing to do with sharpness and detail? After all, our previously mentioned 1985 study involved much fuzzier pans than the present generation. However, if you understand the concept of **saturation,** then you will begin to see the light.

With the advent of digital intraoral sensors, the mA has been lowered from 10 or 15 on older machines to about 7 mA on average. Higher mA levels may cause an artifact called "blooming" in electronic sensors. This artifact produces an overall blackness to the image, which renders the image nondiagnostic. In addition, the digital intraoral exposure time is somewhere between 50% and 75% lower, depending on other factors such as cone length and film speed, if film is being used. The mA plus the exposure time are represented as the mAs, and this factor is responsible for the saturation of the object (the tooth being imaged). The saturation for digital sensors has been significantly lowered while the pan mA may, in some cases, be as high as 14 mA, which results in more saturation of the object but a low radiation dose, primarily because of the thin slit collimation and the speed of the moving pan beam.

ROLE OF TOMOGRAPHY AND TOMOSYNTHESIS: The standard pan BW is a form of a **tomographic** image. This means that only the layer of tissue containing the teeth is in focus and clearly depicted in the image. The minimal filtering effect of the surface tissues during the passage of the thin collimated pan beam permits more saturation of an object such as a tooth than with an imaging technique that involves straight through-and-through radiation such as an intraoral BW. In addition, **tomosynthesis** is a new panoramic technology in which the pan tomographic layer in focus can be further subdivided into multiple separate thin layers within the layer in focus. With the appropriate software, overlapped interproximal contacts in tomosynthesis-generated pan BWs can be opened *after* the exposure, and this feature is presently available on some panoramic machines. Tomosynthesis cannot be done on any form of intraoral film-based or digital intraoral BW without doing a new exposure. This means that variables such as proper pan BW technique, different jaw sizes and shapes, tooth crowding, and tooth orientation before or after orthodontic therapy, which may cause unwanted overlap of the posterior tooth contacts in the standard pan BW, can now be overcome to a significant degree *after* the exposure. With pan BW tomosynthesis, overlapped contacts can, in many instances, be opened and fully visualized after the exposure.

Conclusions

It is important to learn about the new pan BWs as they will become ubiquitous, just as standard pan machines are now ubiquitous. In spite of everything written here regarding the technology advances, the best pan BW technique still requires the use of good technique by the doctor and staff with the objective of obtaining a diagnostic image without further postexposure processing of the image. In other parts of this book, pan error troubleshooting has been well described and illustrated. Still, many practitioners and staff have not mastered the troubleshooting of standard pan errors. Recognition of the cause(s) of pan technique errors allows users to improve techniques. By studying these errors, flawless technique can be achieved on a regular basis. Unlike standard pans, pan BWs require more attention to technique because, without good technique, the contacts will be more difficult to open. Therefore pan BW errors and artifacts are explained in this chapter so that the cause(s) of the technique-error regarding pan BW images can be recognized and corrected. Tomosynthesis is not yet ubiquitous and can only go so far in opening the contacts after the exposure. Therefore good technique is as always best.

Panoramic Bitewing Error Troubleshooting

Panoramic BW errors are very different from intraoral BW errors yet very similar to errors seen on regular pans. However, not all of the full pan errors are seen in the pan BWs. For example, slumping, chin not on the chin rest, and head tilting are quite rare. The most common pan BW errors are head turning, chin down, chin too high, and tongue not against the palate. Did I say "tongue not against the palate"? Yes, this is a very common error, and it can be prevented by telling the patient to swallow and hold their tongue against their roof of their mouth during the exposure.

Overall, the errors are the same for adults and children. However, there is a unique error seen in children. As the machine passes in front of their faces, children have a tendency to rotate their head and follow the machine as it passes; in children the more classic presentation of movement is also seen. Also, blurred or streaked images representing ghost images from the opposite side are seen mostly in adults because, when the patient is in the BW position, the posterior teeth are either on or behind the path of the rotation center, and thus ghost images can be seen. This latter error is rarely seen in children because the growth of the jaw has not been sufficient in a posterior direction so as to impinge on the path of the rotation center.

In summary the pan BW is subject to fewer errors than the full pan; a special unique error occurs in young children, and ghosting is a phenomenon seen mainly in the BW images of adults.

MULTIPLE CHOICE QUESTIONS WITH FIGURES

Instructions

Select the correct choice and check your selection with the correct answer in the Answer Key at the back of the book.

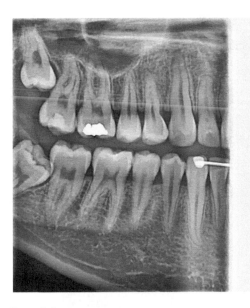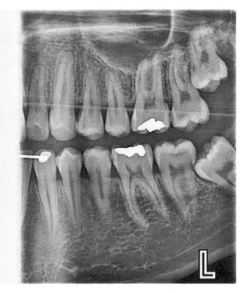

Figure **9-4**

1. This is a panoramic image of an adult patient. This image is:
   A. Diagnostic for interproximal caries
   B. Demonstrating bilateral dens in dente in the maxillary laterals
   C. Almost perfect, except the patient was slightly slumped
   D. All of the above
   E. Only A and B are correct

2. Look again at this panoramic BW (Figure 9-4). You will notice a thin radiolucent line under each of the three posterior occlusal *amalgam* restorations. This line is:
   A. Over-sharpening of the image by the operator
   B. Recurrent caries under leaky amalgam restorations
   C. A unique digital artifact seen in all panoramic BWs
   D. Machine brand/software specific and unavoidable

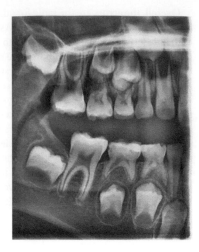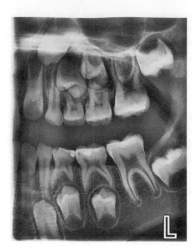

Figure **9-5**

1. This is a special type of panoramic image of a child whose age is _____ years old.
   A. 4.5
   B. 6
   C. 7
   D. 7.5

2. This image is:
   A. A cropped normal pan image
   B. An interproximal mode full pan with edges cropped
   C. A pan bitewing image
   D. A cropped pan image with the patient positioned too far back

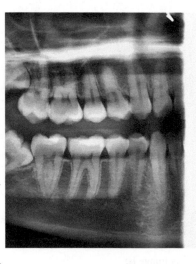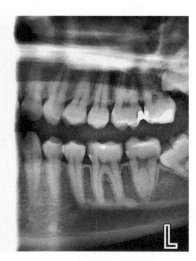

Figure **9-6**

1. The patient positioning for this pan BW image is:
   A. With the chin too high
   B. Too far back in the machine
   C. Too far forward in the machine
   D. An example of a well-positioned patient

2. On the upper left 1st molar there is a dark line under the *composite* restoration. In this case, this appearance may represent:
   A. Over-sharpening of the image
   B. Redecay
   C. A radiolucent liner
   D. A "void" or "pull back" of the restorative material
   E. All of the above

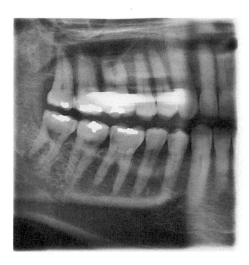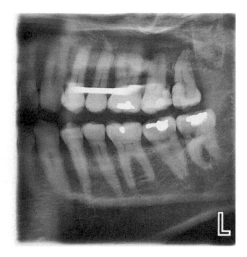

Figure **9-7**

1. The two radiopaque streaks superimposed on the right and left posterior teeth represent ghost images of the:
   A. Metallic earrings that were not removed
   B. Amalgam restorations in the upper teeth
   C. Amalgam restorations in the lower teeth
   D. Amalgam restorations in the lower 3rd molars

2. Ghost image linear streaking results from metallic objects:
   A. Just in front of the path of the rotation center
   B. Right in the path of the rotation center
   C. Just behind the path of the rotation center
   D. Well behind the path of the rotation center

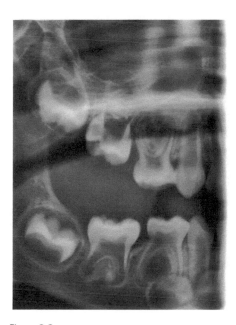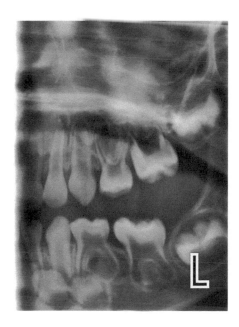

Figure **9-8**

1. The age of this child is:
   A. 2 years
   B. 3 years
   C. 3.5 years
   D. 4 years

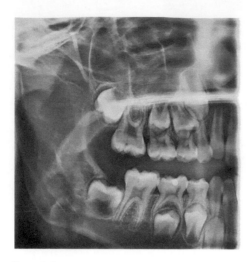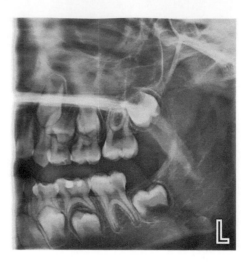

Figure **9-9**

1. This is a panoramic bitewing image of a child of about 6 years of age. There is too much of the ramus in this pan BW image. The reason for this is:
A.   The pan BW setting was for the jaw size of an adult
B.   The machine was in panoramic mode for a small adult
C.   The patient was too small for a bitewing exposure
D.   The patient was too far back in the machine

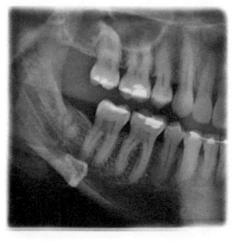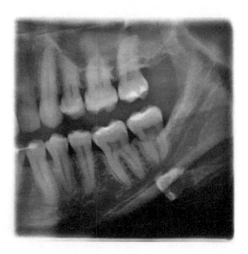

Figure **9-10**

1. The problem with this pan BW is that _____ in the machine.
A.   The jaw was positioned too high up
B.   The jaw was positioned too low down
C.   The patient was "slumped" or "stooped"
D.   B and C are correct
E.   The patient was positioned correctly

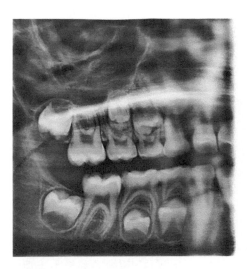
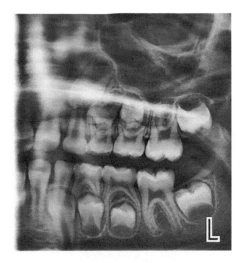

Figure **9-11**

1. The problem with this child pan BW is that the dense radiopaque hard palate shadow is obscuring parts of the developing upper permanent teeth and there is a dark shadow beneath this on the left side. The cause of this is:
   A. The chin was too high
   B. The tongue was not against the palate on the left side
   C. A and B are correct
   D. Actually this is a good pan BW of a child

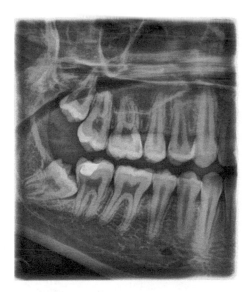
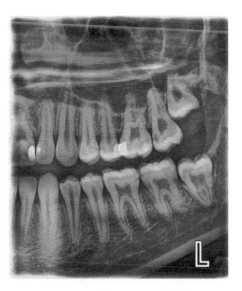

Figure **9-12**

1. Notice how this pan BW demonstrated incipient, deeper enamel and dentinal interproximal caries as well as occlusal caries, but:
   A. There is overlap of the interproximal surfaces on the right side
   B. The lateral incisors on the left side are well visualized while they are only partially seen on the right side
   C. The patient's head was turned in the machine
   D. All of the above are correct
   E. None of the above are correct as this image is within normal parameters

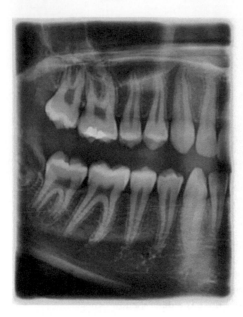
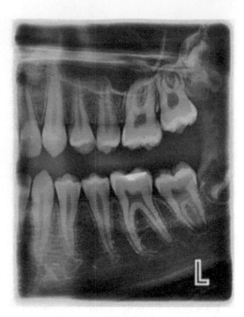

Figure **9-13**

1. Here we see a pretty good example of a pan BW. However:
   A. The patient is about 18 years old and well positioned
   B. The patient is about 12 years old and is slightly "slumped"
   C. The patient is about 18 years old and is slightly rotated
   D. The patient is about 18 years old and is slightly "slumped"

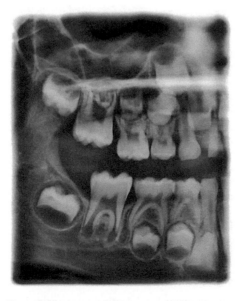
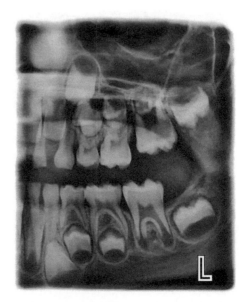

Figure **9-14**

1. This is a pretty good pan BW of a:
   A. Six-year-old child
   B. Patient with the chin just a bit too high
   C. Patient with the tongue not up against the palate
   D. All of the above
   E. None of the above

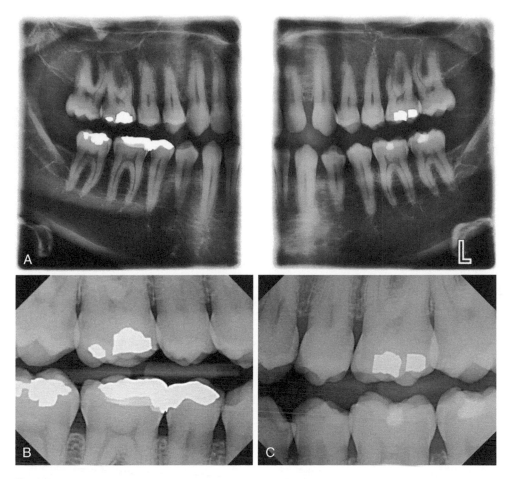

Figure **9-15**

1. Here we see a pan BW and a set of two intraoral BWs of the same patient taken on the same day.
- A. While both image types have overlapped contacts, the intra BWs have more overlapped contacts
- B. While incipient caries on the distal of the lower right 1st molar and the mesial of the lower right 2nd molar can be seen in both image types, caries just past the dentinoenamel junction (DEJ) can only be seen in the pan BW
- C. The patient was slightly slumped for the pan BW
- D. All of the above are true
- E. Only A and B are true

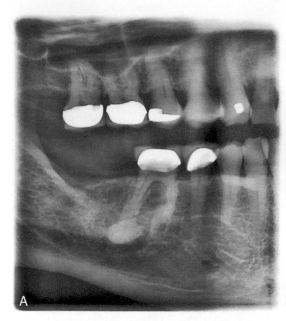
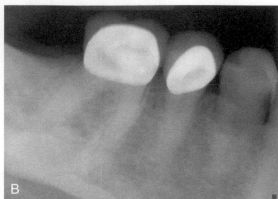

Figure **9-16**

1. Both of these images were taken on the same day; image A is a half of a pan BW on the same patient.
   A. Diagnostically, the pan BW demonstrates an impacted microdont, which cannot be seen in image B of the same region
   B. The pan BW has been over-processed with the software-sharpening tool
   C. The intra BW is underexposed
   D. Only A is true
   E. All of the above are true

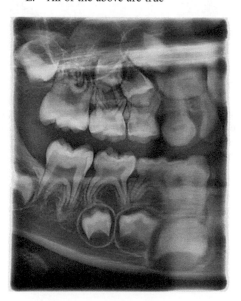
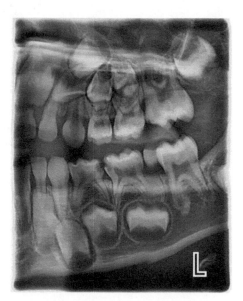

Figure **9-17**

1. This is a pan BW of a child.
   A. This represents a pretty good pan BW of a child
   B. The patient appears to be about 12 years old
   C. The patient followed the machine as it passed in front of his face
   D. There was very slight movement causing a "chink" in the outline of the left mandibular cortex

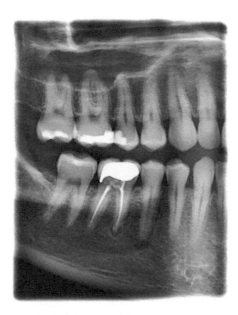
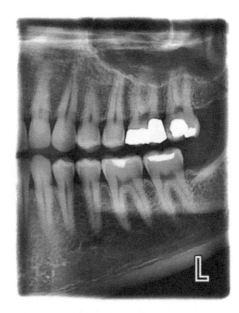

Figure **9-18**

1. Examine the upper left and the lower right 1st molars; there is a thin, dark line beneath the restorations, which appeared sound upon probing with an explorer. The cause of this is:
   A. Over-sharpening with the digital software
   B. Redecay beneath the restorations
   C. Leakage of the cement from under the cast gold restorations
   D. Loose crowns

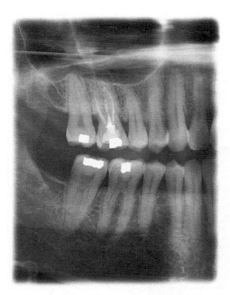
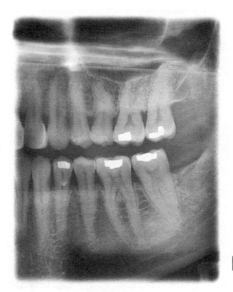

Figure **9-19**

1. This pan BW has a slightly speckled appearance; the cause of this is:
   A. Too much software filtration
   B. Not enough software filtration
   C. Inadequate post-processing with the software
   D. The milliamperage (mA) setting was too low

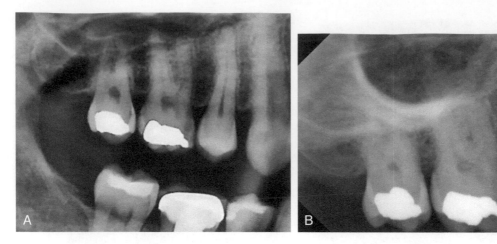

Figure **9-20**

1. Figure A is a cropped pan BW; note the interproximal caries on both upper right molars, which extends to past the DEJ. Figure B is a digital periapical image of the same area taken on the same day. Note the lack of caries on the intra periapical image.

   A.   This finding is true because the pan BW is better for the detection of interproximal caries

   B.   This comparison is inaccurate because interproximal caries should be diagnosed on intra BWs not periapicals

   C.   The digital periapical image is underexposed

   D.   The digital sensor is an early model with not only poor resolution but with limited digital image processing capacity

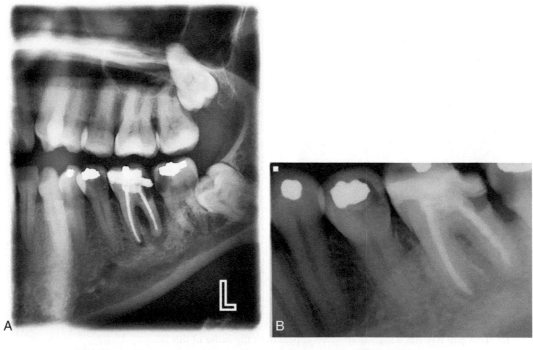

Figure **9-21**

1. Compare A (a half pan BW) and B (a digital periapical image taken with an electronic sensor). The patient has a fever and discomfort in the lower left mandible. Clinically, the tissues were red and swollen, and the placement of the bulky intraoral sensor was difficult and uncomfortable. The poor sensor image was because:

   A.   Of the local sensitivity of the soft tissues

   B.   The coverage of a single sensor image is less than a half pan BW

   C.   The coverage was poor because it was placed on top of the tongue and then pushed down; note the soft tissue image of the tongue

   D.   A single-sensor image may not be as diagnostic as a pan BW due to the greater coverage and comfort of the pan BW in this case

   E.   All of the above

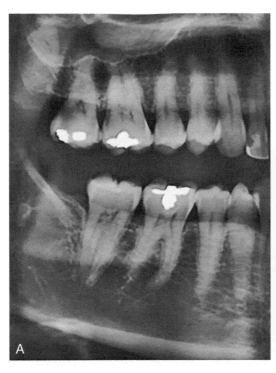
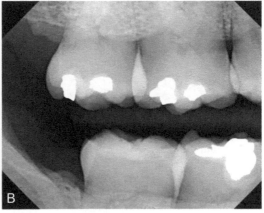

Figure **9-22**

1. Compare A (a half pan BW) and B (a digital periapical image) taken with an electronic sensor on the same patient at the same appointment. While the sensor BW image is somewhat limited compared with the pan BW image, the sensor image:
   A. Is not well executed as it is a bitewing image with grossly overlapped contacts
   B. Of the distal part of the upper 2nd molar can be compared with the same area on the pan BW, which demonstrates a large carious lesion
   C. May not be diagnostic because of poor technique
   D. Has, by its very nature, less periapical coverage than the same region on the pan BW
   E. All of the above

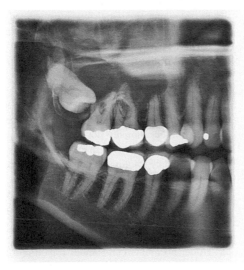
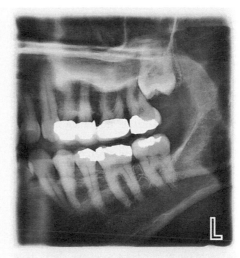

Figure **9-23**

1. This is a pan BW, which has about the same radiation dose as four intra BWs taken with the long, rectangular cone. See if you can identify the pathology that would be impossible to detect on a set of intra BWs.
   A. Impacted upper right and left 3rd molars
   B. The upper right 3rd molar exhibits a dentigerous cyst, which is radiolucent and extends into the lower half of the maxillary sinus
   C. The upper left 3rd molar appears to be associated with a mucositis of the lower half of the left maxillary sinus, which is radiopaque
   D. All of the above

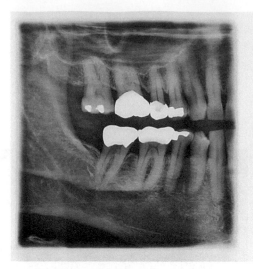
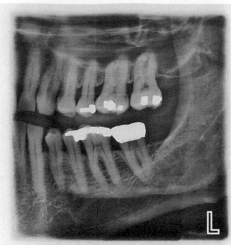

Figure **9-24**

1. Find the cavity.
   A. Distal upper left 1st molar
   B. Distal upper right 2nd molar
   C. Mesial upper right 2nd molar
   D. There is no caries present

MULTIPLE CHOICE QUESTIONS WITHOUT FIGURES

Instructions

Please select the best answer and check your selection with the correct answer in the Answer Key at the back of the book.

1. Which of the following statements is *not* true with respect to pan BWs?
   A. Pan BWs involve a lower radiation dose than intra BWs taken with the long, round cone
   B. With the exception of incipient caries, pan BWs can detect larger interproximal caries
   C. Pan BWs require much less infection control than intra BWs
   D. There is no need to wear protective gloves when taking a pan BW

2. Although pan BW technology has been available since about 2006, it has not been universally accepted in 2016.
   A. The reason for this is not known
   B. Intra BWs are universally accepted as the method of choice for the radiographic detection of interproximal caries
   C. Not all practitioners, schools, and clinics have pan machines capable of generating a pan BW
   D. All of the above
   E. Choices B and C only

3. As opposed to intra BWs, pan BWs can:
   A. Detect periapical lesions
   B. Demonstrate details on impacted 3rd molars
   C. Show the presence of infection in the floor of the maxillary sinus
   D. All of the above
   E. Choices A and B only

4. Pan BWs can demonstrate periapical lesions while a well-positioned and exposed intra periapical image taken at the same time will occasionally not show the periapical lesion.
   A. This is a true statement
   B. Actually intraoral periapical images are the most diagnostic for the detection of periapical lesions
   C. If the lesion is present on the pan, it will be present on the periapical image of the same area taken on the same day
   D. The statement as written is false

5. Under normal circumstances, a panoramic bitewing requires:
   A. No barrier glove protection for the operator
   B. No countertop surface disinfection in the vicinity of the machine
   C. Except for the bite stick, no surface barrier wrapping on parts of the machine or machine part disinfection after the exposure
   D. All of the above
   E. Only A and C are true

6. In terms of exposure of the parotid grand, the pan BW:
   A. Does not expose the parotid gland
   B. Exposes most, if not all, of the parotid gland
   C. May expose small parts of the parotid gland
   D. All of the above
   E. None of the above

7. The reason parotid gland exposure is an issue is:
   A. Parotid gland cancer has been associated with past exposure to both medical and dental radiation
   B. Parotid stones have been associated with past exposure to dental radiation
   C. Parotid gland infection has been associated with past exposure to dental radiation
   D. All of the above
   E. None of the above

8. Given that both the panoramic machine and the intraoral machine and sensors have been paid for:
   A. The pan BW will involve a lower overhead expense
   B. The pan BW will involve a higher overhead expense
   C. The pan BW will not reliably detect incipient posterior caries
   D. The pan BW is a more difficult technique than the familiar intra BW

9. One problem with big pan machines relative to small children is that the pan BW function cannot generally be used on young children below the age of:
   A. 8 years
   B. 12 years
   C. 5 years
   D. None of the above

10. When an adult patient is missing the upper and lower central and lateral incisors, the pan BW is:
    A. Not recommended because proper positioning is difficult
    B. Still possible because the positioning light can be placed a few millimeters anterior to the upper canine tooth
    C. Still possible because the acrylic partial dentures (if available) can be left in place to help with positioning
    D. All of the above
    E. Only B and C are true

11. Because electronic sensors are bulky, the pan BW:
    A. Is especially useful in children
    B. Should only be used for special situations such as gaggers or patients with sensitive oral tissues
    C. Is best used in edentulous patients because they cannot bite on the intraoral bite block
    D. Is nevertheless an unproven application that may lead to missed carious lesions

12. The pan BW involves radiation over a much larger area than a set of four intraoral BWs, therefore:
    A. They should only be used in special circumstances
    B. The radiation dose is much higher than the much smaller intra BWs
    C. It should especially *not* be used routinely in children
    D. None of the above
    E. All of the above

Dental Anomalies

Goal

To understand and recognize dental anomalies as seen in intraoral and panoramic images

Learning Objectives

1. Recognize variations in tooth number
2. Identify variations in tooth size
3. Identify variations in tooth shape
4. Recognize variations in tooth structure
5. Recognize acquired defects in teeth
6. Identify eruption problems
7. Recognize altered tooth positions
8. Classify impactions

GENERAL CASES

Instructions

In this section you will find one or more examples of the conditions listed in the learning objectives. When answering the questions, try first to identify the condition from memory. Most of these conditions are common. Because they can impact patient management, these disorders are important. Of course, the order in which these entities are presented here is scrambled. Compare your answer to the correct answer in the Answer Key at the back of the book.

Okay, here we go!

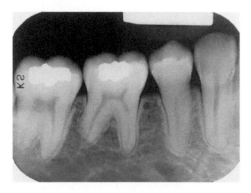

Case **10-1**   Most of this 22-year-old woman's teeth looked like this.
1. What iatrogenic treatment did she receive?
2. What condition is present?

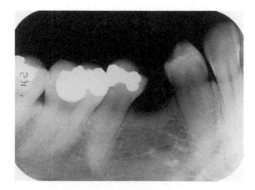

Case **10-2**   This 23-year-old man lost his 1st molar at a young age.
1. What term best describes the abnormal position of the 2nd premolar?

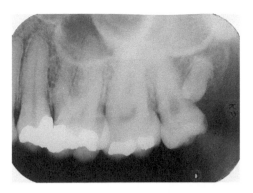

Case **10-3**   Look carefully at this posterior quadrant and notice the tiny tooth.
1.   What two terms used together best describe this anomaly?

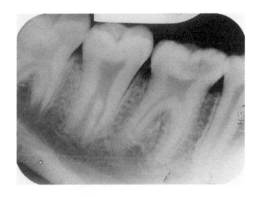

Case **10-4**   Take a look at the lower 2nd molar.
1.   What term best describes its shape?
2.   Is there anything characteristic about the pulp or root canal spaces?
3.   Is this usually a solitary finding, or is it associated with other problems?
4.   Can this condition affect the primary dentition?

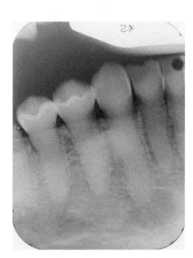

Case **10-5**   This 22-year-old man complains that several of his front teeth have begun to chip.
1.   What condition is present?
2.   List the characteristic radiographic features seen here and several others not seen here.
3.   With what condition of bones is this dental finding sometimes associated?

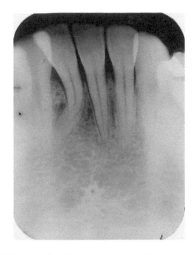

Case **10-6**   Take a look at the right central incisor.
1.   What term describes the altered root shape?
2.   How did it get this way?

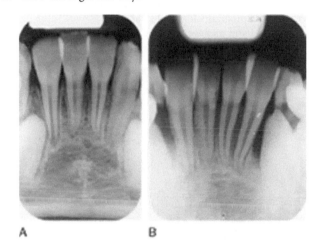

A   B

Case **10-7**   A and B represent two children (Andrew and Billy, respectively) of the same age. One of them is going to have a crowding problem with regard to the eruption of the permanent teeth.
1.   Which one is going to have the crowding problem?
2.   How did you figure that out?
3.   What would you do about it?

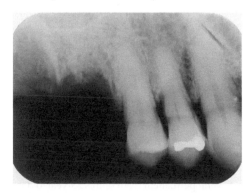

Case **10-8**   Study these teeth carefully. Notice that all three teeth have a radiolucent line in the cervical area. Clinically, the areas appeared V-shaped and were partially subgingival.
1.   What is the differential diagnosis?
2.   What condition do you think is present?
3.   What is the cause, and how is it managed?

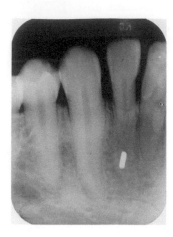

Case 10-9   The lower right lateral incisor of this hockey player was avulsed last year during practice. The tooth was cleaned and sealed with a retrograde amalgam and then reimplanted and splinted with 009 wire and composite for several months.
1.   What has happened to the root of this tooth?
2.   What is the prognosis for the tooth?
3.   How would you manage this case?

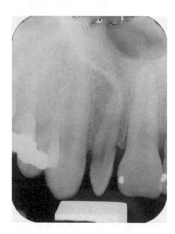

Case 10-10   Take a look at the lateral incisor.
1.   What term(s) best describe(s) this tooth's morphology?
2.   How would you manage this?

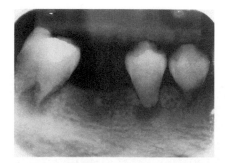

Case 10-11   Several permanent teeth of this 23-year-old man "exfoliated" spontaneously. All of his remaining teeth look like this. Notice the relative lack of root formation, the pulp is completely obliterated, and the apical radiolucencies may develop as a result of periodontal inflammation.
1.   Exactly what condition is present?
2.   How would you manage this?

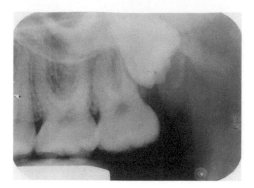

Case 10-12   This patient complained of mild pain associated with the erupting 3rd molar.
1.   See if you can identify the problem.
2.   What would you do about it?

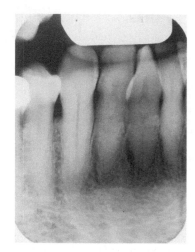

Case 10-13   Note the pulp spaces in the central and lateral incisors. The teeth are vital.
1.   What are these pulpal radiopacities called?
2.   With what developmental dental problem can they be associated?
3.   Does this developmental problem exist here?
4.   What (if any) is the significance of this finding?

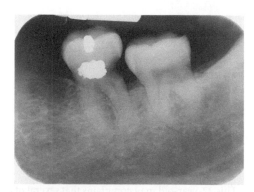

Case 10-14   This middle-aged man has a habit that causes a factitial injury to one of his teeth. Clinically the area on the distal aspect of the 1st molar was hard and shiny and has been a definite "meat catch" for many years.
1.   Comment on the whole situation concerning the 1st molar.
2.   What is the meaning of *factitial*?

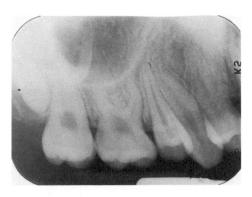

Case 10-15 Study this radiograph carefully.
1. What eruption problem has occurred here?
2. How can this be managed?

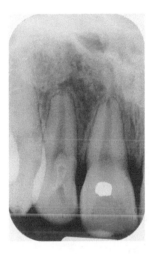

Case 10-16 This patient is a healthy, attractive 15-year-old female. Examine her teeth carefully. Look again before going to the answer.
1. Report what you see. Be complete.

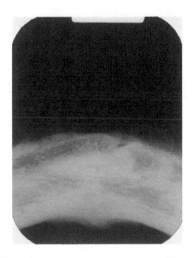

Case 10-17 This older patient wears upper and lower dentures.
1. Exactly what do you see here (if anything)? Be specific.

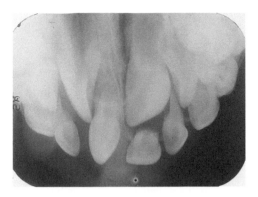

Case 10-18 Gina is the youngest sibling among three others. Mom was a dental assistant before she married the boss (don't laugh, Denyse was my dental assistant!). The appearance of this tiny spiked tooth provoked Mom to take the brood to the dental office to get a radiograph taken.
1. What anomaly did we all discover?
2. What (if anything) should be done about it?

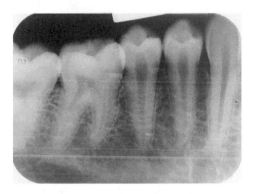

Case 10-19 This patient is a healthy teenager.
1. Comment on the pulps of these teeth. Once again, look closely.

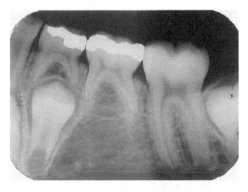

Case 10-20 This patient is a 6-year-old girl.
1. What problem is seen here?
2. What would you report to her parents regarding the present and future management of this problem?
3. What other developmental anomaly would you suspect in this patient?

CASE-BASED **QUESTIONS**

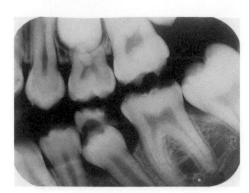

Case **10-21** This 11-year-old boy was sick with high fevers earlier in his life. Now he is normal and healthy.
1. What condition affects the permanent 1st molars?
2. At what time in this boy's life did this occur?

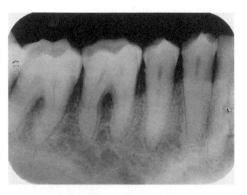

Case **10-22** Believe it or not, this gentleman was 80 years old and had never been to the dentist. He was currently having a little discomfort because of the class 1 furcal involvement and a "meat catch" in the area. He would probably have ignored this but his favorite granddaughter was now a hygienist and insisted upon his dental visit.
1. What anomaly do we see in association with these teeth?

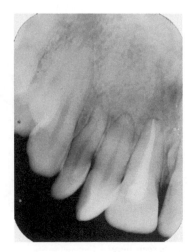

Case **10-23** This patient is being considered for esthetic veneers in the anterior dentition.
1. What anomaly (anomalies) can you see here?

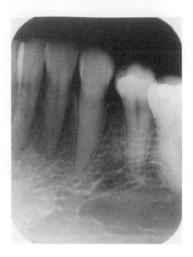

Case **10-24** This patient is in his late 30s. He is asymptomatic.
1. Can you pick out the nonvital tooth?
2. What are the radiographic signs of this nonvitality?
3. How would you treat this?

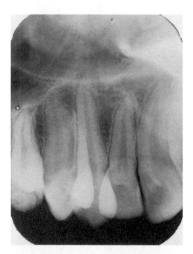

Case **10-25** This patient was given a nickname in high school that referred to this tooth. Now in her mid-20s and a burgeoning chartered public accountant, she has decided to go ahead with the orthodontics.
1. What term best describes the malposition of the canine?
2. What other preventive procedure would you initiate for this patient ASAP? State your reason.

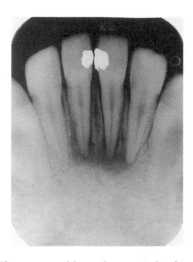

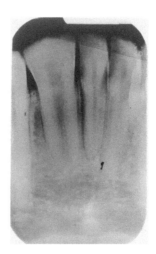

Case 10-26 This 26-year-old man has a couple of unesthetic lower anterior restorations. Note the periapical radiolucencies in the area and the shape of the pulp chambers of the incisors. Right there you have the unique features of this anomaly. (That's a lot of clues!)
1. What anomaly is present? Be specific.
2. What material are the centrals restored with?

Case 10-28 This is a 20-year-old man. He complains that he does not like the looks of one of his bottom front teeth. He has never had an extraction. Starting at the patient's posterior right side (left side of the figure) we see the canine, a very wide incisor, the left central and lateral incisors, and the left canine.
1. Identify the anomaly present in the large incisor.
2. What clinical term best describes the large tooth?
3. Define the term you have selected.

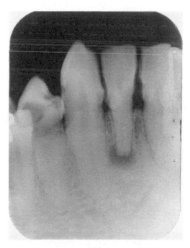

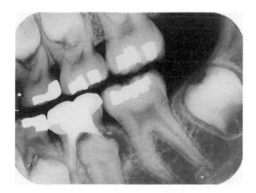

Case 10-27 This 7-year-old boy is in for a check-up.
1. What treatment has the primary 2nd molar received?
2. What condition affects the developing 2nd premolar?
3. Is there any connection between questions 1 and 2? (That's a hint!)

Case 10-29 This middle-aged white man has periodontal disease. The 1st premolar is restored with an older radiolucent composite for esthetics. The right lateral incisor is a dark yellowish brown color, and he wants something done about it.
1. What condition affects the apical region of the right lateral incisor? Be complete.
2. How would you manage this case?

CASE-BASED **QUESTIONS**

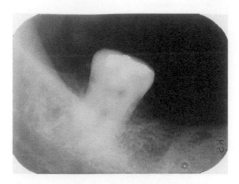

Case 10-30   This patient came in with a broken lower partial denture. He wears a complete upper denture, which he was very satisfied with. Because of this, he was wondering if he should get a complete lower denture. If so, this tooth would need to be extracted.
1. What factor would you consider regarding the removal of this tooth?
2. Of what use (if any) would percussion be in the clinical evaluation of this tooth?

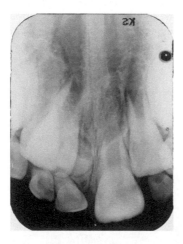

Case 10-31   Just after the big Thanksgiving turkey meal, the mother of 6-year-old Julie noticed that Julie had not lost her 2nd front baby tooth. The tooth was not even loose at this point. "All she wants for Christmas is her two front teeth" quoted Julie's mom to her hygienist several days later.
1. Can you state what the problem is?
2. What would you do?
3. What about the two front teeth for Christmas?

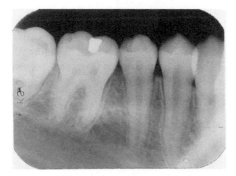

Case 10-32   Lee Ong is a 12-year-old Asian female. Upon looking at this radiograph and subsequently examining the patient, the hygienist reported an unusual finding to the dentist.
1. What unusual finding was reported?
2. What is the significance of this discovery?

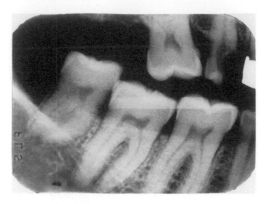

Case 10-33   This patient is a 58-year-old man.
1. What term best describes the position of the lower 3rd molar with respect to the other teeth?
2. What generalized change in the teeth can we see here?

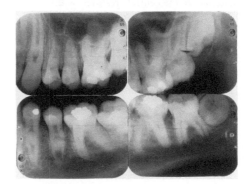

Case 10-34   This patient is a 12-year-old male.
1. What condition affects these teeth?

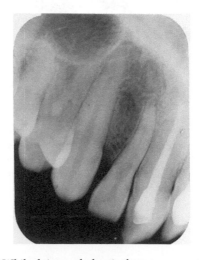

Case 10-35   While doing endodontic therapy on an adjacent tooth, it was discovered that the lateral incisor looked different.
1. What condition affects the lateral incisor?
2. How would you manage this case?

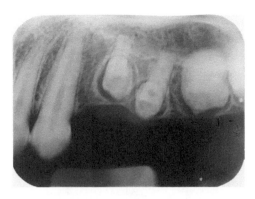

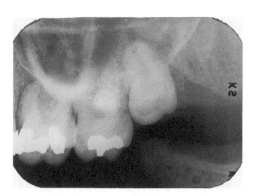

Case **10-36** This patient received radiation therapy. The radiation was collimated to include the posterior maxilla and exclude the anterior jaws.
1. What term(s) best describe(s) the teeth in this area?
2. Will they erupt?
3. How would you manage this case?

Case **10-37** This patient has an anomaly that may be hard to see in this image.
1. Look carefully at these molars and see if you can identify it.

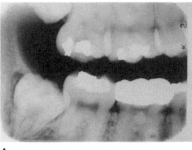
A

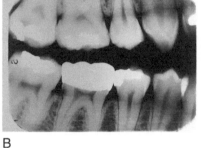
B

Case **10-38** Here's an interesting phenomenon. Follow these instructions carefully: Look at the posterior bitewing (A) and note the round, radiopaque structure (lower 1st molar). Before looking anywhere else, think about what this might be. Now look at the anterior bitewing (B) taken the same day. Presto! The thing you thought you saw has disappeared!
1. What entity did you think the little round radiopacity represented?
2. What is this phenomenon called, and what is the cause?
3. What is the significance of recognizing this phenomenon?

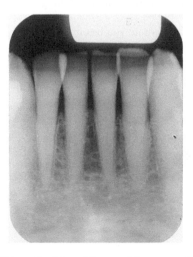

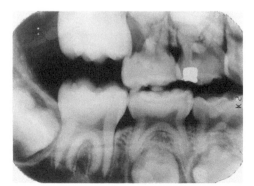

Case **10-39** This patient is a 68-year-old woman. She takes very good care of her teeth these days. The teeth have obliterated pulps in the pulp chamber and upper root canal space.
1. What is the cause of this observation?

Case **10-40** This is a 6-year-old boy whose 1st molars are just erupting. In the newly erupted molar, the root length is about the same length as the crown length. Remember, when an unerupted tooth has a root length longer than the crown length, something is delaying the eruption. In this case there is a different eruption problem.
1. Can you identify the problem?
2. What is the significance of this finding?

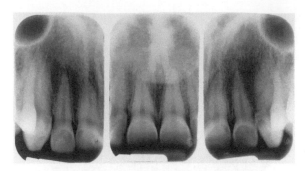

Case **10-41**   This patient is a 32-year-old woman with a behavioral and psychological problem that she has not yet admitted to. The defect is maximal on the lingual aspect of the maxillary anterior teeth.
1.   What dental anomaly do you think is present?
2.   What is the most accurate technical term for this pattern?
3.   How would you manage this case?

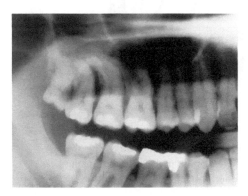

Case **10-42**   This patient has an anomaly.
1.   Identify the anomaly.

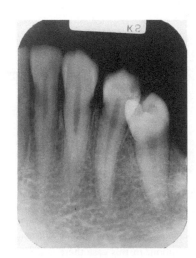

Case **10-43**   Observe this radiograph carefully.
1.   What endodontically significant finding do these teeth demonstrate? These teeth do not require endodontic therapy.

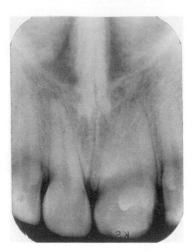

Case **10-44**   Here's a 23-year-old man who says his left front tooth is just too big. Here we see his two central and lateral incisors.
1.   What general term can be used to describe the big tooth?
2.   What specific problem affects this tooth?
3.   Define the term you have selected for your previous answer.

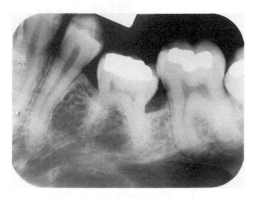

Case **10-45**   This patient is an adult in his 20s, and something needs to be done about this situation.
1.   What terms can we use to describe the primary 2nd molar?
2.   Can you see any problem developing as a result of this situation?
3.   What treatment would you recommend?

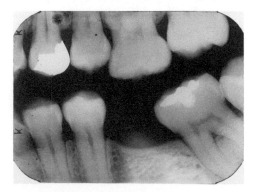

Case **10-46**   This situation is common. The lower 1st molar has been missing for a long time.
1.   What do you see here?
2.   How would you manage this?

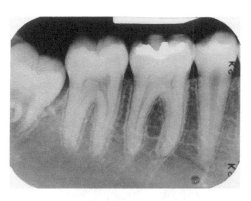

Case **10-47**   Okay. Here's an easy one. Study this radiograph.
1. How old is this patient?
2. Comment on the pulp chambers of the 1st and 2nd molars.
3. What is the significance of this observation?

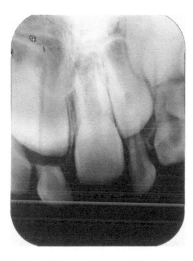

Case **10-48**   This is a 5½-year-old girl. There is an indication she may have crowding of her permanent dentition. To avoid misleading you, note the film was bent and caused distortion in the left central incisor that is not associated with the sign being sought.
1. What sign indicates probable crowding in the permanent dentition?

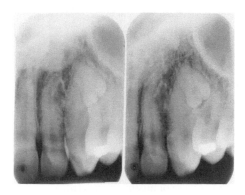

Case **10-49**   This patient is a 28-year-old man. He is asymptomatic. A radiopacity was noted in the apical region of the canine.
1. What anomaly do you think is present clinically?

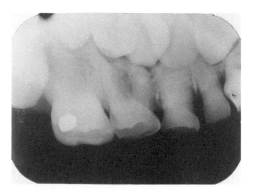

Case **10-50**   This patient is in his late teens with delayed eruption of all his permanent teeth. He has an underdeveloped set of bones in his upper torso, frontal bossing, and hypertelorism.
1. What condition do you think he has?
2. Which bone is underdeveloped?
3. What is hypertelorism, and exactly how do you determine this is present?

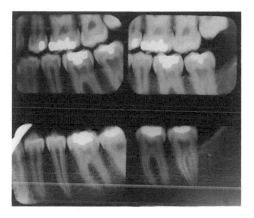

Case **10-51**   This patient is in his late 20s. He has a metabolic problem and takes huge amounts of vitamin D with a poor response. He is small in stature, especially in the lower body. The sign associated with his problem affects most of his teeth.
1. Describe the abnormal dental findings; you need to look carefully.
2. What condition do you think is present?

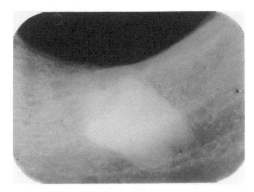

Case **10-52**   This edentulous patient has a radiopaque area in his left jaw.
1. Precisely what is this radiopaque entity?
2. How would you manage this?

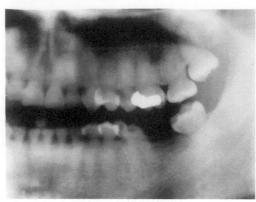 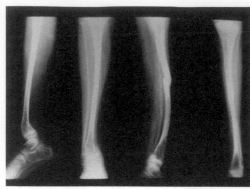

A   B

Case **10-53**   This patient is an 18-year-old white female. She has a problem with her teeth (A) and with her bones (B), and her eyes have a very visible anomaly.
1.   What condition affects the teeth?
2.   What is the overall systemic condition called?
3.   What do you think can be seen in the eyes?

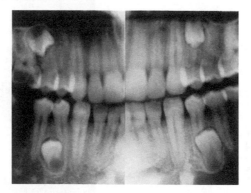

Case **10-54**   Here is a patient with a very apparent finding.
1.   What anomaly is present?
2.   How would you treat this?
3.   What is the most common site of this anomaly?

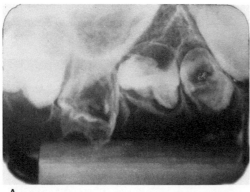 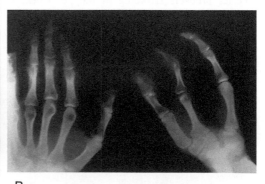

A   B

Case **10-55**   This patient has a syndrome named after the same folks who first reported the jaw cyst basal cell nevus syndrome. (Big clue!) The patient is a young man in his early 20s and had some abnormal looking teeth (A). Among other stigmata, he has a clawlike hand because of missing fingers (B), hypoplasia of the dermis in patches, and skin lesions.
1.   What term best characterizes the appearance of these teeth?
2.   What syndrome does this patient have?

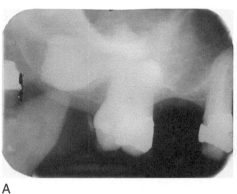

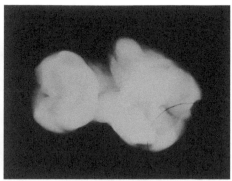

A   B

Case **10-56**   This simulated case demonstrates an impacted 3rd molar (A) whose roots are in proximity to each other. When the 3rd molar was elevated (during extraction), the erupted 2nd molar moved with it. As a result, both teeth were removed (B).

1. What condition affects these teeth?
2. Define the term you have chosen for the above answer.

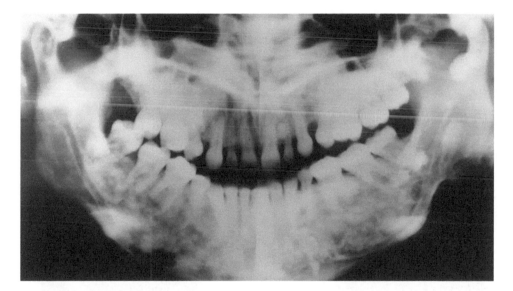

Case **10-57**   This patient is a 27-year-old man who had a large radiopaque mass removed from the left angle area of the mandible.

1. What dental anomaly involving numbers of teeth can you find?
2. What are the radiopaque lesions?
3. What syndrome does this patient have?
4. What important feature of the syndrome would you discuss with this patient?

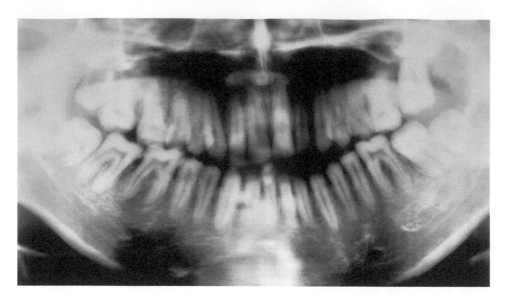

Case **10-58**   Study this radiograph carefully. This patient has a generalized condition affecting all of his teeth. A sibling is also affected the same way.
1.   What condition of the teeth is present here?

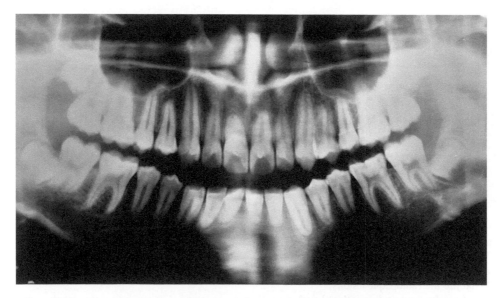

Case **10-59**   Henry is a 12-year-old Hispanic boy. He has never had orthodontic treatment.
1.   Name at least two dental anomalies seen in this case.
2.   What syndrome is present?
3.   What other features are sometimes seen?

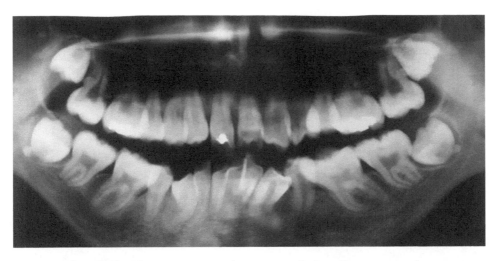

Case **10-60** This teenage patient has an anomaly that affects many teeth.
1. Can you name the anomaly (anomalies) present in this case?
2. Can you quantify your findings?
3. What other anomalies do you see?

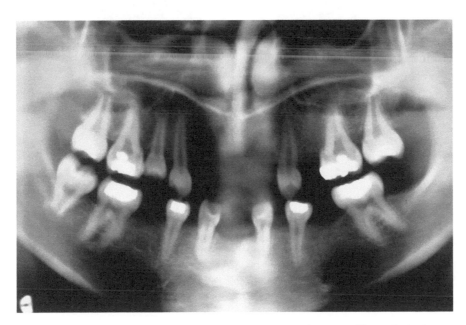

Case **10-61** This patient has fine, sparse, blond hair; he has no eyebrows; and his nails don't grow out because they crumble once they get beyond the nail bed. His complexion is dry and is ruddy and reddish in color. He has one other affected sibling. He has never had any teeth extracted.
1. What condition affects this patient?

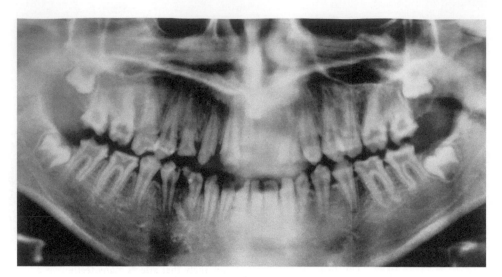

Case **10-62** This patient is a 12-year-old female who rarely smiles with an open mouth or otherwise shows her teeth.
1. What condition affects her teeth?

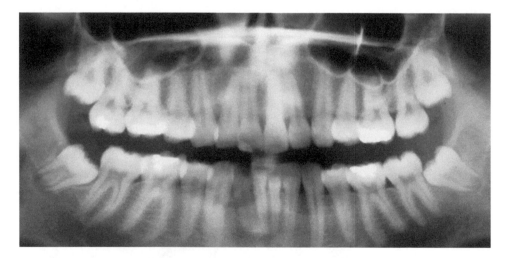

Case **10-63** This patient is a 19-year-old male. He has just completed a full course of orthodontic therapy with extraction of all four 1st premolars.
1. Should we consider the developing 3rd molars as impacted and extract them or leave them alone because they are still erupting?
2. Do you think the erupting 3rd molars can cause a regression of the original crowding?

SPECIAL SECTION ON THIRD MOLAR IMPACTIONS

Study Figure 10-1, A to F, which demonstrates classification for impacted 3rd molars. Having a classification is important in medico-legal record keeping and confirms that the dentist has thoroughly evaluated the tooth's position in relation to the adjacent tooth, to the potential space available, and to structures like the maxillary sinus. The relationship to the inferior alveolar canal will be considered separately. This classification is based on the work of Pell and Gregory as well as Winter and Archer.

Mandibular Impactions (Figure 10-1, A to C)

FACTOR I: Space (distance) between the distal of 2nd molar and ramus:

Class 1: Equal to or greater than m-d diameter of 3rd molar crown.
Class 2: Less than m-d diameter of 3rd molar crown.
Class 3: All or most of 3rd molar is in ramus.

FACTOR II: Depth of 3rd molar in bone:

Position A: Most superior aspect of 3rd molar level with or above occlusal plane of 2nd molar.

Position B: Most superior aspect of 3rd molar below occlusal plane but above cervical line of 2nd molar.
Position C: Most superior aspect of 3rd molar below cervical line of 2nd molar.

FACTOR III: Position of long axis of 3rd molar relative to long axis of 2nd molar:

Vertical	Mesioangular
Horizontal	Distoangular
Inverted	Buccoangular
Rotated	Linguoangular

Mandibular Impactions

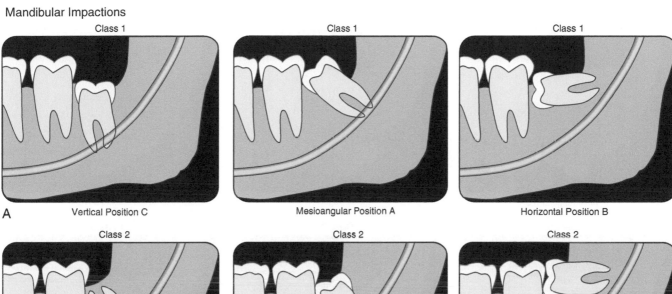

Class 1

A Vertical Position C

Class 1

Mesioangular Position A

Class 1

Horizontal Position B

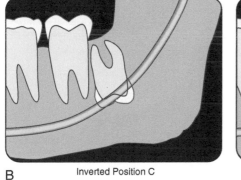
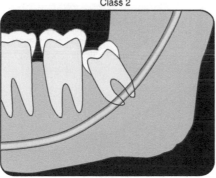
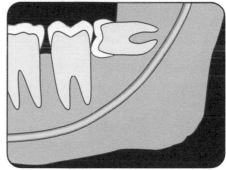

Class 2

B Inverted Position C

Class 2

Mesioangular Position B

Class 2

Horizontal Position A

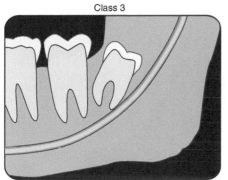
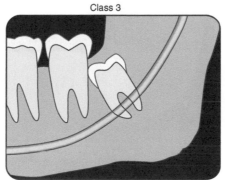
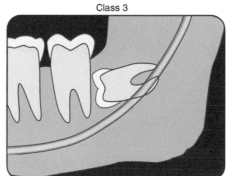

Class 3

C Distoangular Postion B

Class 3

Mesioangular Position C

Class 3

Horizontal Postion C

Figure **10-1** A, B, C

CASE-BASED **QUESTIONS**

Maxillary Impactions (Figure 10-1, D to F)

FACTOR I: Depth of 3rd molar in bone:

Class A: Most inferior aspect of 3rd molar crown is on level with or below occlusal plane of 2nd molar.

Class B: Most inferior aspect of 3rd molar crown is between occlusal plane and cervical line of 2nd molar.

Class C: Most inferior aspect of 3rd molar crown is at or above cervical line of 2nd molar.

FACTOR II: Position of long axis of 3rd molar relative to long axis of 2nd molar:

Vertical	Mesioangular
Horizontal	Distoangular
Inverted	Buccoangular
Rotated	Linguoangular

FACTOR III: Relationship of 3rd molar to maxillary sinus:

Sinus approximation (SA)

No sinus approximation (NSA)

Maxillary Impactions

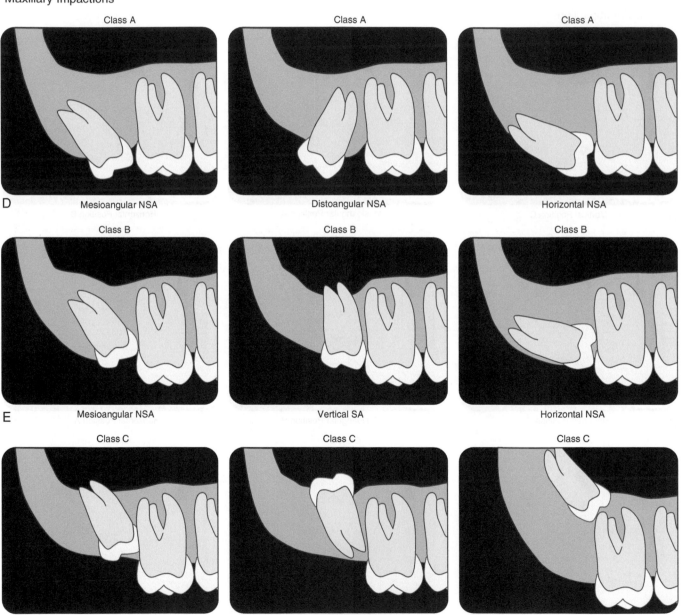

Class A — Mesioangular NSA   D

Class A — Distoangular NSA

Class A — Horizontal NSA

Class B — Mesioangular NSA   E

Class B — Vertical SA

Class B — Horizontal NSA

Class C — Mesioangular SA   F

Class C — Inverted SA

Class C — Distoangular SA

Figure **10-1**   D, E, F

Instructions

All of these patients have impacted 3rd molars. Classify the impacted 3rd molars for each case. Some cases include upper and lower 3rd molar impactions. Compare your answer to the correct answer in the Answer Key at the back of the book.

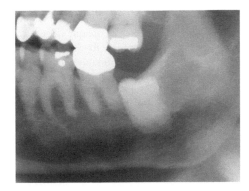

Case **10-64**

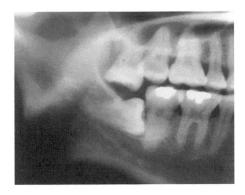

Case **10-67**

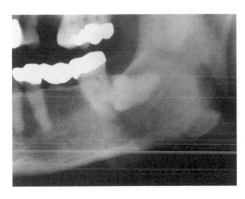

Case **10-65**

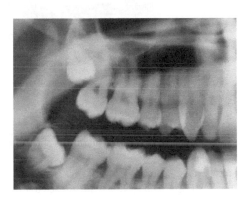

Case **10-68**

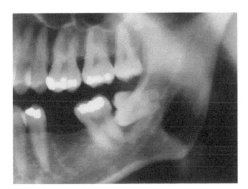

Case **10-66**

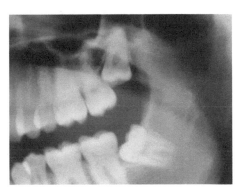

Case **10-69**

SPECIAL SECTION ON LOCALIZATION

There are three "rules" for the localization of objects toward the buccal or lingual within the jaws using two periapical radiographs taken at different angles.

- First described by C. Clark in 1909, this rule requires a fixed vertical angulation and a different horizontal angle of the beam for the two radiographs. If the object in question moves in the same direction as the horizontal shift of the tube head, it is toward the lingual; if the object moves in the opposite direction, it is on the buccal. This is where the SLOB rule comes from: Same on Lingual; Opposite on Buccal. The problem for many is that it is hard to figure out which way the tube head moved in the two comparison radiographs.
- The *buccal object rule* was first described by Richards in 1952. Here the buccal object will move with the angulation change of the BID (cone), including up, down, mesial, or distal when the two radiographs are compared. This rule is easier because students can recognize the effects of vertical and horizontal changes in the BID.
- The *known object rule* was first popularized by Langlais in the early 1980s. In this instance there is no need to figure out which way the tube head or BID has moved. The only requirements are the two comparison radiographs taken at different vertical or horizontal angles and a known object you can identify as buccal or lingual. The known object will have moved either up or down or mesially or distally in the two comparison radiographs. Some known objects are the buccal cusps; the buccal malar process of the maxilla; the lingual mandibular and palatal tori, and the incisive foramen; the buccal mental foramen and external oblique ridge; the lingual genial tubercles and internal oblique ridge, etc. Now look at the unknown object and compare its movement to the movement of the known object. If the unknown object moves in the same way as the known object, it is located in the same place (either buccal or lingual); if it moves in the opposite direction as the known object, it is opposite in location. If it does not move, it is in the middle of the jaw in question. If the movement is in the same direction as the known object but not as much, it is not as far out on the side (buccal or lingual) of the known object.

Instructions

Compare your answer to the correct answer in the Answer Key at the back of the book.

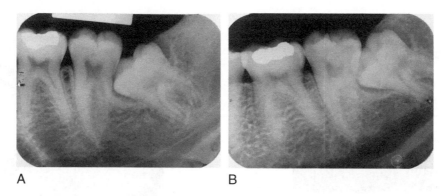

A   B

Case **10-70**   Notice the impacted 3rd molar. Look at the lingual cusps of the 2nd molar; they can be used as the known object.
1.   On which side of the mandible is the impacted 3rd molar located?

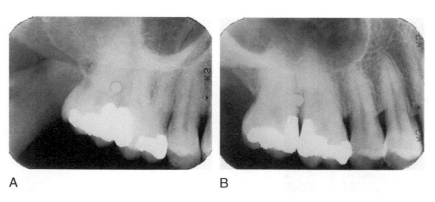

A   B

Case **10-71**   Notice the enamel pearl on the maxillary 2nd molar.
1.   Because you suspect an associated periodontal defect, toward which side (the buccal or lingual) will you probe for the enamel pearl?

SPECIAL SECTION ON PERIODONTAL ASSESSMENT

Instructions

The following cases are presented in no particular order. All of the selected cases demonstrate some radiographic finding(s) that may be associated with periodontal disease. Compare your answer to the correct answer in the Answer Key at the back of the book.

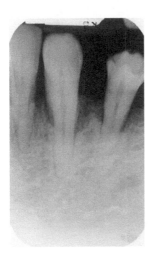

Case 10-72 Here we are interested in the canine and 1st premolar teeth.
1. Describe your findings associated with the canine.
2. Describe your findings in association with the premolar.

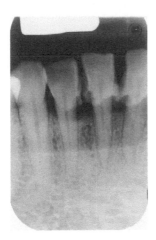

Case 10-73 This is the lower anterior region of a periodontal patient.
1. What term is used to classify this calculus regarding its location above the gingiva?
2. What term describes such copious amounts of calculus?
3. What periodontally significant factor can such copious amounts of calculus mask?
4. Classify the type of bone loss in association with these teeth.
5. What periodontal disease do you think is present?
6. What is the horizontal radiopaque line at the apical region of all these teeth?

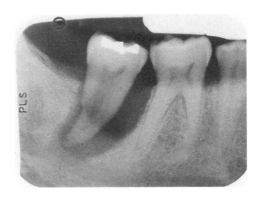

Case 10-74 Note this patient's molars.
1. What term describes the periodontal status of the 2nd molar?
2. In this circumstance, what other disease(s) must be ruled out?
3. Describe the periodontal defect associated with the 2nd molar.
4. What finding suggests this tooth has been mobile for a long time?
5. Is there anything that may suggest the cause of this mobility?
6. What do we see in the furcal area of the 1st molar?

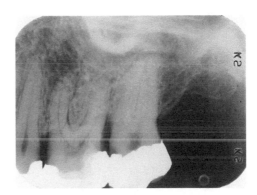

Case 10-75 This radiograph is part of the patient's routine radiographic examination.
1. Report your findings in association with the 1st molar.
2. Report your findings in association with the 2nd molar.

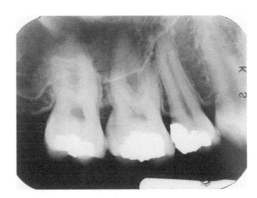

Case 10-76 This patient is in her early 30s.
1. List one periodontally significant finding associated with each of the three most posterior teeth seen here.

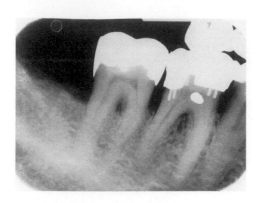

Case **10-77** Take a look at these two molars.
1. What would you report?

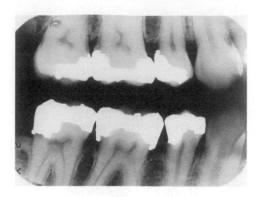

Case **10-79** Here we have a lot of periodontally significant defective restorations.
1. Identify the defective restorations, describe the defect, and suggest how each should be managed.

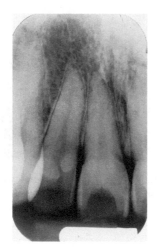

Case **10-78** Look at this radiograph closely and note the shovel-shaped incisors. (Prominent marginal ridges, deep lingual pit, and tendency for class III caries.) There is some horizontal bone loss. The lamina dura is much more prominent for the lateral than for the central incisor.
1. In this area, and especially in this case, what further additional periodontally significant finding would you look for in this radiograph? Explain.

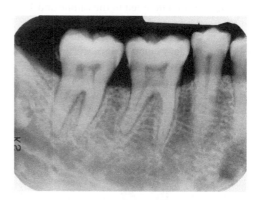

Case **10-80** Look at the two molars and the 2nd premolar.
1. What periodontally significant findings can you see?

SPECIAL SECTION ON CARIES AND CARIES SEQUELAE

Caries can be classified and/or described in many ways. It can be described by the standard classification: class I is occlusal; class II is interproximal, usually involving the contact point(s) of adjacent posterior teeth and sometimes including the distal portion of the canines; class III is anterior interproximal caries involving the contact points; class IV involves the incisal edge of an anterior tooth; class V is usually located on the buccal or lingual surface of any tooth; class VI involves a cusp tip only.

Caries may also be referred to as incipient caries when it is less than halfway through the enamel, enamel caries when it involves half or more of the depth into the enamel but not into dentin, dentinal caries, or pulpal caries. Caries can be acute or chronic.

Here are some further descriptive terms:

* **Bottle caries** is seen in young children who are bottle-fed fluids with high sugar content.
* **Rampant caries** is often seen in teenagers and is associated with dietary, hygiene, and hormonal factors. Caries affects many teeth and advances at a rapid rate.
* **Xerostomia caries** is a form of rampant caries associated with xerostomia secondary to factors such as drugs and age; it often affects the roots of teeth.
* **Radiation caries** is similar to xerostomia caries, but the etiology is different and multifactorial, involving radiation effects on the oral ecology, immune factors, quantity of saliva, and dietary factors in postirradiation patients. It ultimately results in a rubbery, circumferential caries and eventual fracture of the tooth.
* **Recurrent caries** is seen at the margin or under a restoration.
* **Arrested caries** is when the caries process has ceased and the affected area becomes hard and remineralized and often stained a brownish or blackish color, and the caries advancement may be anywhere from incipient to very advanced.
* **Root caries** is seen on any surface of the root; when on the interproximal, it must be distinguished from class II caries by its location below the cemento-enamel junction. A special form of root caries is associated with overdentures.

Caries sequelae include space loss; periapical conditions of pulpal origin such as abscess, radicular cyst, periapical granuloma, and the rare cholesteatoma; also a lateral periodontal cyst can develop from a lateral canal in the root of a nonvital tooth; pulp polyp and residual cyst can remain upon extraction of the tooth; and Turner's **enamel hypoplasia** is a sequela of caries or trauma to a developing permanent tooth.

Radiographically, other conditions may resemble caries such as:
* **Abfraction**
* **Toothbrush abrasion**
* **Abrasion** from a partial denture clasp
* **Adumbration,** or cervical burnout, especially seen at the cervical aspect of anterior teeth, the distal aspect of canines, and upper aspects of 1st and 2nd molars
* Mach band effect seen in the dentin immediately beneath enamel and disappears when the enamel is covered with an opaque material like the paper wrap from a film packet
* Some forms of **erosion**
* Older, radiolucent, tooth-colored filling materials, radiolucent cements, and pulp capping materials
* Developmental defects such as the various presentations of enamel hypoplasia

* The so-called controversial pre-eruptive caries, whereby a tooth becomes "carious" before eruption, when not exposed to the oral environment by, for example, a periodontal defect; such cases most likely represent external or internal resorption

Instructions

Compare your answer to the correct answer in the Answer Key at the back of the book.

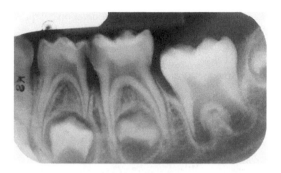

Case **10-81** This patient is a 6-year-old boy with an erupting 1st permanent molar. Note how root formation does not exceed crown length when the tooth first emerges into the mouth; the apical half of the root will develop from first emergence until the tooth is in occlusion. This is important in the early identification of delayed eruption.
1. Classify the caries in the two primary molars.
2. What caries sequela must we avoid in this situation?
3. When will these teeth be shed?
4. How would these teeth be treated?

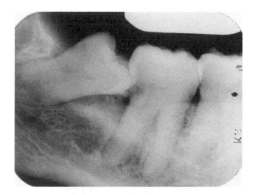

Case **10-82** This is a patient with a toothache. It is relieved by a cold drink. He is now in his 40s and has never needed to go to the dentist. The tooth is sensitive to percussion. This is a common situation in people with a partially erupted 3rd molar that was not extracted.
1. What periodontally significant factor(s) can you see in association with the 3rd molar?
2. Is there any problem with the 2nd molar? Explain.

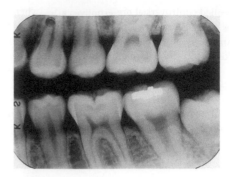

Case 10-83   This is a patient under consideration for preventive treatment.
1.   Which one surface would you not seal as the only treatment? Why?
2.   On which one tooth can cervical burnout be most clearly seen?

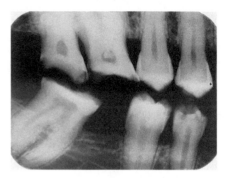

Case 10-84   This patient's molars are rock-hard on the occlusal surface, which is dark brown in color, smooth, and shiny.
1.   What type of caries has affected the molars?
2.   What is the radiolucent area on the distal aspect of the mandibular 1st premolar?
3.   Do you see any occlusal caries anywhere?
4.   Classify the caries on the mesial aspect of the lower 2nd premolar.

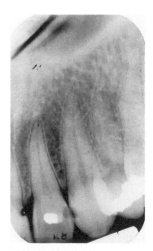

Case 10-85   Here we are interested in the lesions on the lateral and canine.
1.   Classify the caries on these two teeth.
2.   What would you conclude if no caries could be found upon clinical examination?
3.   With what material is the lingual pit restored?

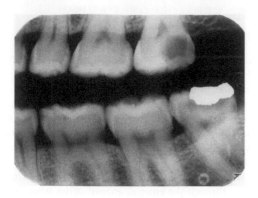

Case 10-86   This patient has a number of carious lesions.
1.   Classify the caries in the following teeth:
   Maxilla:
   •   1st premolar
   •   2nd premolar
   •   2nd molar
   Mandible:
   •   1st molar
   •   2nd molar
   •   3rd molar
2.   On which one surface is the most obvious cervical burnout?

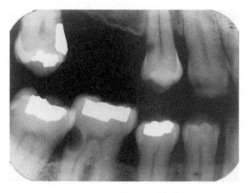

Case 10-87   This patient has two very obvious carious lesions of interest to us here.
1.   Classify the lesions on the upper 1st premolar and on the lower 1st molar.
2.   Comment on the etiology (cause).

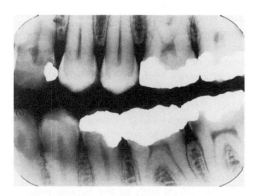

Case 10-88   This case is short and sweet.
1.   Where is the recurrent caries?

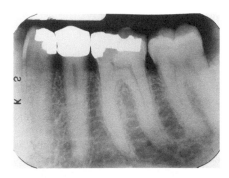

Case **10-89** This is a common situation. This patient does not have any clinically detectable caries though the problem was easily seen during the clinical examination.
1. What problem do you think affects the lower 1st molar?
2. What treatment would you recommend?

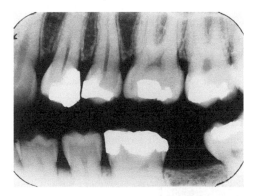

Case **10-90** This is an important and somewhat frequent situation. This patient complains of a slight twinge or sensitivity in one of his teeth on this side, which he just cannot seem to localize. This sensation comes and goes, never stays for long, and is absent for long periods. He also complains of a "meat catch" in the upper premolar area but is not certain the pain he is speaking of comes from there. The problem is actually obvious if you know what to look for.
1. Which one tooth would you suspect as the source of the problem? Explain.

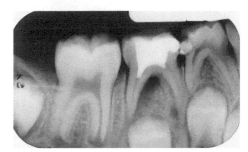

Case **10-91** Here we see an important set of circumstances that must be recognized. The pulpotomy was done six months ago at the last dental visit. A gum boil still comes and goes. Note that the root formation is only about two-thirds complete; thus eruption of the 1st molar is still in progress. Remember, the occlusal plane of the permanent dentition is higher than that of the primary dentition.
1. What problem relative to the mandibular 2nd premolar do we need to prevent?
2. What treatment would you suggest?

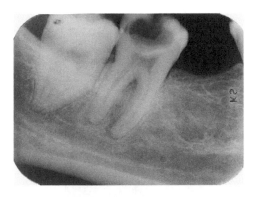

Case **10-92**
1. Comment on the mandibular 2nd molar vitality status.
2. How would this case be restored?

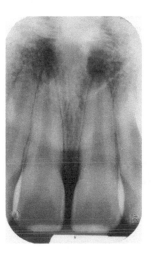

Case **10-93** This 8-year-old boy fell off his skateboard and traumatized his upper lip. The teeth did not appear fractured clinically; however, this radiograph was taken to make sure.
1. What problem(s) (if any) do you see?

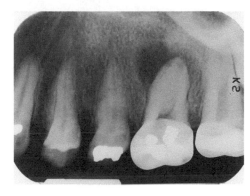

Case **10-94** Here we are interested primarily in the maxillary 1st molar.
1. Comment on the vitality status of this tooth.
2. What condition is present at the apex?
3. What type of crown is on the 1st molar?
4. What condition affects the 2nd molar?

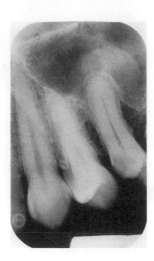

Case **10-95**   This is an unusual periapical radiograph of the premolars. It is actually a botched canine radiograph. The tooth in question is the 2nd premolar.

1. Classify the caries in the 2nd premolar.
2. Comment on the root shape of this tooth.
3. What periapical reaction (if any) do we see here?
4. How would this tooth be managed? Comment on extraction.

SPECIAL SECTION ON THIRD MOLAR RELATIONSHIP TO THE MANDIBULAR CANAL

Depicted are some of the most important means of determining a very close relationship of the 3rd molar root to the inferior alveolar canal. The suspicion of this intimate relationship is important to incorporate into the treatment plan because neurogenic symptoms, such as a numb or burning lower lip, or vascular problems, such as severe bleeding, can occur if the structures within the canal are damaged during the procedure. More recently, the validity of these findings has been questioned. However, it is certainly desirable to be cautious whenever these findings are seen. In Case 10-96A, note that one or both walls of the canal are not apparent in the region of the roots; here the roots may have resorbed or thinned the canal wall. In B, a radiolucent band is on one or more roots where the canal crosses the roots; here there may be a groove in the roots, making this area more radiolucent caused by the proximity of the canal during root development. In C, the canal is narrowed where it crosses the roots; here we may actually have the canal going right between the roots or being completely or partially enveloped by the roots. Also, any two or three combinations are an even stronger suggestion that the 3rd molar roots are close to the canal.

Instructions

Compare your answer to each question to the correct answer in the Answer Key at the back of the book.

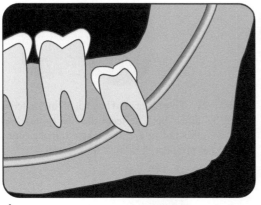

A   Interuption of canal wall

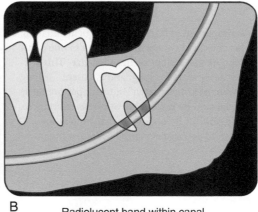

B   Radiolucent band within canal

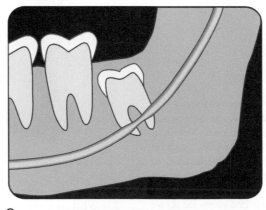

C   Constriction of canal diameter

Case **10-96**

1. Having studied the above diagrams, can a close relationship of the 3rd molars and the mandibular canal be suspected with any of these three appearances?

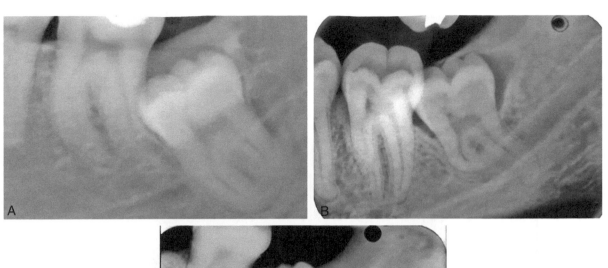

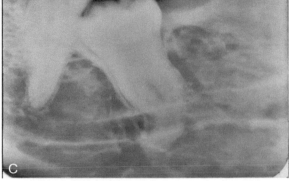

Case **10-97**

1. What feature(s) cause(s) you to suspect a close relationship between the 3rd molar and the inferior alveolar canal?
2. Match the diagrams in Figure 10-96 with the periapical images in Figure 10-97.

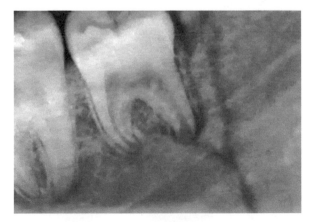

Case **10-98**

1. What feature(s) cause(s) you to suspect a close relationship between the 3rd molar and the inferior alveolar canal?
2. The actual history on this patient of Dr. Langlais' when he was in general practice was that this young man heavily bumped his jaw on the refrigerator door which he opened a little too vigorously in his quest for another glass of champagne at a wedding reception. He felt a little pain at first, but somewhat more when he woke up the next morning around 10 AM. He presented 2 days later with a toothache and continuing pain in his jaw, which was exacerbated when eating. What do you see?

SPECIAL SECTION ON SINUS PNEUMATIZATION

In Case 10-99 you can see the stages (A to C) by which pneumatization of the maxillary sinus develops. This concept is more important than ever as implant therapy is common.

The pneumatization process seems to vary over time and from one person to another. It may be most prominent in persons with chronic sinus problems such as allergies or sinusitis. In any case, the available alveolar bone for an implant in this area may alter over time, and the patient should be informed.

Instructions

Compare your answer to the correct answer in the Answer Key at the back of the book.

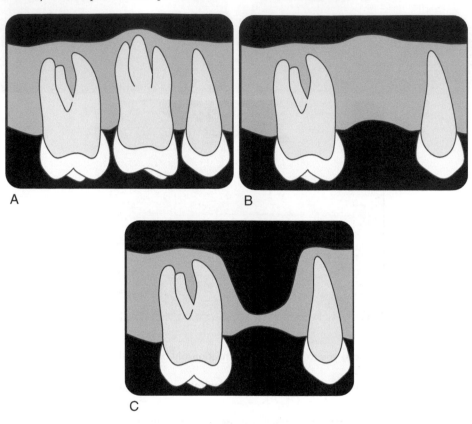

Case **10-99**
1.   Based on the diagrams, can pneumatization be seen in periapical radiographs?

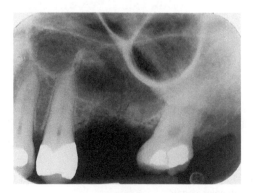

Case **10-100**   This patient wishes to have the edentulous space replaced with several implants. This radiograph was taken as part of the initial assessment.
1.   How do things look for one or more implants here? (Good, not bad, or bad)
2.   What pathology do you see in the edentulous area?
3.   What condition affects the sinus?
4.   Is there anything that can be done if the patient insists on exhausting every possibility in order to have implants?

Chapter 11

Assessment/Interpretation of Pathology of the Jaws

Goal

To know how to assess and/or interpret radiographic images for the presence of disease

Learning Objectives

1. Recognize abnormal features in the jaws
2. Recognize cysts of the jaws
3. Know the features of tumors of the jaws
4. Recognize developmental or genetically related disorders
5. Identify fibro-osseous conditions
6. Recognize inflammatory disorders and infections
7. Recognize the most common pathologic abnormalities affecting the jaws

CASE INTERPRETATION

Instructions

The questions are short and to the point. They contain clues such as the age and sex of the patient, laboratory values, and even in the patient's fictitious name! So watch for the clues. Compare your answer to each question to the correct answer in the Answer Key at the back of the book.

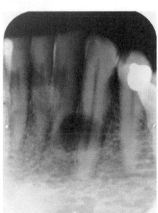

Case **11-1**   Bill is an asymptomatic 47-year-old who presented for routine dental treatment. This radiograph was taken as part of the full mouth survey.
1. On what side of the mandible (buccal or lingual) is the radiolucent lesion in the canine area located?
2. What developmental anomaly do you think this finding represents?
3. What treatment (if any) would you recommend?

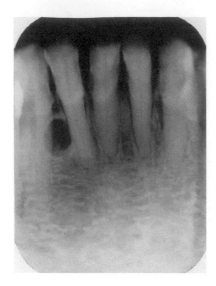

Case **11-2** Mary is a 67-year-old who was referred to the periodontist. As part of the radiographic examination, this small radiolucent lesion was detected. The teeth were vital.

1. Give a differential diagnosis for this lesion. Include three conditions, stating your most likely choice first and least likely last.
2. Considering the patient's age and the location, size, and clinical findings, what is your diagnostic impression?
3. What treatment would you recommend? Why?

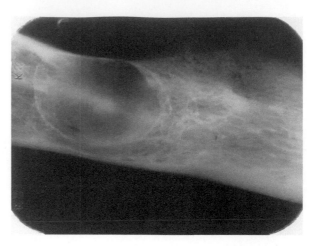

Case **11-4** This 72-year-old woman presented with loose 20-year-old dentures and slight intermittent pain under the lower denture. She stated she had her teeth extracted because of severe untreated caries and abscessed teeth. The radiolucent lesion was detected on a radiograph of the painful area.

1. Describe the lesion.
2. What is your diagnostic impression?
3. Name several other lesions that could look like this.
4. What treatment would you recommend?

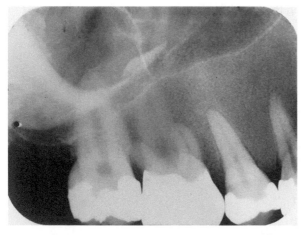

Case **11-3** This is a 35-year-old asymptomatic woman who has slight buccal and palatal enlargement of the alveolar bone in this area. Other studies indicated portions of the zygoma were involved. This condition was first detected at age 19 years and is slowly progressive. Her alkaline phosphatase was normal to high-normal, and her serum calcium was normal.

1. Describe the significant radiographic findings.
2. Give a differential diagnosis consisting of three conditions, with your best choice first.
3. What is your diagnostic impression?
4. What treatment (if any) would you recommend?

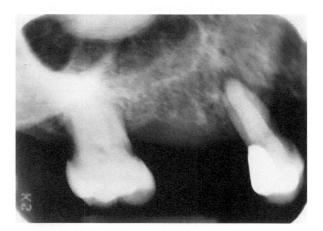

Case **11-5** Mary is a 55-year-old who is about to have dentures made.

1. Study this radiograph and determine what significant factor might affect the treatment plan.

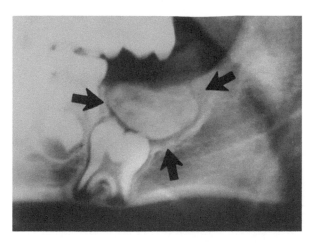

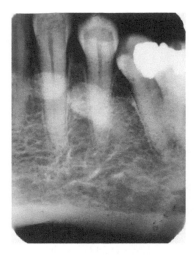

Case 11-6   This 6-year-old boy presented with intermittent pain in the left posterior mandible. A clinically missing lower left 1st molar was noted, and the other three 1st molars were erupted. No bony expansion was in this area (arrows); however, the tissue at the crest of the ridge was slightly reddish and swollen.
1. What is the cause of the patient's pain?
2. Describe the lesion causing the delayed eruption.
3. Give a differential diagnosis of four conditions.
4. What is the most probable diagnosis?
5. Upon removal of the mass, will the 1st molar erupt?

Case 11-8   This patient is missing all of his lower molars bilaterally, and a removable partial denture is being planned.
1. What (if any) treatment plan modification(s) would you consider after studying this radiograph? Comment on the prognosis of your treatment plan.

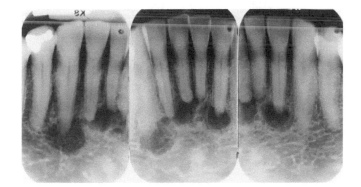

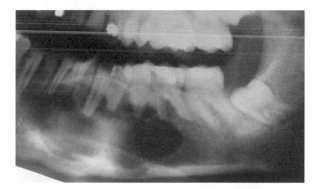

Case 11-7   This asymptomatic patient is a 45-year-old woman. Her routine radiographs indicated several periapical radiolucencies in the lower anterior region.
1. What is the probable race of this patient?
2. What condition is present?
3. In all likelihood, are the teeth vital?
4. If applicable, what stage(s) is (are) present?
5. What treatment (if any) would you recommend?

Case 11-9   This is a 16-year-old female with a lesion in the left mandible. All of the teeth are vital.
1. Describe the lesion.
2. Give a differential diagnosis of five conditions in descending order of certainty.
3. State your diagnostic impression.
4. Discuss the certainty and prognosis of your diagnostic impression.

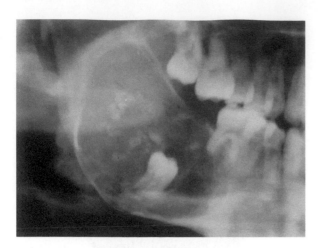

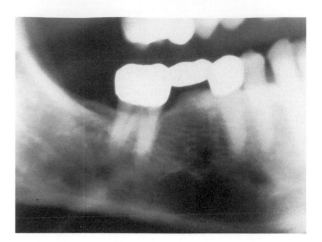

Case **11-10**   Terry is a 12-year-old boy with intermittent pain and swelling in the right posterior mandible.
1. Describe the lesion.
2. Give a differential diagnosis.
3. State your diagnostic impression.
4. What is the treatment? State the prognosis.

Case **11-12**   George is a 41-year-old with slight discomfort in the area of this 15-year-old bridge. Clinically, the gingiva beneath the pontic was red and swollen.
1. What condition do you think is present?
2. What is the treatment and prognosis?

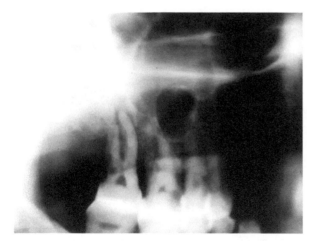

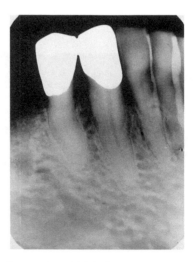

Case **11-11**   Clara is a 72-year-old who reports pain and slight facial swelling in the right maxilla. Clinically, you could see swelling at the mucobuccal fold between the 1st molar and 2nd premolar. Her history revealed she had a Caldwell-Luc procedure performed on the right maxillary sinus some 20 years ago.
1. Based on this history and radiographic findings, what lesion is present?
2. Briefly describe the three variations in location with which this lesion presents.

Case **11-13**   Ollie is 64 years old. He has a removable partial denture with bilateral free end bases, which he has worn for years. Look at the most distal tooth in the lower right quadrant; it was the only tooth affected.
1. What condition affects the root of this tooth?
2. What is the characteristic radiographic appearance?
3. With what systemic disease is this associated, and do you think this case applies?
4. Comment on how this may have developed.
5. Has the dilacerated root developed in association with this condition or its history?

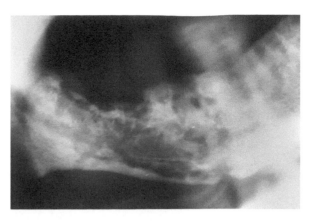

Case **11-14** Mr. X is a 59-year-old homeless person. He recently had his remaining mandibular teeth extracted for tenderness, redness, swelling, and intraoral and submandibular fistula formation in the right quadrant. However, the pain has not regressed. Now paresthesia has developed in the lower right lip. The radiograph revealed a possible partially healed fracture of the mandible in the right canine region, the cause of which the patient could neither affirm nor deny.
1. Describe the radiographic findings.
2. State your diagnostic impression.
3. In normal extraction socket healing, how long does it take for the lamina dura to disappear?
4. How would you treat this?

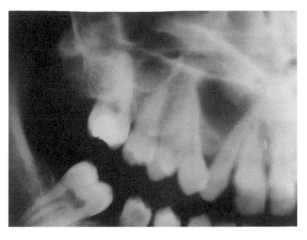

Case **11-16** Denise is a 27-year-old who complained that her "front tooth" seemed to be getting "crooked." The radiolucency in the right maxilla was a serendipitous finding.
1. Regarding the lesion, what diagnostic test would you perform?
2. What is your diagnostic impression?
3. How would you manage this case? Remember the chief complaint!

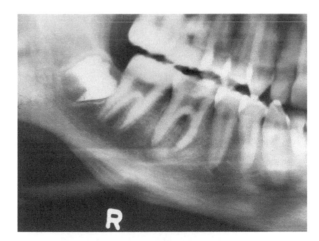

Case **11-15** Dennis is a 13-year-old boy with a slightly swollen face on the right side. Clinically, a nontender, bony, hard swelling was in the mucobuccal fold adjacent to the 1st molar. There was a history of past toothache, but it went away.
1. Describe the significant radiographic findings.
2. State your diagnostic impression.
3. How would you treat this?
4. With successful treatment, how long would you expect it to take for the swelling to go away?
5. Describe the radiographic evidence of resolution.

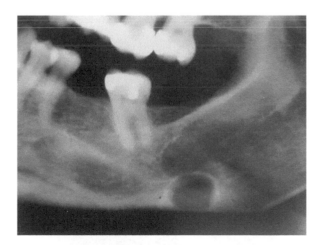

Case **11-17** This 52-year-old man gave us the okay for a fixed prosthesis to replace the lower left molar. Everybody was surprised to find the radiolucent lesion at the inferior border of the mandible.
1. What is your diagnostic impression?
2. How would you manage this lesion?
3. About the bridge, can the angular relationship of teeth (such as abutment tooth parallelism) be assessed accurately from a panoramic radiograph?

CASE-BASED **QUESTIONS**

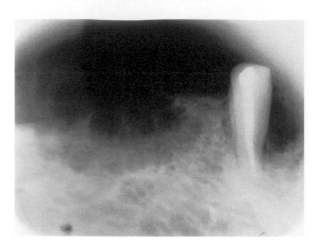

Case **11-18**   Mrs. Sally S. is 42 years old. She complained that her overdenture no longer fit well and chewing was painful. Clinically, a reddish, slightly swollen area was at the crest of the edentulous ridge in the right posterior mandible.
1.   Describe the lesion.
2.   What is your diagnostic impression?
3.   How would you manage this case?

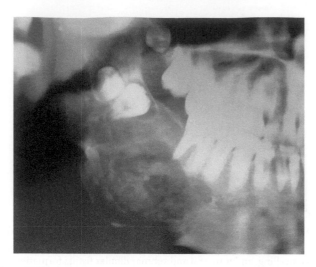

Case **11-20**   Normie is an 11-year-old boy who presented with a slowly progressive facial swelling over the past 6 to 8 months and mild pain on chewing.
1.   Describe the lesion.
2.   Give a differential diagnosis.
3.   State your diagnostic impression.
4.   How would you manage this case?

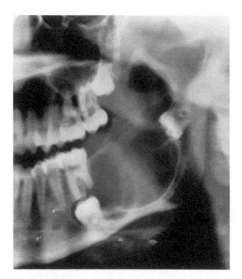

Case **11-19**   This patient is a 16-year-old male. He complained of pain on chewing, and his mother noticed the left side of his face seemed a bit swollen. He had never been to the dentist. At surgery, some straw-colored fluid could be aspirated.
1.   Describe the lesion.
2.   Give a differential diagnosis of five lesions.
3.   State your diagnostic impression.
4.   How would you manage this case?

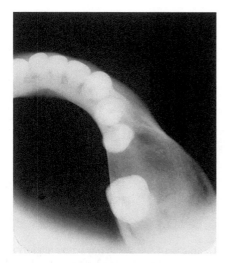

Case **11-21**   While working up this patient for a bridge, this lesion was noted. There is a radiographic feature here that almost certainly suggests the diagnosis.
1.   Describe the "pathognomonic" (almost certain) feature.
2.   What is the diagnosis?

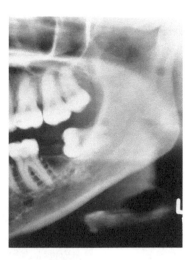

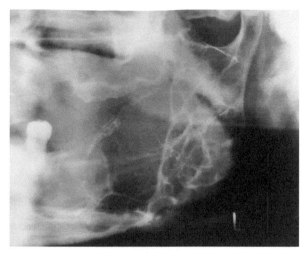

Case **11-22**   This patient has not seen a dentist in 10 years. There are two radiologically distinct conditions affecting the mandible.
1. Name the two conditions.
2. What is the significance of these two findings (if any)?
3. What is the probable sex of this patient?

Case **11-24**   This patient is a 32-year-old man. The maxilla is edentulous, but he does not wear a denture. At surgery, the lesional tissue was an amber, gelatinous, gooey material.
1. What is the overall radiographic pattern of the lesion in the left posterior mandible?
2. Clinically, what does this pattern suggest regarding the nature and behavior of this lesion?
3. Describe the lesion.
4. Give a differential diagnosis.
5. What is your diagnostic impression?
6. Comment on the 2nd premolar.

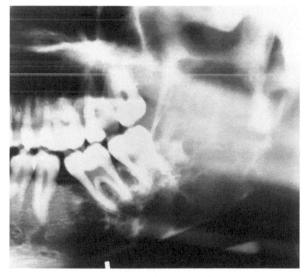

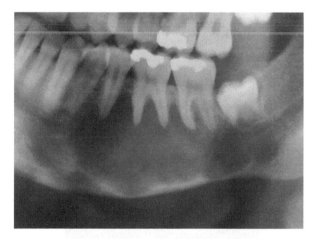

Case **11-23**   Okay, this is a hard one… but this general group of lesions is really important to recognize in x-rays. As with all of the histories given with the cases, watch for the clues! Sang is a 20-year-old woman who reports a rather recent development of swelling and pain in the left side of her face. There was a deep carious lesion in the upper left 2nd molar, but the tooth proved to be nonvital. The lower 2nd molar displayed +2 mobility. There was a "welling up" of blood when the lesion was incised at surgery.
1. What basic radiologic pattern does this lesion display?
2. What radiographic features can you see that, when correlated with the history, suggest a diagnosis?
3. State your diagnostic impression.

Case **11-25**   Solitaire is a 14-year-old member of the all-girl softball team. She remembers the ball slamming into her jaw several months ago when the sun got into her eyes and she missed a pop fly.
1. What is the radiographic pattern of this lesion?
2. Describe this lesion.
3. State your diagnostic impression.

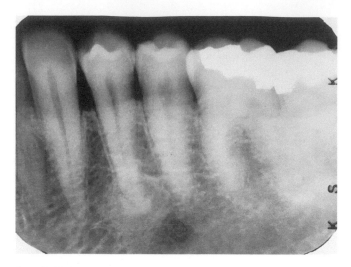

Case 11-26 Jenny A. is a 38-year-old asymptomatic white woman. There is a radiopacity at the apex of the 1st premolar and a radio-lucency at the root end of the 2nd premolar.

1. Are these findings part and parcel of the same condition (yes or no)?

Answer either question #2 or #3:

2. If yes, state the condition and explain your choice.
3. If no, identify the two conditions.

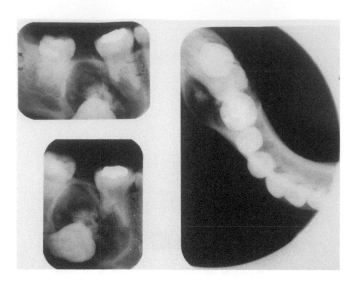

Case 11-28 This patient is a 27-year-old woman with swelling in the right mandible.

1. What radiographic pattern characterizes this lesion?
2. Give a differential diagnosis for this lesion.
3. State your diagnostic impression.

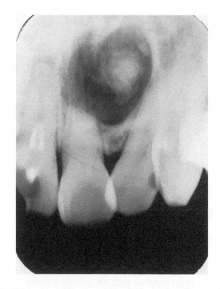

Case 11-27 Monsieur Phantome is a 45-year-old Frenchman who noticed his front tooth has been getting crooked. Clinically, a slight bony swelling was at the mucobuccal fold and on the palate. The associated left central and lateral incisors were vital.

1. Give a differential diagnosis for this lesion.
2. Notice the root resorption; what, in general, does this indicate regarding the nature of the lesion?
3. Can you take a guess as to the diagnosis?

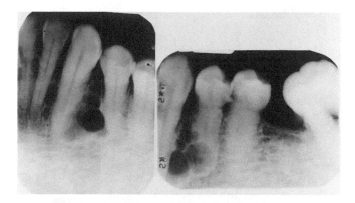

Case 11-29 This patient is a 50-year-old man. Clinically, a slight swelling was between the left canine and 1st premolar.

1. Classify the radiographic appearance of this lesion.
2. Give a differential diagnosis.
3. State your diagnostic impression.
4. How would you manage this case?

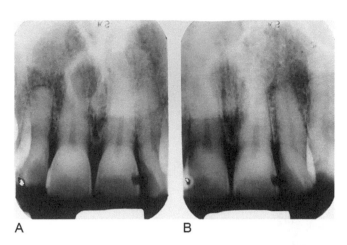

A B

Case **11-30** This patient is a 37-year-old woman. She reported a vague, slight discomfort in the maxillary anterior area and a more definite, transient salty taste. The lesion in question is in the maxillary midline.
1. What is your diagnostic impression?
2. Can you make any comment(s) on the radiographic appearance of this case?
3. With what anatomic structure might this pathologic entity be confused?
4. What previous dental treatment has this patient had?

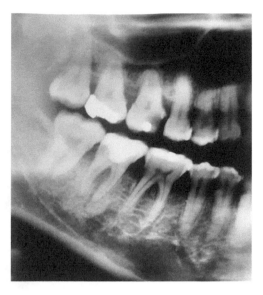

Case **11-31** This 40-year-old man has restorations, active small and large caries, periodontal disease with horizontal bone loss with calculus, and erupted 3rd molars. The asymptomatic mandibular right 2nd molar is the main focus of this case: note the large and apparently deep restoration and the radiopaque area at the apex.
1. What is your diagnostic impression of the condition affecting the mandibular right 2nd molar?
   What important clinical test would you perform to confirm your diagnosis?
2. What treatment (if any) is needed? Does this condition regress?
3. In passing: Do you see any caries in association with the lower 3rd molar? Explain.

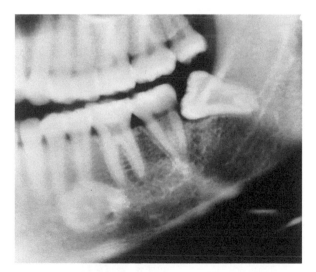

Case **11-32** This 42-year-old man has had little need for dental treatment for either caries or periodontal disease. The asymptomatic mandibular left 2nd premolar is the main focus of this case. Note the lack of caries or restorations and the radiopaque area at the apex.
1. What is your diagnostic impression of the condition affecting the mandibular left 2nd premolar? What important clinical test would you perform to confirm your diagnosis? In this case, why do any test at all?
2. What treatment (if any) is needed? Does this condition regress?
3. In passing: Do you see any caries in association with the lower 3rd molar? Explain. Can you classify the 3rd molar impaction?

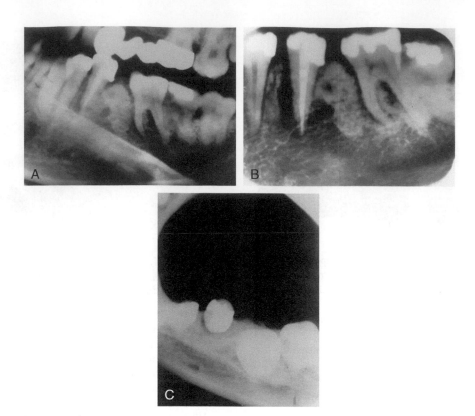

Case **11-33**   This 32-year-old woman complained of toothache on the right side of her mandible. A panoramic radiograph (A) was taken, and the radiopaque area was discovered on the other (left) side. Upon consultation, there was disagreement as to whether this lesion was idiopathic osteosclerosis (can be seen in nonapical areas) or if it represented something else. As a result, the additional intraoral periapical (B) and occlusal (C) radiographs were taken. Clinically, the upper fixed prosthesis appeared to have been constructed to occlude with the lingually displaced 2nd premolar about 12 months ago by a dentist in Germany.

1.   Looking at all three radiographs, what is your diagnostic impression? Explain.
2.   Look at the 2nd premolar: In the panoramic radiograph it appears to be supraerupted, whereas in the periapical view it is on the same occlusal plane as the adjacent teeth. Explain this apparent contradiction.

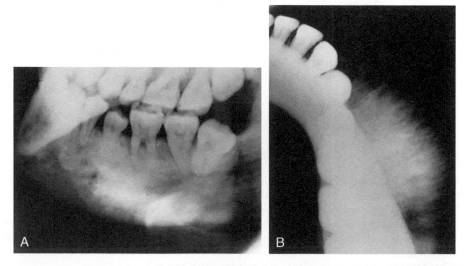

Case **11-34**   This patient, a 28-year-old man, had never been to the dentist. The left side of his face has become noticeably swollen lately. Now he is experiencing deep bone pain in his jaw, paresthesia in the lower left lip, and a loosening of his lower 1st molar.

1.   Describe the radiographic findings.
2.   What is your diagnostic impression?

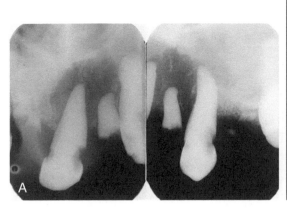

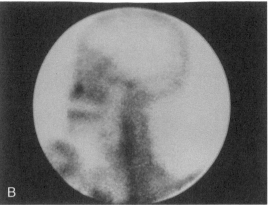

Case **11-35**   This is a person who has neglected himself. He abuses alcohol, smokes two to three packs of cigarettes a day, and has poor oral hygiene. Though he has had difficulty breathing, especially on exertion, he has no known lung disease. The technetium scan you see in B was taken before biopsy and in association with a nuclear scan of the lungs.
1.   What radiographic pattern can we ascribe to this lesion?
2.   Describe the lesion.
3.   State your diagnostic impression.

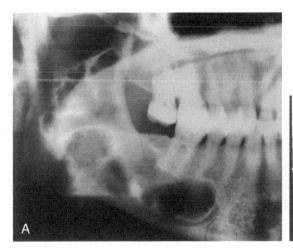

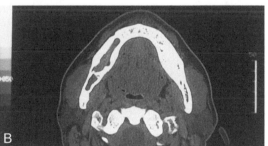

Case **11-36**   This patient is a 52-year-old man with no clinically visible swelling. However, he had pain because his extruding maxillary 2nd molar was traumatizing the opposing mandibular edentulous ridge. If you have been getting discouraged with these hard cases, this one is classic if you know your stuff!
1.   What radiologic pattern do we see here?
2.   Correlate the findings between the panoramic and CT images.
3.   Give a differential diagnosis.
4.   State your diagnostic impression.

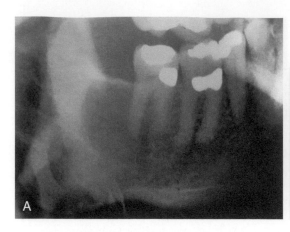

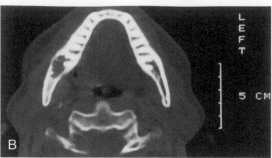

Case 11-37   This is a 57-year-old woman who complained of pain in her right jaw and paresthesia in the right lower lip. Clinically, she had ever-so-slight right facial swelling that she noticed but that was hard to see by the clinicians who saw her. The radiograph and CT image were taken at the time of presentation to the oral and maxillofacial radiology clinic.

1.   Describe the radiographic findings.
2.   Do you have any idea as to what is going on here? If so, state your diagnostic impression.

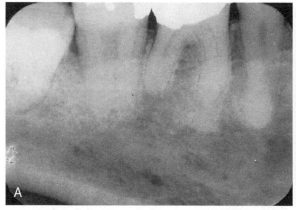

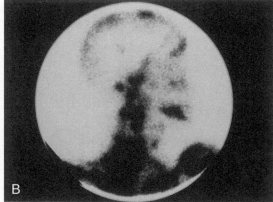

Case 11-38   This is a 75-year-old man on medication for frequent nocturia. He has pain in his right mandible and subsequently had the technetium scan done.

1.   Describe the radiographic findings in A.
2.   What is your diagnostic impression without considering B?
3.   What do you see in B?
4.   Considering the history and the findings in A and B, what is your diagnostic impression?

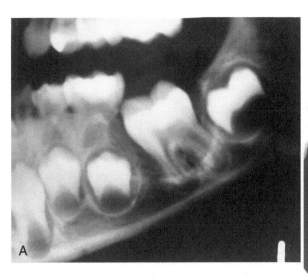

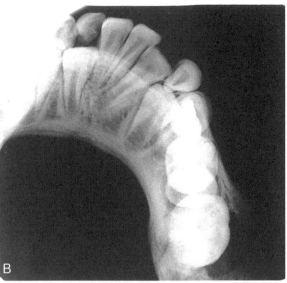

Case **11-39**   This patient is a 6½-year-old boy from Toronto, Canada, where they told his mom he needed some treatment. He had pain in the area and slight facial swelling that was relieved following an initial course of antibiotic treatment. The family was transferred to the United States where the problem was not immediately recognized. Ultimately the radiologist saw him; this is what was found.

1. Panoramic radiograph (A): describe what you see.
2. What is the eruptive potential of the mandibular 1st molar?
3. Occlusal radiograph (B): describe what you see.
4. Give a differential diagnosis.
5. State your diagnostic impression.
6. What treatment would you recommend?

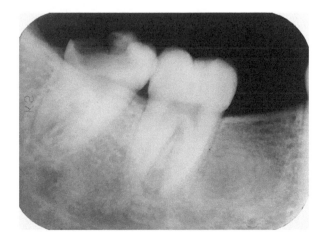

Case **11-40**   This patient is a 38-year-old woman who has had acne since age 12. This is a radiograph of her buccal mucosa.

1. State your diagnostic impression.

Case **11-41**   This patient is a 45-year-old Hispanic man.

1. State your diagnostic impression regarding the targetlike lesion mesial to the molar.

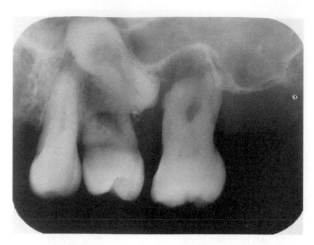

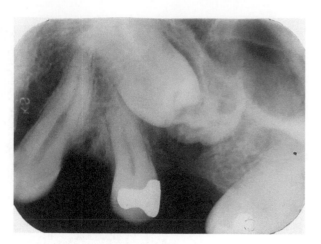

Case 11-42   This patient is a 60-year-old man with a history of having teeth extracted as they become bothersome. This molar has now become loose, it hurts, and he wants it extracted. Interestingly, he is taking an antibiotic for an aching sinus on this side. The medical doctor did not examine his teeth.

1. First, what pattern of bone loss do you see in association with the molar?
2. What is the etiology of this molar problem?
3. Report as much as possible about what you can see regarding the unerupted tooth.
4. How would you manage this case?

Case 11-43   This case involves "what do you see" sorts of questions. The patient complains of sensitivity to hot and cold in this area.

1. Describe what you see in association with the 1st premolar.
2. How about the 2nd premolar?
3. Do you see anything in the sinus?

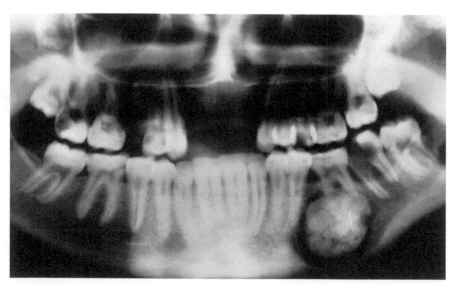

Case 11-44   This patient is a 17-year-old male who complained of pain and swelling in the left side of his jaw.

1. Describe the lesion at the apex of the left 1st molar.
2. What is your diagnostic impression of the lesion?
3. What do you see regarding the mandibular left 2nd molar? (*Hint:* you've seen this before.)
4. Why are the roots of the maxillary teeth obscured?

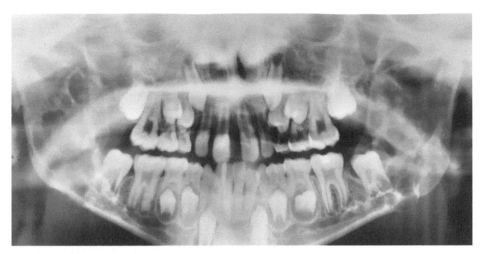

Case 11-45   Jill is an 11-year-old with a bilateral, painless facial swelling that has been present since about age 5 years. When looking straight ahead, her eyes appeared "turned upward to heaven."
1. What condition is present?
2. What is the cause of the eye problem?
3. How would you manage this case?

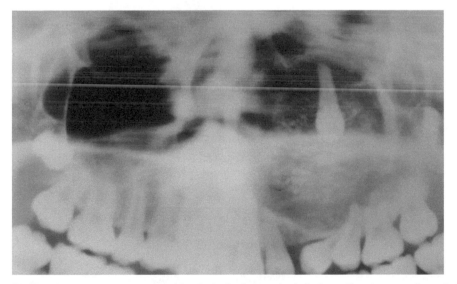

Case 11-46   This patient is a 13-year-old girl. She had surprisingly little swelling but complained of a space between her teeth on the left side and several crooked teeth.
1. What condition is present?
2. How should this be managed, and what is the prognosis?

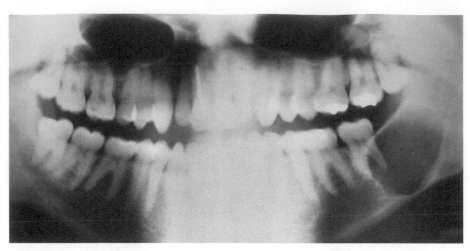

Case **11-47**   This is a 27-year-old man who was asymptomatic. However, you noted a very slight buccal swelling on the left side. Study this entire radiograph carefully.

1.   What is your diagnostic impression?
2.   Histologically, what would you expect the pathologic diagnosis to be?
3.   How would you manage this case?

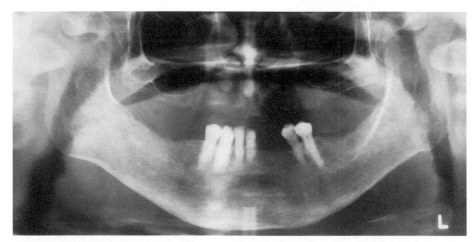

Case **11-48**   Take a good look at this entire radiograph of a 63-year-old woman of British descent.
1.   In this case the radiologic diagnosis being sought is a systemic problem.
2.   What features did you observe to come to this conclusion...or did you just guess?

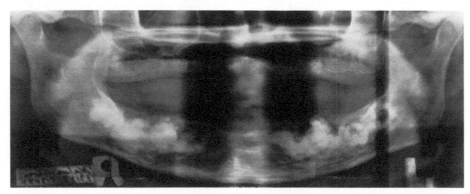

Case **11-49**   This edentulous 65-year-old black woman came in complaining of pain beneath her lower denture. The tissue in the mandibular premolar area appeared red and ulcerated with a bony spicule clinically visible at the base of the ulcer.
1.   What condition affects her jaws?
2.   What specific complication of this condition has occurred?

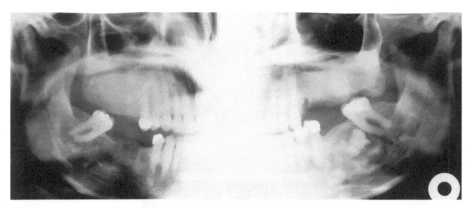

Case 11-50 Elizabeth J-L, age 37 years, has kept both her maiden and married names. On her torso she has several café au lait spots whose outline resembles the coast of Maine. Her problem was first discovered when she complained of pain in her hip after a long day of shopping. Her alkaline phosphatase is a little bit elevated.

1. What does "café au lait" mean anyway?
2. What condition do you think is present?
3. Comment on the lesions in the jaws.
4. What is the radiopaque area in the middle of the radiograph?

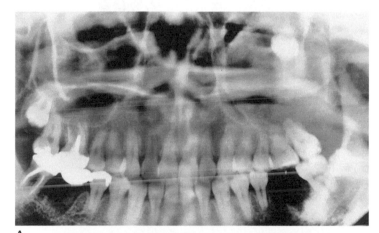

A

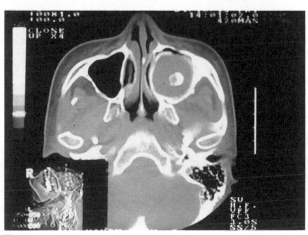

B

Case 11-51 This is a 20-year-old man who has had a lot of work done for his age. Note that the maxillary right 3rd molar appears to be still erupting as the apex is open. The problem is with the upper left 3rd molar.

1. Study the images and give your diagnostic impression.
2. Why does the left 3rd molar appear to be in the orbit (above the infraorbital margin) on the panoramic radiograph and well below the orbit in the CT image?

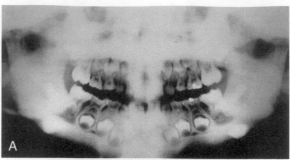

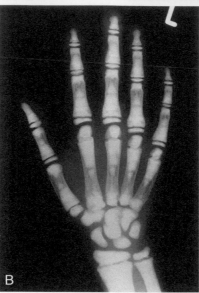

Case **11-52**   Peter is a 6-year-old boy with a problem that made it difficult for us to get a good panoramic radiograph. The hand film demonstrates the "bone within a bone" feature, especially in the metacarpals and in some phalanges.
1. What condition affects this patient?
2. How would you manage this case?

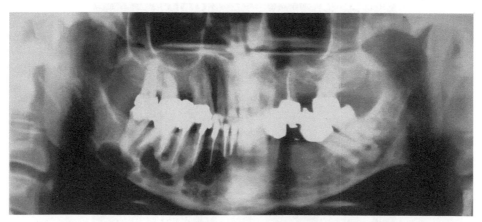

Case **11-53**   This patient is a 42-year-old black woman. She has continuing mild-to-moderate pain in the right mandible. She has had one surgery on the radiolucent lesion in the right canine area and endodontic treatment of the adjacent teeth. The area did not heal but actually enlarged after the surgery. Meanwhile, several other radiolucent lesions developed in the same quadrant.
1. Believe it or not, this history and radiograph are typical of this condition. See if you can state your diagnostic impression.
2. How would you manage this case?

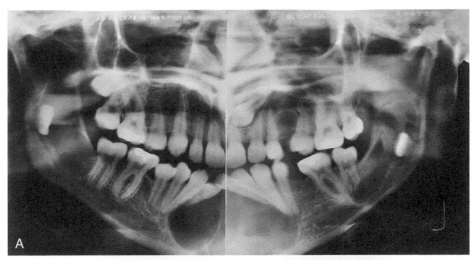

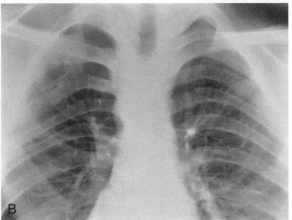

Case **11-54**   This is a 14-year-old teenager. She has several anomalous ribs, although you can see the clavicles are present (B). She has no facial swelling, although she does have several small skin lesions.   *Jaw lesions: (A)*

1.   What is your diagnostic impression?
2.   The lesion in the left mandible appears to contain some radiopaque material. Can you state what that is?
3.   How would you manage these lesions?
     Skin lesions:
4.   What skin lesions do you suppose she has?
     Ribs: (B)
5.   Name three rib deformities on the right (left side of photo) side of her chest.
     Diagnostic impression:
6.   State the diagnosis. By now bells should be ringing loud and clear!
     Bonus questions:
     Forget about the details of this case for a moment. If, in another patient, the finding was hypoplastic or missing clavicles:
7.   What condition would you suspect?
8.   What would you look for in the jaws?

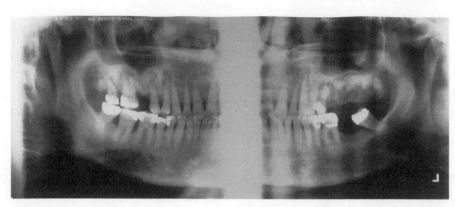

Case 11-55   This 56-year-old white man from England now lives in the United States. He takes medication to lower his alkaline phosphatase levels and to curb progression of his disease. He has one family member back in England with the same condition.

1. Describe the radiographic findings.
2. What is your diagnostic impression?
3. What anomaly affecting the roots of the teeth might we watch for in this patient?
4. If we make a removable maxillary partial denture, would we warn the patient about it getting loose over time?
5. On long-term follow-up, what else would we look for (if anything) in his jawbones?

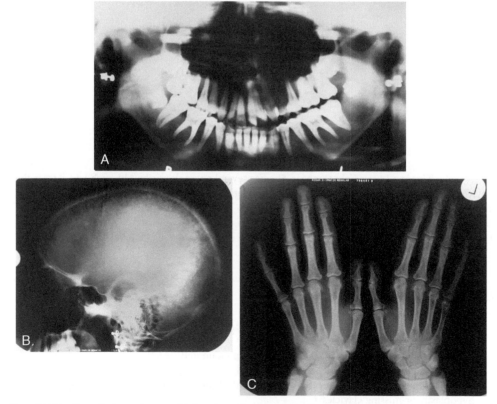

Case 11-56   Rene P. is a 13-year-old female with a systemic disease characterized by glandular and organ components. She has a high serum calcium and high urinary calcium when placed on a low-calcium diet. The radiographs were all overexposed (too dark) on the normal settings. Her desire was to have orthodontic treatment.

1. Radiographically, what do you see in the panoramic radiograph (A)? Focus on the mandibular posterior areas only. (No, this is not a trick; the rest is not readable.)
2. Radiographically, what do you see in the skull (B)?
3. Radiographically, what do you see in the hands (C)?
4. State your diagnostic impression.
5. Can you state the tetrad of features that characterize this disease?
6. How would you manage this case? Don't forget the ortho!

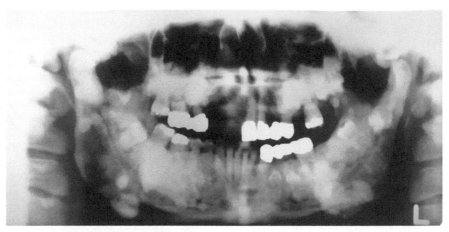

Case **11-57**   Getting tired of hard cases? This one should be easy, but it is important.
Mary Quitecontrary is 35 years old. She is aware of her diagnosis.
1.   Describe the radiographic findings.
2.   What is your diagnostic impression?
3.   Relative to her diagnosis, what serious counsel would you offer?

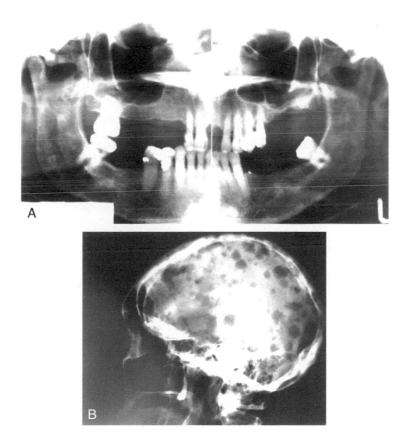

Case **11-58**   This is a 62-year-old man with a disease that affects the jaws, skull, and other bones
in the skeleton. His primary complaint is back pain caused by involvement of the vertebral column.
Bence Jones protein was found in the urine, and the serum calcium and alkaline phosphatase
were elevated.
1.   What findings can you see in the panoramic radiograph? (Findings are subtle.)
2.   What findings can you see in the skull?
3.   What is your diagnostic impression?

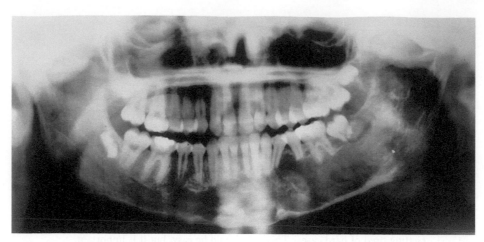

Case **11-59**   This patient is a 12-year-old girl who presented with a slight swelling in her left submandibular area and in the midline mental region. There was no pain or systemic disease.
1.   Describe the radiographic findings.
2.   What is your diagnostic impression?

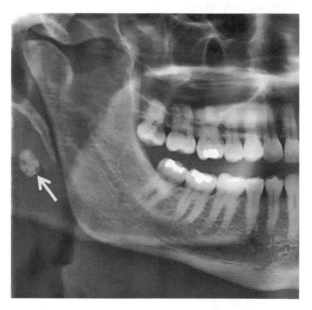

Case **11-60**   This patient is asymptomatic, although there has been a history of a chronic pericoronal infection associated with the 3rd molars. He also suffers from chronic sinus infections.
1.   What do you think the radiopacity, as indicated by the yellow arrow, represents?

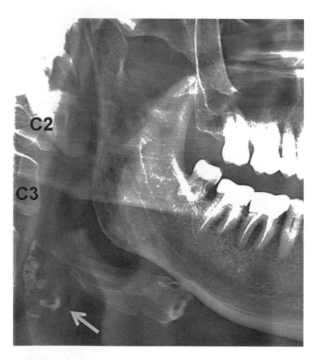

Case **11-61**   This is a 62-year-old male. His upper 3rd molar was removed some years ago. Presently he has sensitivity to hot and cold in the back of his mouth, on the right side.
1.   Comment on what you see in association with the lower 3rd molar.
2.   What, in your opinion, does the calcification as indicated by the orange arrow represent?
3.   What further follow-up/treatment would you recommend for this patient?

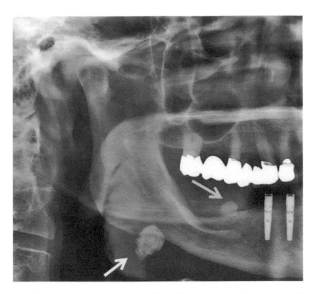

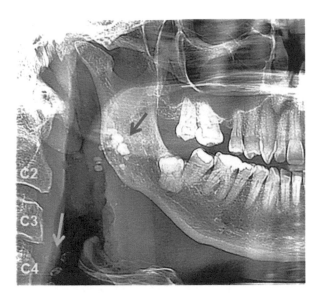

Case **11-62**   This is a 65-year-old female who is undergoing implant therapy.
1. Describe the radiopacity as indicated by the yellow arrow.
2. Comment on what you think about the radiopacities as indicated by the yellow and orange arrows.
3. What else do you see?

Case **11-63**   This patient is a 68-year-old male. Although he has no significant history of periodontal disease, he does have a lot of ear, nose, and throat infections apparently associated with the air quality in the factory where he worked for 42 years.
1. Describe what you see at the red arrow.
2. Describe what you see at the orange arrow.
3. What assessment or diagnosis would you suggest?

Chapter (12)

Cone Beam Computed Tomography (CBCT)

Goal

To understand the concepts of CBCT

Learning Objectives

1. Understand the basic principles of CBCT
2. Know the difference between a pixel and a voxel
3. Understand some differences between medical CT and dental CBCT
4. Identify the image planes in a 3D volume

INTRODUCTION

Cone beam computed tomography (CBCT) is a relatively new *low-dose* 3D dental x-ray technology that can image any selected location within the hard tissues of the head and neck including the jaws. While intraoral, panoramic, and cephalometric x-ray devices produce 2D radiographic images, CBCT produces 3D x-ray scans. For example, an intraoral periapical image can only display the height and mesiodistal width of a tooth but cannot show the buccolingual width of the tooth. In addition, the 2D image, such as the periapical in Figure 12-1, is magnified and is often distorted (unequal magnification). Distortions such as an elongation or foreshortening of a tooth may sometimes not be detected if the distortion is minimal. In contrast, CBCT technology does not distort the anatomic findings—it displays structures in all three dimensions, and all measurements, both linear and/or volumetric, as well as angular relationships, are accurate. This provides great utility for general dentists and specialists. For example, endodontists can make linear or curvilinear measurements to properly plan a root canal; orthodontists can measure spaces as well as the angular relationships of teeth; and surgeons or periodontists can calculate the volume of bone needed to raise the floor of the maxillary sinus to accommodate a maxillary implant. These and many other applications exist for CBCT within the practice of dentistry.

Figure 12-1 shows intraoral periapical images of three different patients: A, film; B, photostimulable phosphor (PSP) plate; and C, electronic sensor.

Periapical radiographs lack some of the advantages of CBCT. For example, periapical radiographs as shown here can demonstrate the height and mesiodistal widths of a tooth; however, measurements such as those used to determine root canal length for endodontics will almost always be subject to inaccuracies. PSP plates (B) need to be scanned into the computer after they are exposed, which requires time and additional machinery. As illustrated in Figure 12-1, electronic sensors have approximately 25% to 33% less image size than intraoral film or PSPs, thus they may miss the periapical region, as shown in C. Sensor dimensions are larger and thicker than film or PSP plates and involve an attached wire, thus adding difficulty to intraoral imaging.

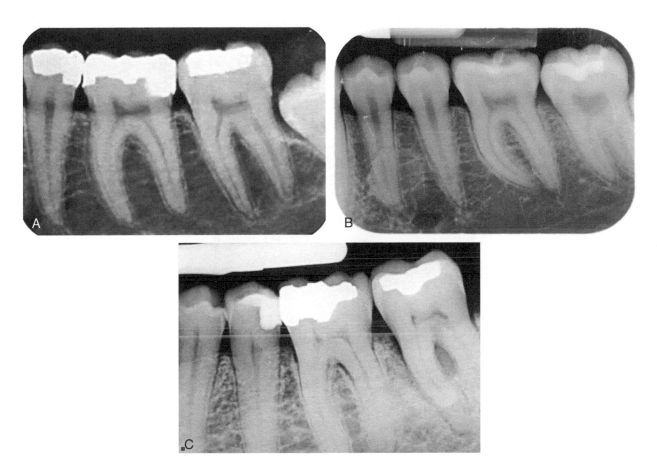

Figure **12-1**   A, Acceptable periapical film-based image; B, Foreshortened film-based periapical image; C, Electronic sensor based periapical image with 25% to 30% less imaging area, making the apical areas difficult to capture.

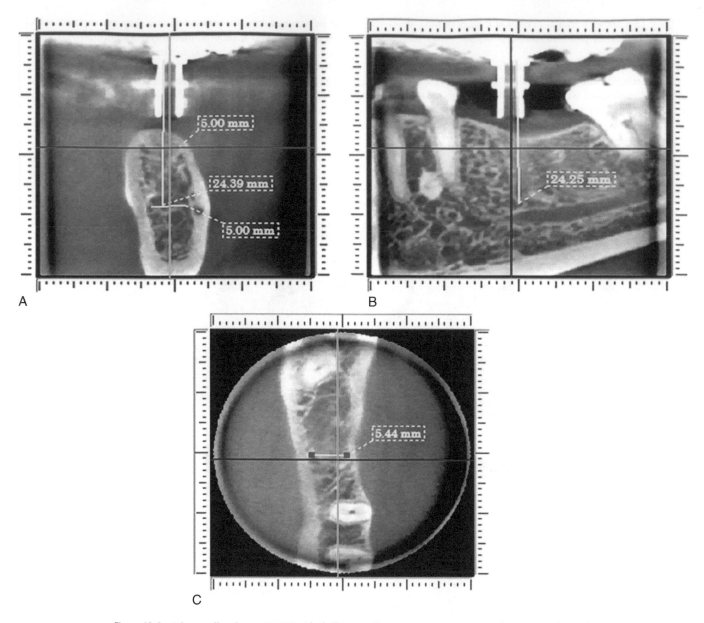

Figure **12-2**   The small-volume CBCT with drilling guide measuring 4 × 4 cm can be seen on the scale at the sides of the image: A, Cross-sectional view at right angles to the area of interest; B, Sagittal view; C, Axial view of exactly the same location.

In Figure 12-2, the CBCT images demonstrate the ability to see anatomic structures in 3D. Here an edentulous space is viewed in all three dimensions and accurate measurements can be obtained. In this case the measurements are for implant selection and surgical placement. These measurements are essential to the proper selection of an implant of the correct size and shape, which is discussed in great detail in Chapter 13.

HOW DOES CBCT WORK?

The CBCT scan involves a circular movement pattern of both the x-ray beam on one side of the selected volume and a corresponding movement of the sensor on the opposite side. It is usually best if the area of interest is scanned from all sides by the x-ray beam. The simplest scanning motion involves a symmetric circular path used for smaller volumes. An asymmetric path is used for larger volumes and results in a lower dose than a symmetric scan (Figure 12-3).

Scanning motion of the x-ray beam and sensor with respect to the volumes is outlined in red in Figure 12-3: A, symmetric scanning motion for small volumes; B, asymmetric scanning motion reduces the dose for larger volumes

CBCT scanners are digital and use a sensor to capture the scan. In 2D digital imaging, the image consists of a "matrix" that is made up of an array of **pixels** arranged in vertical columns and horizontal rows. The individual pixels are usually square in shape. The smaller the pixels in a given matrix, the sharper the image will appear, and very fine details can be visualized. In CBCT imaging, the image volume is composed of *voxels,* which are cubic in shape and together they make up the volume (Figure 12-4).

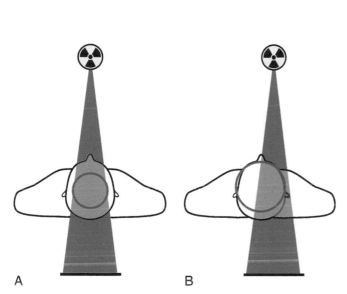

Figure **12-3** The scanning motion of the x-ray beam and sensor with respect to the volumes is outlined in red. A, Symmetric scanning motion for small volumes; B, Asymmetric scanning motion reduces the dose for larger volumes.

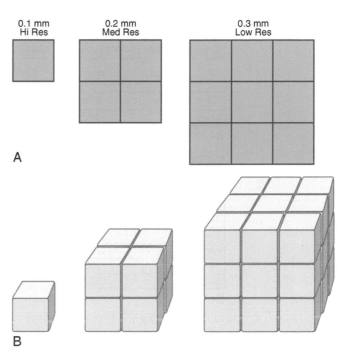

Figure **12-4** Figure 12-4 shows voxel sizes: A, Different voxel sizes can be selected for a given volume; B, The three-dimensional nature of the voxels is illustrated with diagramatically stacked sugar cubes; voxel sizes of 0.1 mm, 0.2 mm, and 0.3 mm are demonstrated.

CBCT RADIATION DOSES

At the very outset the author wishes to state categorically that the full dose for the 4×4 cm CBCT scan, as illustrated in Figure 12-2, would be less than 50 µSv (Figure 12-5), and in Ultra Low Dose (ULD) mode, the dose could be as low as 3 µSv (Figure 12-5) or about the same dose as a set of four bitewings (BWs) using photostimulable phosphor plates (PSPs) or "F"-speed film and a long rectangular cone (Figure 12-6), and the small-volume CBCT dose is less than the same BWs with a long round cone. In CBCT, one way of lowering the dose is to increase the voxel size as illustrated in Figure 12-4. Increasing the voxel size allows the scan to be taken with less mA (milliamperes), which is the factor most directly responsible for dose. The increased voxel size decreases the image resolution (sharpness and detail) but does not generally affect measurement accuracy or structural relationships. Therefore to find a hairline crack in a tooth, the smallest voxel size is needed because fine image detail will be needed (Figure 12-5). To view a large tumor or cyst or even to make implant measurements, the large voxel size (low-dose, low-resolution mode) will often be adequate (Figure 12-5). In either case, the orientation of structures to one another will remain accurate.

Brand X Digital Hybrid Panoramic/CBCT Scanner Model A					
Program/region	FOV (mm)	Normal mode (µSv)	Normal mode ULD (µSv)	Low dose (µSv)	Low dose ULD (µSv)
Tooth maxilla incisors	Ø50x50	50	12	13	3
Tooth incisors	Ø50x80	91	21	20	5

Brand X Digital Hybrid Panoramic/CBCT Scanner Model B					
Program/region	FOV (mm)	Normal mode (µSv)	Normal mode ULD (µSv)	Low dose (µSv)	Low dose ULD (µSv)
Tooth incisors	Ø50x50	51	12	13	3
Teeth	Ø50x80	161	38	41	10

A

Brand X Digital Hybrid Panoramic/CBCT Scanner Model C					
Program/region	FOV (mm)	Normal mode (µSv)	Normal mode ULD (µSv)	Low dose (µSv)	Low dose ULD (µSv)
Tooth maxilla incisors	Ø50x55	74	17	13	4
Teeth	Ø100x90	261	74	70	20
Face	Ø130x130	229	54	58	16
Skull lower	Ø230x160	154	60	95	29
Skull full	Ø230x260	212	75	140	43

B

Figure **12-5**   Varying selectable dose levels for different sized volumes in various anatomic locations.

John B. Ludlow DDS. MS. DFS RCSEd			
Table 7. Conventional dental radiography dose calculations following ICRP 2007 Recommendations			
Technique	Effective dose in µSv	Dose as multiple of average panoramic dose	Days of per capita background
FMX with PSP of F Speed film and Rectangular Collimation	34.9	2.2	4.3
BWs with PSP of F Speed film and Rectangular Collimation	5.0	0.3	0.6
FMX with PSP of F Speed film and Round Cone	170.7	10.6	21
FMX with D Speed film and Round Cone	388		
Panoramic-CCD	16.1		
PA Cephalometric-PSP	5.1		
Lateral Cephalometric-PSP	5.6		

Figure **12-6**   Figure 12-6 shows some intraoral and pan imaging doses for comparison with CBCT doses as seen in Figure 12-5. (From Ludlow JB, Davies-Ludlow LE, White SC. Patient risk related to common dental radiographic examinations: The impact of 2007 International commission on radiologic protection recommendations regarding dose calculation. *JADA* 2008;139(9):1237-1243, with permission from American Dental Association.)

Figure 12-5A shows that the full (normal) dose for a 5×5 cm CBCT volume is 50 µSv; however, this dose can be lowered to 13, 12, or 3 µSv, depending on the desired resolution as indicated by the Normal mode, Normal-mode ULD, Low-Dose, and Low-Dose ULD columns. Figure 12-5B shows CBCT doses for different volume sizes as reported by the University of Helsinki in Finland. All of the CBCT doses are lower than a full-mouth survey using "D"-speed film and the long, round cone, as can be seen in Figure 12-6.

It should be noted that in the author's experience, only a few dental offices among hundreds of dental practices surveyed during presentations over the past 5 years have admitted to using the rectangular cone. Therefore the most likely BW dose would be in the range of 25 µSv (5×5 µSv, as illustrated in Figure 12-6, using a multiple of $5\times$) or approximately double this dose (50 µSv) in practices still using "D"-speed film and the long round cone, as calculated using the data in Figure 12-6. Also the reported doses in Figure 12-6 will be higher if a 12- or 8-inch cone is used as opposed to a long, 16-inch cone. Even a CBCT scan of the whole head (Figure 12-5B) can be acquired with no more radiation dose than a digital or "F"-speed film full-mouth survey (FMX) using a long round cone (170.7 µSv, Figure 12-6) and much less dose than an FMX with "D"-speed film and a long round cone (388 µSv, Figure 12-6). Note in Figure 12-5B that the full skull (23×26 cm volume size) CBCT dose is 212 µSv, and other dose options for this same volume include 140, 75, and 43 µSv, depending on the desired resolution.

The bottom line is that students and practitioners alike should not shy away from acquiring a CBCT machine or individual scans based on the dose, because most CBCT doses for everyday use in smaller volumes can be well within the range of intraoral and panoramic doses, and in some instances, much lower than the dose of a full mouth survey.

Before 1990, dental radiation doses were generally reported as measured without consideration of the sensitivity of the different tissues within the x-ray beam. In 1990, tissues were assigned a sensitivity factor as a multiple of the measured dose, and thus new values were established. In 2007 the International Council on Radiation Protection (ICRP) assigned higher tissue sensitivity values resulting in higher effective doses (Figure 12-7). Using the

2007 values as published by Ludlow et al. (Figure 12-6), the FMX with PSP or "F"-speed film and round cone was five times more dose (170.7 µSv) than the baseline value of 34.9 µSv for the FMX using PSPs or "F"-speed film and rectangular collimation and 11 times more radiation (388 µSv) when "D"-speed film was used (Figure 12-6). In 2007, the BW dose using PSPs or "F"-speed film and rectangular collimation was 5 µSv. This dose will be much higher if the round cone and PSPs or "F"-speed film is used and higher still if "D"-speed film is employed. The maximum dose for a digital pan is 16.1 µSv, thus the pan BW dose will be slightly less and much lower than all of the full-mouth surveys using different combinations of image capture device and long cone shape, as illustrated in Figure 12-6. The pan BW is discussed in detail in Chapter 9.

CBCT vs. Medical CT

CBCT is currently limited primarily to the visualization of hard tissues such as bone, teeth, and calcified soft tissues, although pathologic soft tissues impinging on an air space such as the sinuses or parts of the airway can be seen. Also the gray scale can be measured in CBCT Hounsfield units. In medical CT, this measurement, when applied to a known or an unknown tissue, can be suggestive of its nature. In current CBCT technology, the Hounsfield number of a tissue can be displayed, but it is only a relative density measurement compared with other tissues in the scan. In dentistry, CBCT Hounsfield numbers do not correspond to the tissue identification norms as established for medical CT. In the near future, a new cadmium telluride photon counting (CaTePC) CBCT sensor will be introduced in North America. With this sensor, soft tissues will be capable of being studied separately from the hard tissues, and the Hounsfield number of a tissue may correspond to the norms as established for medical CT. Also, the new CBCT sensor should result in significantly lower doses than current CBCT values.

The mA setting is another way to illustrate the lower dose obtained by CBCT compared with CT doses. For example, for CBCT, the mA will be somewhere between 2 and 14, whereas for medical CT, the mA may be in excess of 250 mA (Figure 12-8).

TYPE OF EXAMINATION	EFFECTIVE DOSE (microsieverts)		CHANGE IN EFFECTIVE DOSE 1990-2007 (%)
	ICRP 1990 Tissue Weights	ICRP 2007 Tissue Weights	
FMX with PSP or F-Speed Film and Rectangular Collimation	12.2	34.9	186
BW with PSP or F-Speed Film and Rectangular Collimation	1.0	50	422
FMX with PSP or F-Speed Film and Round Cone	58.4	170.7	192
FMX with D-Speed Film and Round Cone	133	388	192
Panoramic Brand XX (CCD)	4.3	14.2	231
Panoramic Brand XXX (CCD)	7.1	24.3	241
Posteroanterior Cephalometric (PSP)	3.9	5.1	32
Lateral Cephalometric (PSP)	3.7	5.6	51

Effective dose for commonly used dental radiographic examinations: comparison of International Commission of Radiological Protection (ICRP) methods from 1990 and 2007.

Figure **12-7**   Figure 12-7 shows effective dose increases from the 1990 tissue weighting factors to 2007 using increased tissue weighting factors. For intraoral BW images using PSP or "F"-speed film and rectangular collimation, the effective dose increase was 422%.

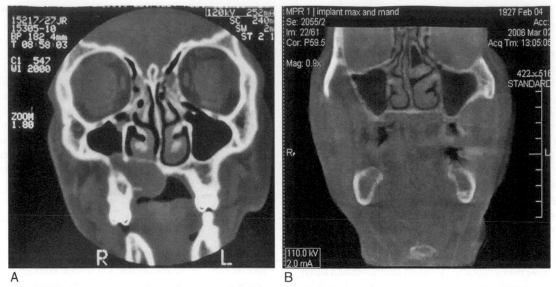

Figure 12-8   Figure A is a medical coronal view taken using 252 mA, as seen in the top right corner of the image (patient's left); Figure B is a CBCT coronal view taken using only 2.0 mA, as seen in the yellow box at the bottom left hand corner of the image.

Medical CT has traditionally consisted of the acquisition of individual axial slices, and a volume is created in the software from those axial slices. Coronal and sagittal views are reconstructed from that volume, but they are not as sharp as the axial views. The sharpness of the reconstructed medical CT slices will depend on the selected axial slice thickness at the time of acquisition and any physiologic or other movement of the patient during the relatively longer acquisition time. However, the sharpest CT reconstructed views will necessitate very thin axial slices, which in turn, significantly increase the already high CT dose. In CBCT, the volume is acquired with a relatively short exposure time and then the axial, coronal, sagittal, cross-sectional, and custom views are reconstructed from the volume. This means that in medical CT the best images are the axial views whereas in CBCT all reconstructed views are equally sharp and detailed as is the volume. This conceptual difference is illustrated in Figure 12-9.

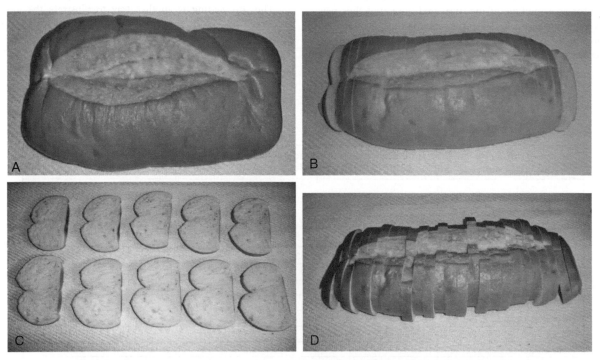

Figure 12-9   Figures A and B represent simulated slices from a CBCT volume; Figures C and D represent simulated CT volume from the slices.

CBCT SOFTWARE

CBCT software can display the axial, sagittal, and coronal views as well as 3D reconstruction with the hard tissues displayed in clear and sharp detail. Also the slice thickness can be selected, which in this case is 1.5 mm. Each of these three views can be scrolled by moving the colored lines (Figure 12-10).

In Figure 12-10, the InVivo software by Anatomage displays the axial (top left), sagittal (top right), and coronal views (bottom left). A 3D reconstruction of the whole volume is displayed (bottom right). The orientation lines are in red, green, and blue.

If, for example, we move the red orientation line as seen in Figure 12-10 superiorly in the coronal or sagittal view, the axial view, which is the upper left panel (i.e., the image that does not show a red line), will display the structures in a new image at the new anatomic level of the red line (Figure 12-11). In this case, the red line has been moved to the level of the temperomandibular joint (TMJ) condyles and the maxillary sinus.

In Figure 12-11, the red orientation line has been moved superiorly to the level of the TMJ condyles, which can be seen in the axial view (top left).

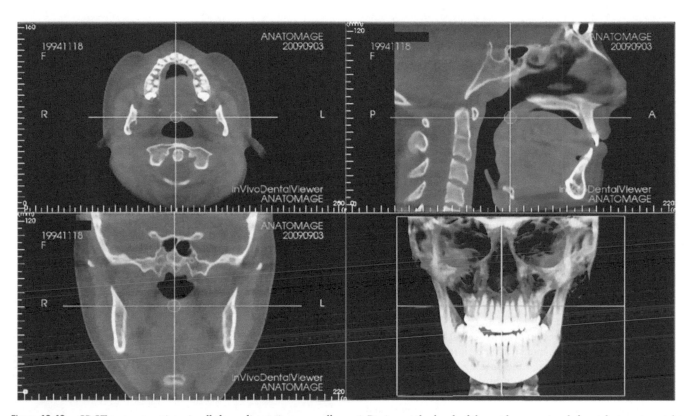

Figure **12-10**   CBCT reconstructions in all three dimensions as well as a 3-D view at the level of the mid ramus; top left axial view; top right sagittal view; bottom left coronal view; bottom right 3-D reconstruction.

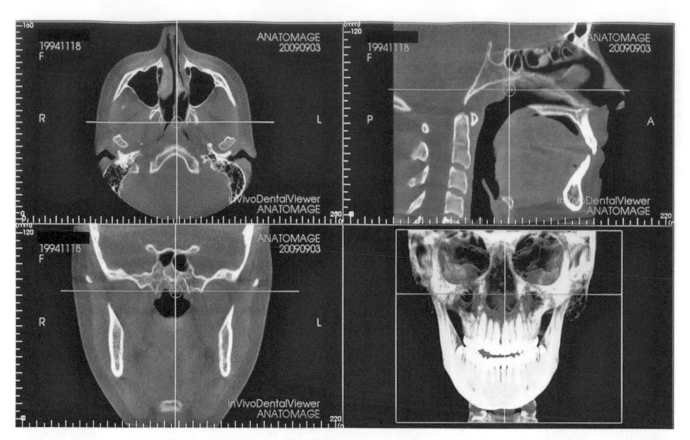

Figure **12-11** CBCT reconstructions in all three dimensions as well as a 3-D view at the level of the TMJ; top left axial view; top right sagittal view; bottom left coronal view; bottom right 3-D reconstruction.

Other anatomic structures that can be seen at this level are the clivus, the mastoid air cells, and structures in the ear; the medial and lateral pterygoid plates; and the opening of the nasolacrimal duct, which is under the inferior turbinate in the nose, as well as the nasal septum, which is deviated (Figures 12-11 and 12-12). Additional anatomic structures can be seen in the sagittal and coronal views. The identification of anatomic structures in various CBCT views and at different levels are illustrated. Note that while it is difficult to make out some of the soft tissue features, others such as swelling, assymmetry, interuption of an air space, or calcification within the soft tissue may be seen. In larger scans, many normal calcifications in normal brain locations can be identified, and a significant number of brain tumors contain calcifications. Any brain calcification in a child should be investigated. Muscles and tendons may contain calcifications as a result of trauma. Other calcifications including sialoliths, vascular wall calcifications, pheboliths, calcified lymph nodes, scar tissue, and tonsilloliths may show up on a CBCT scan.

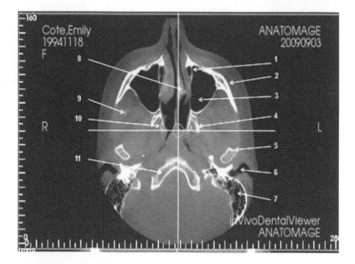

Figure **12-12** The structures seen at the level of the TMJ in the axial view are as follows: (1) nasolacrimal duct; (2) malar process or root of the zygomatic arch; (3) maxillary sinus; (4) lateral pterygoid plate; (5) TMJ condylar head; (6) external auditory canal; (7) mastoid air cells; (8) deviated nasal septum; (9) tip of the coronoid process of the mandible; (10) medial pterygoid plate; (11) clivus.

CBCT Reports

It is important to note that the dentist is responsible for identifying any pathology in all parts of the volume, even unfamiliar anatomic regions in the scan or in areas of the scan that are not in the direct interest for which the scan was taken. Also, the dentist must write a report that includes: (1) reason for taking the scan, (2) all relevant (i.e., any pathologic) findings as seen in the scan, and (3) diagnoses. This information must be included in the patient's chart. If the dentist does not feel comfortable with this responsibility, the CBCT scan (i.e., volume) can be sent to an oral and maxillofacial (OMF) radiologist or an OMF radiology reporting service to obtain a report. Many reporting services are available online. It is for this reason that the dentist should select the smallest volume suitable to the task at hand so that the structures and any pathology identified are more likely to be familiar and easily recognized. It may also be said that the smaller the scan volume, the lower the radiation dose (Figure 12-13).

Figure 12-13 shows the pathology at an implant site. In Figure 12-13A, the 2D sagittal view is reconstructed from the whole volume; in Figure 12-13B, the sagittal view through a thin slice centered on the implant imaging guide that can be used as a drilling guide is shown. There is inadequate bone and possible pathology and foreign material at the implant site. Thus the selected implant site requires further treatment before an implant can be inserted. A smaller volume could have been used for this purpose.

CBCT has been a boon to dental practices. In general, CBCT image acquisition is not technique sensitive. If the patient is not perfectly positioned, as long as the area of interest is included in the volume, the volume and/or slices can be subsequently re-aligned on any plane in order to view an anatomic site in any desired orientation and in any plane (i.e., axial, coronal, and sagittal views). The volume can be reoriented for custom views such that a cross-sectional right-angle view or other custom slices can be created (Figure 12-14).

One of the biggest advantages of CBCT is that more accurate diagnoses can be made. In fact, some diagnoses would be difficult to make without CBCT, and these diagnoses do not involve complex problems or exotic diseases. These more accurate diagnoses can be made on a very regular basis to the point that some practitioners have wondered what they did before they had CBCT. Just as panoramic radiology was not commonly seen in dental offices before the 1980s, so too CBCT is predicted to become ubiquitous in dental practices in the next decade.

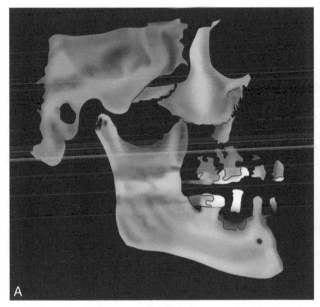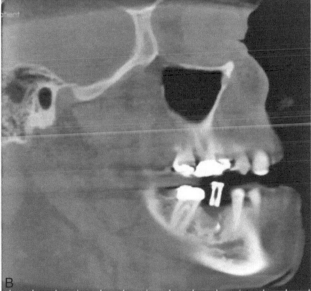

Figure **12-13** Figure A demonstrates in detail the anatomic location and orientation as seen in Figure B with a drilling guide in place and clearly demonstrates a possible lesion and foreign material at the implant site.

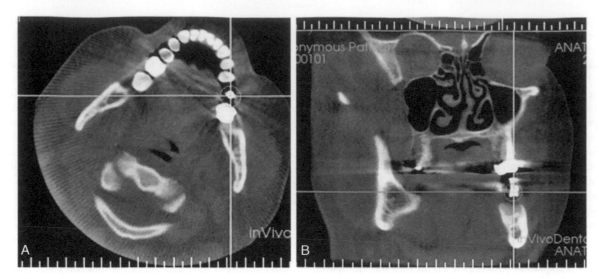

Figure **12-14**   Figure A, a cross-sectional view of the implant site is seen; the orientation of the volume to produce the cross-sectional view is seen in Figure B.

CBCT imaging was introduced in the United States in approximately 1999. At that time our department at the University of Texas Dental School in San Antonio received their first CBCT machine from the J. Morita company of Japan. It was a great honor for us as Mr. Ricky Morita owner and CEO of the J. Morita Company in Kyoto, Japan, delivered the machine himself along with his staff. Actually, the first machine went to the University of the Pacific in San Francisco, and several days later we received ours. Even in the dental school setting, the technology was not immediately accepted or understood. Folks continued to do endodontics, 3rd molar removal, and implant placement as well as nameless other dental procedures without the aid of CBCT. Nowadays, the department receives referrals for CBCT scans on a continuous basis, and other departments have acquired their own machines. In the beginning (1999) the CBCT devices could only do CBCT scans. Now the technology

has advanced to the point that new models of pan machines are also capable of acquiring a CBCT scan as well as standard pan and pan BW and cephalometric images. The net result is that dentists can make better, more accurate, and more complete diagnoses, some of which could not have been possible without CBCT.

SHORT ANSWER QUESTIONS WITH FIGURES
Instructions

Answer the questions based on a CBCT image. Compare your answer to the correct answer in the Answer Key at the back of the book.

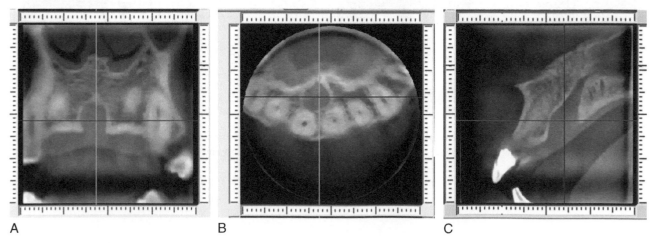

A   B   C

Figure **12-15**

1. What type of machine captured these images?
2. Each of these images has a designated identifier according to the view; for example, in intraoral radiography, you have periapical and BW views. Identify each of the above views.
3. The colored cross hairs in each view are centered on an anatomic structure. Name this structure.
4. Anatomically, where does this structure begin and end? Or you could ask, what two anatomic regions does it connect?
5. What function does this structure have?

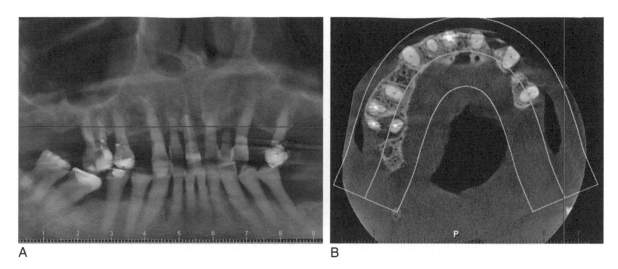

A   B

Figure **12-16**

This is a patient who was being evaluated for a very mobile upper right 1st molar.
1. What type of image is seen in A?
2. What type of image is seen in B?
3. What view do we see in B?
4. What does the green line in B represent?
5. In B, what does the area outlined in yellow represent?
6. What do we see in B that we cannot see in A?

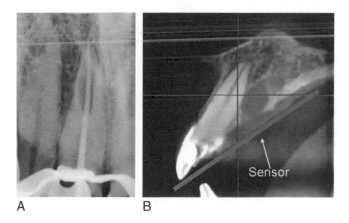

A   B

Figure **12-17**

1. What type of image is seen in A?
2. What do you think about the radiolucent area within the root canal space in A? The patient was asymptomatic, and the tooth undergoing root canal therapy was vital. Looking at A, what do you think the preliminary diagnosis was?
3. What type of image is seen in B? Image B is from the same patient as image A.
4. What was the final diagnosis for the radiolucency in the root of A?

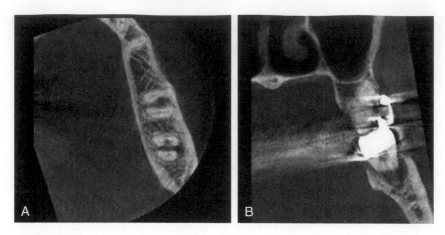

Figure **12-18**   This is a periodontal patient. Upon probing, the furcation area of the lower left 2nd molar was sensitive.
1. What type of image is seen in A and B?
2. What views are seen in A and B?
3. What is the cause of the patient's pain on probing?
4. What material is the lower 2nd molar crown made of?
5. What is the black shadow adjacent to the crown?
6. In B, what is the whitish, horizontal blur spreading across the image on both the buccal and lingual sides of the coronal portion of the tooth?

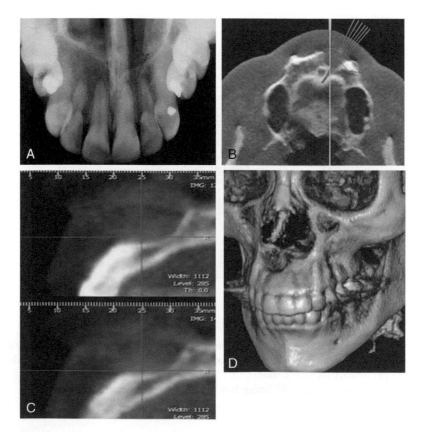

Figure **12-19**
1. What type of image do we see in A?
2. What do you see in A? The patient's right ala of the nose was elevated; the naris was slightly deformed, as was the nasolabial fold.
3. What types of images are B, C, and D?
4. What was the diagnosis?

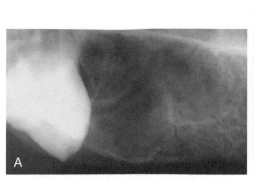
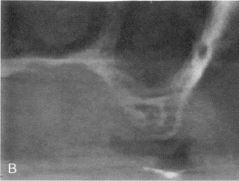

Figure **12-20**
1. What type of image is seen in A?
2. Identify the landmark we see in A as a curved, radiolucent line bound by a thin, radiopaque line on each side.
3. What type of image do we see in B?
4. So anatomically, where is the landmark seen in A?
5. What is the significance of this landmark in certain types of treatment?

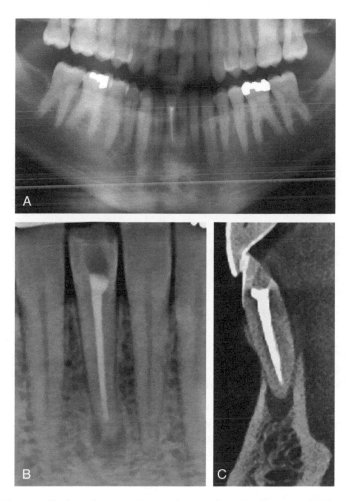

Figure **12-21**   The mandibular right central incisor became devitalized as a result of trauma. The incisal edge was completely fractured off, and the tooth is no longer in occlusion. Endodontic treatment was done about 1 year ago, and the tooth is still sensitive and somewhat painful on masticating food.
1. What types of images do we see in A, B, and C?
2. Looking at image B what do you think is the cause for the continuing discomfort?
3. Now look at image C, is this image helpful in any way?

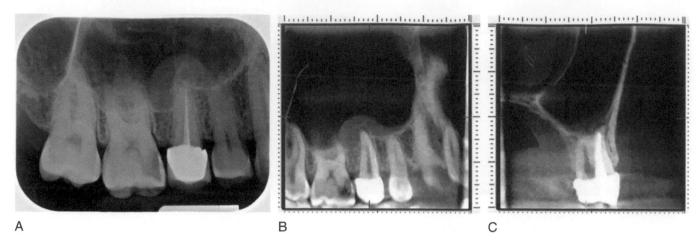

A   B   C

Figure **12-22**   This patient had a sensitivity to hot and cold and sweets in the upper right premolar-molar area. The 2nd premolar was thought to be the cause of the patient's symptoms due to the sinus reaction at the apex. Electric pulp testing was not carried out; however, the tooth was slightly sensitive to percussion. After the endodontic treatment the symptoms persisted. The periapical image in A was taken when the patient returned with continuing symptoms.

1.   What CBCT views do we see in images B and C?
2.   Why was electric pulp testing not carried out?
3.   In the periapical view, describe the reaction you can see at the apex of the 2nd premolar.
4.   Give a differential diagnosis of two possibilities for the soft-tissue density in the maxillary sinus; state your most likely choice.
5.   Compare A and B. Remember the CBCT scan was taken after the periapical image in A.
6.   What do you think is the source of the patient's symptoms?

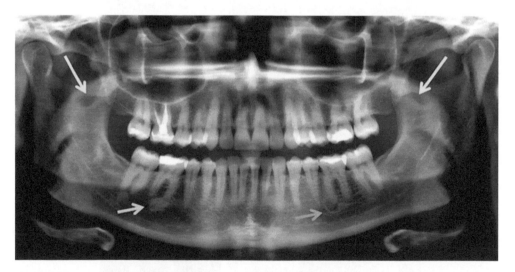

Figure **12-23**   This is a panoramic radiograph of an asymptomatic patient. Each of the colored arrows points to an entity that has a diagnosis. The yellow arrows point to a bilateral anatomic landmark. The first molars associated with the green and orange arrows are vital. This case is included to emphasize the fact that not all cases require CBCT for a diagnosis, although these cases show how very useful CBCT can be.

1.   What structure do the yellow arrows point to?
2.   How about the green arrow?
3.   And the orange arrow? Remember the teeth are vital.

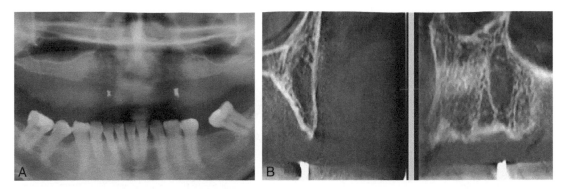

Figure **12-24**   Here we see a trimmed panoramic image in A. The radiopaque markers are sites for implant placement for an implant retained denture. The bilateral radiolucent regions just above the radiopaque markers represent air within the nose.
1.   Look closely at the pan and see if you can find any problem at the implant sites.
2.   In B, what type of images are these, and what views do they represent?
3.   What is your diagnosis?

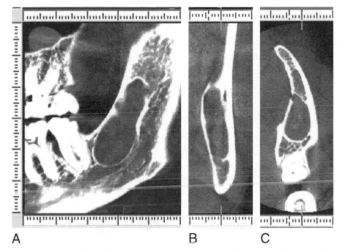

Figure **12-25**   This is a case involving two cystic lesions; one in the jaw and one in the maxillary sinus.
1.   What CBCT views are these (A, B, and C)?
2.   Where is the jaw cystic lesion?
3.   Do the relative lack of expansion and faint radiopaque material within the lumen, representing desquamated epithelium, help at all with the diagnosis of the cystic jaw lesion?
4.   How about the one in the sinus?

MULTIPLE CHOICE QUESTIONS WITH FIGURES

Instructions

Please select the best answer and check your selection with the correct answer in the Answer Key at the back of the book.

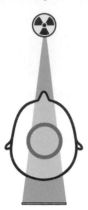

Figure **12-26**

1. Here we see a CBCT imaging diagram with the blue circle being the path of the rotation center as the machine rotates around the patient's head. This movement pattern is used to capture the volume. What term best describes the path of the rotation center?
    A. Circular
    B. Concentric
    C. Eccentric
    D. Volumetric

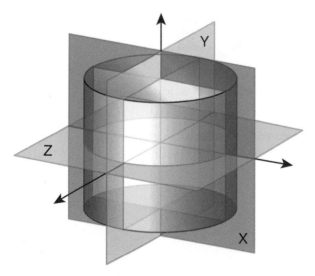

Figure **12-27**

2. This diagram depicts a CBCT volume that is usually cylindrical in CBCT imaging. The three letters X, Y, and Z are color coded and represent:
    A. Individual planes, which can be viewed in the volume
    B. The panels are X for sagittal, Y for coronal, and Z for axial
    C. Single cuts along these planes can all be viewed simultaneously
    D. A and B only
    E. All of the above

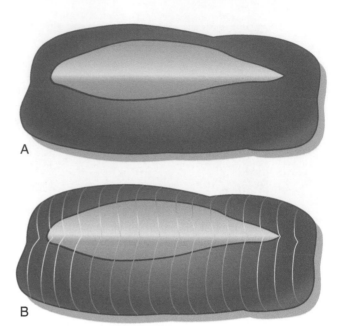

Figure **12-28**

3. The loaf of bread in image A represents the volume; the sliced loaf in image B represents slices through the volume. Note the slices are perfectly aligned with the rest of the volume.
    A. This accurate alignment of the slices with the volume can only be done with CBCT
    B. This accurate alignment of the slices with the volume can only be done with CT
    C. This accurate alignment of the slices with the volume can be done equally with CBCT and CT
    D. This accurate alignment of the slices with the volume can be done with neither CBCT nor CT

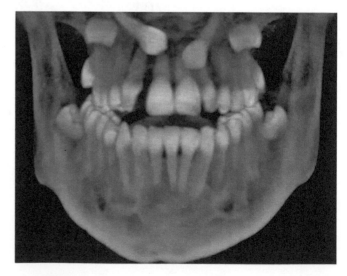

Figure **12-29**

4. What type of image is this? Choose the one most accurate statement.
    A. An image of the upper and lower jaws
    B. An image of the upper and lower jaws and impacted teeth
    C. A CBCT 3D reconstruction of the jaws
    D. A colorized, volumetric CBCT reconstruction of the jaws

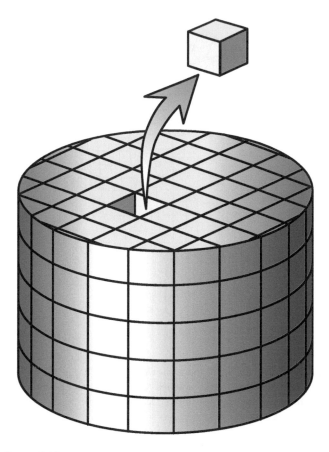

Figure **12-30**

5. Here we see a diagram associated with CBCT. Select the best answer. The diagram represents:
   A.   The image and a pixel
   B.   The cylindrical slice and a voxel
   C.   A voxel, also termed a volume element
   D.   The cylindrical volume and a voxel

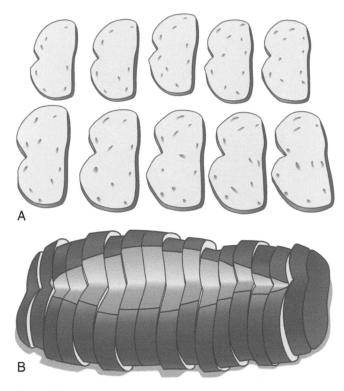

A

B

Figure **12-31**

6. Here we see individual slices of bread in image A, and the rest of the slices have been assembled back into a loaf, representing the volume in image B. This type of alignment of the slices is seen in:
   A.   CBCT before the "realignment" software kicks in
   B.   CBCT after the "realignment" software kicks in
   C.   Medical volumetric CT images
   D.   Both medical CT and CBCT 3D reconstructions

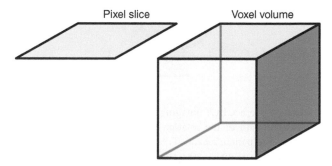

Pixel slice   Voxel volume

Figure **12-32**

7. The elements that make up some specific types of digital x-ray images are depicted here. Select the most accurate and complete statement.
   A.   The left is a pixel and the right is a voxel
   B.   The left is a picture element and the right is a volume element
   C.   The pixel is two-dimensional and the voxel is three-dimensional
   D.   All of the above
   E.   None of the above

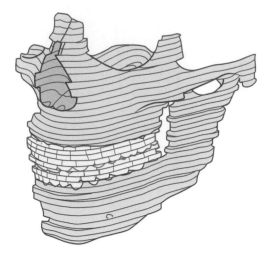

Figure **12-33**

8. Select the most accurate statement. This picture represents:
   A. A medical CT 3D reconstruction of the mandible
   B. Individual stacked slices as captured
   C. An example of 3D modeling using medical CT
   D. An early CBCT volume

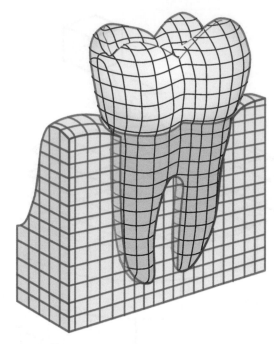

Figure **12-35**

10. This diagram is all about showing the 3D nature of CBCT. Although the little squares appear two-dimensional, a three-dimensional reconstruction is possible because these squares are:
    A. Voxels
    B. Only stacked-up pixels
    C. A way of displaying digital images
    D. All of the above

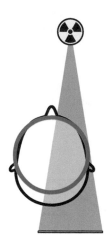

Figure **12-34**

9. Here we see a CBCT imaging diagram with the blue circle being the path of the rotation center as the machine rotates around the patient's head. This movement pattern is used to capture the volume. What term best describes the path of the rotation center?
   A. Circular
   B. Concentric
   C. Eccentric
   D. Volumetric

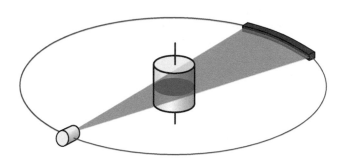

Figure **12-36**

11. This is a diagram of the fan beam used in medical CT. The cylinder in the center represents the volume of tissue to be imaged, and the beam passing from the tube head through the volume to the sensor represents the acquisition of a single slice in the volume. Which of the following statements is *not* true?
    A. In order to obtain a volume, multiple axial slices must be acquired
    B. Physiologic movements, such as breathing or swallowing, affect volume resolution
    C. Multiple slices mean a longer total exposure time
    D. Because the slices are so thin, the dose is low

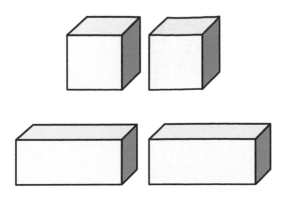

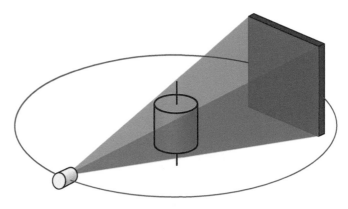

Figure **12-37**

12. These are voxels. The top row illustrates those used in cone beam CT, and the bottom ones are those used in medical CT. Select the most accurate statement.
    A. The square, isotropic voxels require a higher dose
    B. The rectangular, anisotropic voxels produce less sharp images
    C. Both voxel types are used in CBCT
    D. Depending on volume size, both medical and dental CT use both voxel types

Figure **12-38**

13. Here we see the whole volume being scanned with one rotation of the scanner-sensor apparatus. This type of scan:
    A. Is used in CBCT
    B. Involves a lower radiation dose than medical CT
    C. Is designed for use in the dental office
    D. Results in greater image resolution than medical CT
    E. All of the above

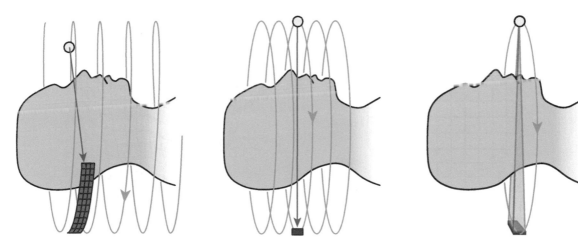

Figure **12-39**

14. In order to acquire a volume, we can see the progression of the sensor as the region of the head is being imaged. Which of the following statements is *not* true?
    A. This is a helical scan used in medical CT slice acquisition
    B. This type of medical scan allows for the reconstruction of a volume
    C. With this type of scan, the dose is similar to dental CBCT scanning
    D. Because of physiologic movements, sharpness and detail may be adversely affected

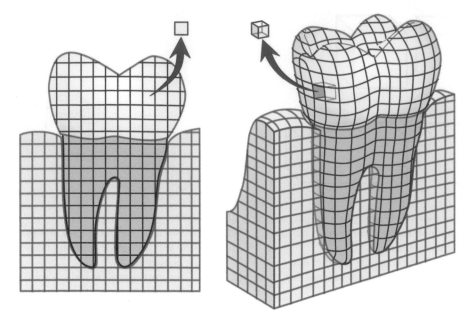

Figure **12-40**

15. Let's take another look at a comparison set of diagrams. Here we are concerned with the image on the *left*.
    A. The image on the left is a 2D image consisting of voxels
    B. The voxels are aligned in a digital image matrix
    C. This matrix consists of vertical rows and horizontal columns
    D. All of the above are true
    E. None of the above is true

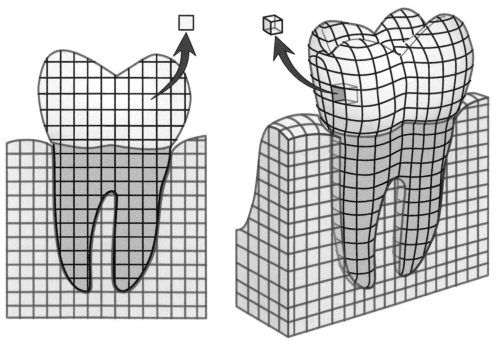

Figure **12-41**

16. Let's take a second look at a comparison set of diagrams. Here we are concerned with the image on the *right*.
    A. The image on the right is a 3D image consisting of voxels
    B. The voxels make up the 3D volume
    C. The 3D volume can be sliced to produce 2D images
    D. All of the above are true
    E. None of the above is true

MULTIPLE CHOICE QUESTIONS WITHOUT FIGURES

Instructions

Please select the best answer and check your selection with the correct answer in the Answer Key at the back of the book.

1. In some cone beam CT devices, the type of x-ray beam used is _____ and results in _____ dose.
A. Continuous and less
B. Pulsed and less
C. Pulsed and more
D. Heterogeneous and less

2. In cone beam CT, tube current modulation is a feature that:
A. Results in less dose
B. Improves image quality
C. Involves the dynamic adjustment of mAs
D. Is used because of different attenuation properties of various tissues in the scan
E. All of the above

3. One problem with CBCT is:
A. Beam scattering blurs the image
B. Large volume doses are always high
C. Multiple slice acquisition causes image blurring
D. The AC type radiation source results in noise

4. Let's say you are capturing a small volume of 8 × 8 cm in a patient with a very large head.
A. Getting the patient into the machine may be a problem
B. The patient may have to stoop during the scan
C. A referral for medical CT may be necessary
D. The anatomy outside of the volume may degrade the image quality

5. In CBCT, when the image slices are not parallel to the beam:
A. An undesirable artifact may occur above the image
B. This relationship makes no difference in CBCT
C. It is possible that some measurements may be inaccurate
D. More dose may be required

6. In comparing CBCT to medical CT, which of the following is untrue?
A. CBCT is faster
B. CBCT has a lower dose
C. CBCT has smaller volumes
D. CBCT is less expensive
E. None of the above

7. In comparing CBCT to medical CT, which of the following is untrue?
A. CBCT has better image quality
B. CBCT has higher resolution
C. CBCT is more convenient
D. CBCT has special dental applications
E. None of the above

8. In some CBCT imaging applications, there is a stroboscopic effect, which results in:
A. Longer pulses during the scan
B. Slight blurring of image quality
C. Increased dose
D. 400 to 600 images during the scan

9. The idea of asymmetric off-set scanning is that during the scan:
A. The whole volume is not always in the beam
B. More magnification is produced
C. The scan angle is limited to about 200 degrees
D. Fewer frames are captured

10. In CBCT, the volume is a cylinder of tissue; for most volume sizes, the cylinder contains about _____ million voxels.
A. 1
B. 20
C. 100
D. 400

11. Voxel size usually increases with the selected volume size; of the following dimensions, which is the smallest *available* voxel size:
A. 0.075 × 0.075 × 0.075 mm
B. 0.1 × 0.1 × 0.1 mm
C. 0.15 × 0.15 × 0.15 mm
D. 0.2 × 0.2 × 0.2 mm

12. The isotropic voxel is used:
A. Only for small-volume CBCT
B. For small- and medium-volume CBCT
C. Mainly for large-volume CBCT
D. For all CBCT volume sizes

13. In spiral medical CT, the pitch is:
A. The angle of the beam
B. The distance between the spiral rounds
C. The dot pitch within the volume of different sizes
D. The relationship of the sensor to the beam

14. In spiral medical CT, the pitch:
A. Is a variable feature, which is desirable
B. Causes undesirable vibrations
C. Causes distortion in any 3D measurements
D. Varies throughout the scan

15. In medical CT, the layer thickness is
A. 0.5 to 0.8 mm
B. 0.10 to 0.15 mm
C. 0.15 to 0.2 mm
D. 0.2 to 0.25 mm

Chapter 13

Implant Imaging

Goal

To understand the principles and procedures for successful implant therapy

Learning Objectives

1. Know the limitations of standard imaging modalities
2. Know the factors for a proper assessment of the implant site
3. Understand why imaging guides are used
4. Correlate imaging guide information for the construction of a drilling guide
5. Recognize signs of implant failure

INTRODUCTION

In terms of dental radiology, one of the most important facets of implant dentistry is the role of x-ray imaging. Before any of the following implant-specific information, the first step is to ensure that pathology is not present at the implant site. The second step is to ensure that there is sufficient bone to support the implant. In the preoperative planning phase, radiographic images are helpful in assessing both bone quality and bone quantity. As stated before in this text, panoramic images are not the best choice for assessing bone quality and quantity; instead cone beam computed tomography (CBCT) should be used. A new cadmium telluride photon counting (CdTePC) sensor has been introduced in some CBCT machines. This sensor can match the current low doses and has the potential to analyze bone density in a manner similar to the dual energy absorptiometry (DXA) equipment, which is the current gold standard in medical practice for assessing osteoporosis. To help with the planning process, an imaging guide can be created in the dental office laboratory. The guide represents the calculated best path (trajectory) for drilling into the bone to create a cylindrical cavity for the placement of the implant. Some imaging guides can be used as surgical guides to help the doctor accurately drill a hole in the bone, exactly where the most ideal location for the implant placement is, as determined preoperatively. This information is very helpful with implant selection for length, width, shape, and vertical orientation of the implant to obtain the best possible outcome. Once the implant has been placed, radiographic images can be used to determine osseous integration of the implant, and in rare instances, to detect and confirm implant failure.

The problem with intraoral periapical and occlusal images is that, in many cases, there is distortion, which can be defined as unequal magnification (Figure 13-1). This can result in inaccurate measurements.

As Figure 13-1 demonstrates, distortion may occur when the sensor or film is not parallel to the tooth, even if the x-ray beam is perpendicular to the tooth. Distortion is unequal magnification of the object being imaged.

Distortion is virtually unpredictable and/or unmeasurable. Clinical examples of distortion consist of elongation and foreshortening of structures in the image. In implant imaging applications, distortion can result in longer or shorter measurements of the available bone, which in turn, results in an implant of less than ideal size. In contrast, CBCT measurements are accurate.

In the example of distortion shown in Figure 13-2, the endodontic measurement of the palatal root canal would be longer, and the buccal root canals would be shorter. The beam must be perpendicular to both the tooth and the film or sensor; otherwise distortion occurs. The same principle applies to structural relationships in implant imaging.

If the beam is not properly aligned, the implant measurement and the implant itself may be too short or too long for the best outcome (Figure 13-3).

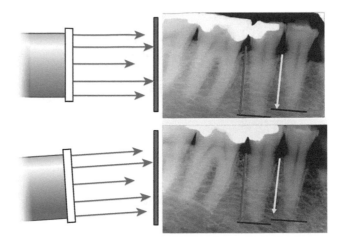

Figure **13-3**   Vertical bone height and root length distortion in interoral radiographs.

Note in Figure 13-3, the two periapical images of the same area. Both red lines are the same length and both yellow lines are the same length; only the angle or direction of the beam was altered—the sensor was not moved for these two images. Note the significantly different measurements illustrated between the upper and lower images.

In addition to the above concepts, intraoral images are two-dimensional and demonstrate length only. That is why an occlusal radiograph is used as a supplemental image to add the dimension of width. However, an occlusal radiograph will not always demonstrate a dip in the bone as well as it does the vertical orientation of the bone in space. Also the beam may not always be perpendicular to both the mandible or maxilla and the film/sensor. In other words, the jaws are not always perfectly vertical and of consistent thickness buccolingually at the site of implant placement.

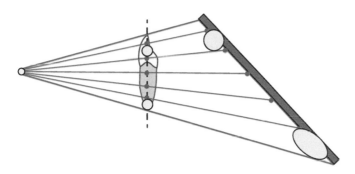

Figure **13-1**   Distortion (unequal magnification) in intraoral radiographs.

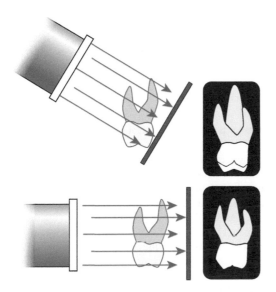

Figure **13-2**   Root length distortion of molar roots in intraoral radiographs.

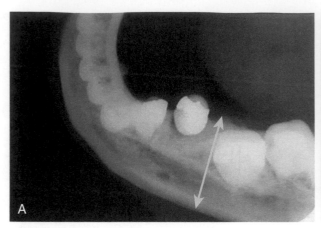

Figure **13-4** Variability of bone width measurements in occlusal radiographs.

In Figure 13-4, the angulation of the beam in an occlusal image can change the buccolingual width of the mandible, as we see in this case.

As we have seen in the panoramic chapter, the problem with measurements derived from these images is that, in panoramic radiography, the beam is directed at an upward angle through the jaws and is therefore not perpendicular to the jaws or to the film or sensor. In implant imaging, this may cause erroneous measurements.

Figure 13-5 shows the upward angle of the panoramic beam as it traverses through the jaws and surrounding structures.

As an anatomic consideration, it is known that the path of the inferior alveolar canal may travel toward the buccal or lingual in an unpredictable manner because it runs from the mental foramen on the buccal aspect and posteriorly to the lingual foramen, which is on the lingual aspect of the mid-ramus. Anatomic studies have shown the inferior alveolar canal may be buccal, lingual, or centrally placed in an unpredictable manner as illustrated in Figure 13-6.

The location of the inferior alveolar canal is important when placing an implant in the mandible. The problem with panoramic imaging for implant placement is that a structure, such as the inferior alveolar canal, can be either buccal or lingual to the center of the alveolar crest, and thus it can be projected higher or lower in the image than it really is in the patient. For example, if the inferior

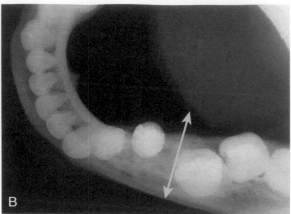

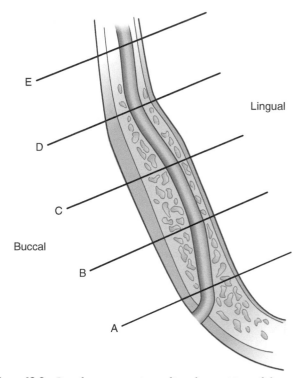

Figure **13-6** Based on anatomic studies, the position of the mandibular canal is variable in a bucco-lingual direction (aspect) causing unpredictable measurements on panoramic images.

alveolar canal is buccal to the crest of the ridge, it will be projected downward with respect to the ridge crest, making the measurement between the crest of the alveolar ridge to the inferior alveolar canal longer than it actually is, even after taking magnification into account. The opposite will occur if the canal is to the lingual of the ridge crest. In this latter case, the available length for the implant will be seen as less than what is really available (Figure 13-7).

In the panoramic images depicted in Figure 13-7, an inaccurate assessment of the position of the canal may result in inaccurate measurements. In contrast, in each of the two cross-sectional image diagrams (as would be seen on CBCT), the distance between the inferior alveolar canal and the crest of the edentulous ridge at an implant site is accurate; however, note how the buccolingual position of the canal is different in the two cases.

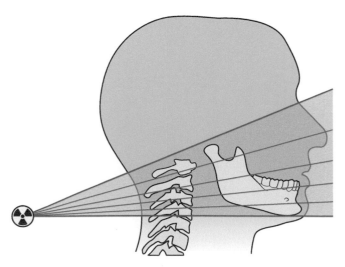

Figure **13-5** The negative projection angle of the panoramic beam causes inaccurate structural relationships.

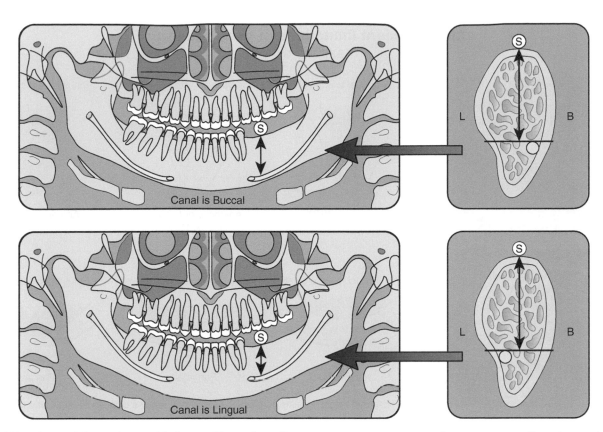

Figure **13-7** The variability in the mandibular canal bucco-lingually causes variations in pan vertical measurements of bone but not in CBCT images as depicted on the right side of the illustration.

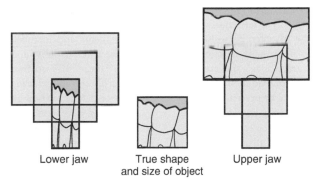

Lower jaw   True shape and size of object   Upper jaw

Figure **13-8** Because of the negative vertical angulation of the pan beam (Figure 13-5), vertical measurements of structural relationships vary based on mandibular vs. maxillary locations.

Another factor in panoramic imaging is that the degree of separation of buccal and lingual objects is greater for structures in the maxilla than in the mandible, as seen in Figure 13-7. This phenomenon is due to the widening of the beam as it traverses the maxilla compared with the mandible, as illustrated in Figure 13-5.

Demonstrated in Figure 13-8, the vertical separation of buccal and lingual objects is greater in the maxilla than in the mandible. Also buccal objects are narrowed and lingual objects are widened with respect to objects in the middle of the structure. Therefore magnification and structure localization are hard to predict in panoramic images for implant assessments in both the maxilla and mandible.

Another example of inaccurate panoramic measurements occurs in the posterior maxilla. In CBCT, the distance between the crest of the edentulous ridge at the implant site is the same when the floor of

the sinus is buccal, centered, or lingual to the ridge crest. In panoramic imaging, this measurement varies depending on the position of the sinus floor and the ridge crest, as seen in Figure 13-9. Other similar anatomic structures so affected are the anterior branch (incisive) of the inferior alveolar nerve and the floor of the nose, if visible in the panoramic image.

In Figure 13-9, the area of interest is within the yellow colored oval in both diagrams. In the CBCT image (upper) the measurement remains constant when the relationship of the sinus floor changes from buccal to lingual in relationship to the ridge crest. However, in panoramic imaging (lower), the measurement of the available bone in the image varies with the relationship of the ridge crest to the floor of the sinus. Thus CBCT is more accurate for implant measurements.

Measurement limitations of pan radiology
(maxillary sinus)

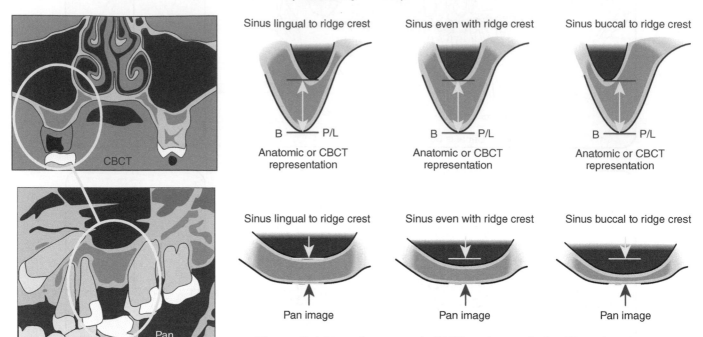

2 views of same patient anatomy

Figure **13-9** In panoramic imaging the maxillary bone depth in relation to the maxillary sinus varies with the bucco-lingual relationship of these two structures.

The trabecular pattern of the bone as seen in the intraoral images, and possibly panoramic radiographs, is mostly a reflection of the trabecular pattern in the cortex vs. the alveolar bone located between the cortices. Trabecular patterns are usually described as dense (lots of trabeculae) or loose (few trabeculae) and are well or poorly mineralized (high density/more radiopaque or low density/more radiolucent), suggesting the absence or presence of osteoporosis. However, since the implant will ideally be placed in the alveolar bone between the cortical plates, the above information, though helpful, is incomplete and more importantly, is unpredictable. Another problem with panoramic imaging is that angular relationships are inaccurate if technique factors or structural relationships are not perfectly centered within the panoramic focal trough (layer of tissue in the image). This may be significant in orthodontic applications as appliances are often designed based on plaster models and a panoramic image. In implant imaging, the angular relationship of teeth adjacent to an implant site or of a drill guide trajectory, as it relates to adjacent structures, may be inaccurate if panoramic imaging is used.

In summary, two-dimensional imaging, such as intraoral periapicals, occlusals, and panoramic radiographs, do not provide fully accurate linear and angular measurements; they do not demonstrate predictable proper relationships of anatomic structures in space either. Additionally, the density of the intercortical alveolar bone in which the implant will be placed is difficult to assess. Structural relationships may be inaccurate. There is an answer to these problems. The solution is CBCT imaging. CBCT provides accurate linear and angular measurements, accurate structural relationships in space, and accurate assessment of the thickness of cortical bone. Additionally, the space and degree of trabeculation in the alveolar

bone between the cortical plates can be assessed more accurately. Finally, most CBCT software allows for the necessary implant measurements and includes an implant library that contains the complete specifications of available implants from most manufacturers. Using CBCT software, implants can be selected from the implant library and placed at the planned site within the CBCT volume to determine best fit.

CBCT can also be used to verify the functionality and quality of the selected implant site. Kits are available to construct an imaging guide in the dental office that can later be used as a surgical guide such that an implant of a perfect size can be placed exactly in the selected best location in terms of depth, width, and trajectory of implant placement. As may occur, the original clinical assessment of the implant site can be revised once information from the CBCT image is assessed. In addition, volumetric calculations can be made to ensure that just the right supply of bone grafting material can be available at the time of the procedure for a sinus floor lift or to correct a subperiosteal defect or inadequacy of alveolar bone at a selected implant site.

Beam Hardening

In the postoperative assessment of some metallic implants, an artifact termed "beam hardening" may cause an appearance of a low-density (radiolucent) area beside the implant simulating bone loss. "Spray" or "star" artifact is high density (radiopaque). The beam hardening artifact may mimic bone loss around an implant or may obscure the bone in some areas adjacent to the implant, as seen in Figure 13-10.

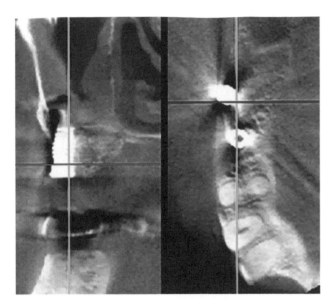

Figure **13-10** Low-density beam hardening (black) metallic and high-density (white) spray artifacts in CBCT imaging.

In Figure 13-10, the low-density (black) artifact is "beam hardening" and is caused by metals in the CBCT volume. The high-density (white) artifact is "spray" artifact and is caused by metals in the CBCT volume. This artifact may mimic bone loss adjacent to the implant.

In the differential diagnosis of beam hardening artifact, actual bone loss must be considered. Because beam hardening artifact does not occur in 2D intraoral and pan imaging, the true nature of the low-density area seen in the CBCT images can be determined by one of these imaging modalities. In Figure 13-11, the low density areas adjacent to the implants may have some contribution from beam hardening; however, the panoramic image of this case, as seen on the left in Figure 13-11, confirms that there is bone loss adjacent to the implants. These findings are consistent with failing implants.

In the panoramic image on the left in Figure 13-11, the radiolucent areas adjacent to the implants represent bone loss. The middle and right images are CBCT cuts of the same case in the sagittal and

coronal planes. The coronal plane on the right corresponds to the plane of the blue line in the center image. The bone loss mimics beam hardening, however the panoramic image confirms bone loss and a failing pair of implants.

Because the same CBCT machine can be used to capture standard panoramic, pan bitewing, pan periapical, and pan cephalometric images, these functions also help to financially absorb the cost of CBCT availability in the dental office. It must be remembered that CBCT imaging involves exposure factors resulting in at least the same low radiation doses as standard intraoral, panoramic, and cephalometric x-ray imaging, as was seen in Chapter 12.

At the time of writing of this book, the assessment of bone density with CBCT is done by visual analysis by the clinician or dental radiologist. Technologically, medical CT can be used to accurately assess bone density by obtaining a simple readout of the Hounsfield number at any point in the image using the mouse. The disadvantage of medical CT is that the dose is many times higher and is not directly accessible by most dentists without a medical referral. In CBCT imaging, a readout of the CT number in Hounsfield units can be done easily; however, these numbers are relative and are not an accurate measure of bone density. That is to say, for example, the inferior cortex of the mandible will have a higher CBCT Hounsfield number than the alveolar bone. However, this does not tell us the absolute degree of mineralization either in the cortex or the alveolar bone, only the relative difference between the two structures. With the advent of the cadmium telluride photon counting (CdTePC) sensor for use in CBCT, absolute bone density measurements similar to those obtainable from medical CT are now possible. In addition, the DXA examination is commonly used for the detection and quantification of osteoporosis. The CdTePC sensor is capable of "binning" the incoming photon energy into three separate bins, thus allowing for "windowing" of hard and soft tissues as is currently possible with medical CT but generally impossible with CBCT. Part of the advantage of binning is that bone density can be measured accurately with this sensor. This means that for the first time in dental radiology we will be able to make accurate assessments of the true quality of the bone at an implant site. And as an extra bonus, the radiation dose of the CdTePC sensor–equipped CBCT machines has the potential of being three to five times lower than some current CBCT doses.

In summary, the CBCT machine circles the patient's head in an arc of at least 180 degrees up to a full circle of 360 degrees. The milliamperage setting ranges from about 10 up to 14 mA and the kilovoltage peak ranges from about 90 to 110 kVp. The rotation may be symmetric or asymmetric, and the rotation time is approximately 12 to 20 seconds. Because the x-ray beam is in pulses, the actual exposure to radiation is 3 to 8 seconds during a single rotation. The sensor captures some 250 to 500 pulses, and the software creates the 3D volume of the selected anatomic area being imaged. The software then slices the volume in all three dimensions into a total of 300 to 500 images. These three dimensions are the axial, sagittal, and coronal planes. Any anatomic location within the CBCT volume can be viewed in all three dimensions, and both angular and linear measurements are accurately obtained. Finally, with the CdTePC sensor, qualitative measurements of bone density are possible.

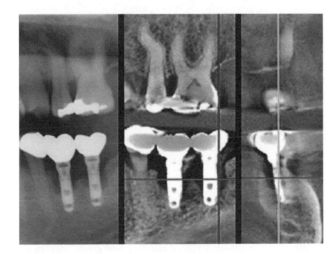

Figure **13-11** CBCT beam hardening artifact may mimic bone loss; intraoral imaging confirms bone loss.

SHORT ANSWER QUESTIONS WITH FIGURES

Instructions

The following questions involve an image or diagram related to CBCT imaging. By answering the following questions, the reader will have a broader knowledge of the most important factors involved in implant imaging. The authors believe that CBCT implant imaging and the associated factors relating to this technology are the foundation on which successful implant therapy is based. Compare your answer to the correct answer in the Answer Key at the back of the book.

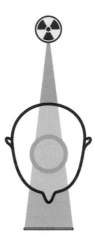

Figure **13-12** Study the above CBCT diagram.
1. What part of this diagram depicts the volume to be imaged?
2. What type of rotation pattern is depicted here?
3. In terms of increased volume size, does the dose increase or decrease?

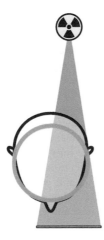

Figure **13-13**
1. What part of this diagram depicts the volume to be imaged?
2. What type of rotation pattern is depicted here?
3. In terms of increased volume size, does the dose increase or decrease?

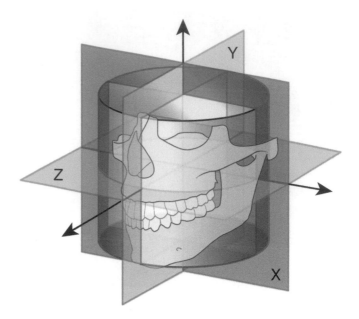

Figure **13-14** This diagram depicts the three planes within a CBCT volume. These planes are labeled "X," "Y," and "Z."
1. Name the "X" plane.
2. Name the "Y" plane.
3. Name the "Z" plane.
4. In CBCT, what shape does the volume have?
5. Within this volume, which measurements are accurate?

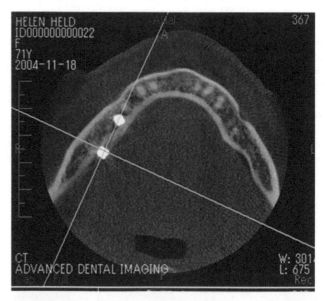

Figure **13-15**
1. What view (plane) is this image?
2. What type of dental restorative device do the green and blue lines intersect?
3. What anatomic structure do we see depicted here?
4. What anatomic level does this image display?
5. Where does this object appear to be located?
6. Identify the planes that the green and blue lines depict.
7. Why has the clinician placed the blue and green lines on the object in question?

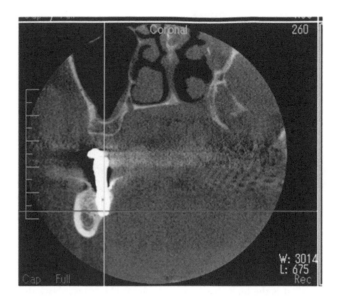

Figure **13-16**

1. What view (plane) is this?
2. What anatomic structure(s) do we see depicted here?
3. What anatomic level does this image display?
4. What do the orange hash marks on the left side of the image represent?
5. Where does this object appear to be located?
6. Identify the planes that the green and blue lines depict.
7. Why has the clinician placed the blue and green lines on the object in question?
8. What medical condition does the patient have that is displayed in this image?

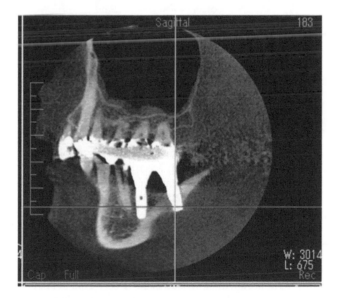

Figure **13-17**

1. What view (plane) is this?
2. What anatomic structure(s) do we see depicted here?
3. What anatomic level does this image display?
4. Where does this object in question appear to be located?
5. Identify the planes that the green and red lines depict.
6. What is the prognosis for this implant?
7. What medical condition does the patient have that is displayed in this image?

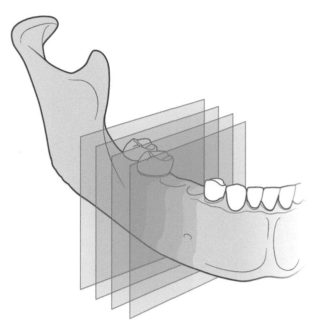

Figure **13-18** In this figure, we see multiple slices within a volume as it relates to the patient's right mandible. These slices are not exactly coronal views; they are a reorientation of the coronal view to be at right angles to a structure of interest as a part of implant planning for one or several lower left implants replacing the second premolar and first molar.

1. Because these cuts are not sagittal, coronal, or axial in orientation, in what plane are they? Remember what is being planned here.
2. Most CBCT machines have a selectable volume size up to the maximum capacity of the machine. Approximately what volume size is depicted here in blue?
3. What is the "rule" with respect to a selectable volume size?

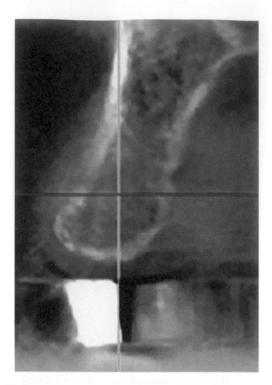

Figure **13-19** Here we see a cropped small-volume CBCT image. It was taken as part of the planning process for the placement of an implant.
1. What view is this?
2. Anatomically, what is the location of this image?
3. What plane does the red line represent?
4. What plane does the green line represent?
5. For what purpose is the radiodense (radiopaque) material represented in this image?
6. Can this radiodense material (gutta-percha) be drilled out and used as a surgical guide in this case?

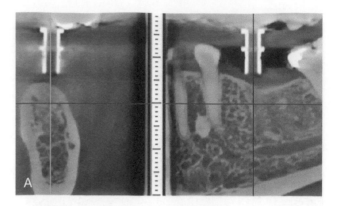

Figure **13-20A** These are two CBCT views for a planned dental procedure.
1. What is the orientation of the left view?
2. What is the orientation of the right view, and to which colored line in the left view does it correspond?
3. What is the high-density (radiopaque) object just above the crest of the ridge?
4. Anatomically exactly what location do these images represent?

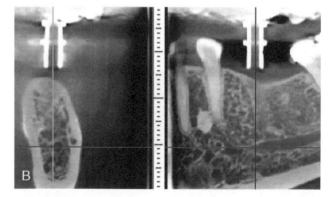

Figure **13-20B** Look at the left image and study the green line closely. There are two radiolucent areas along the green line that are surrounded by a radiopaque margin. Either one of these could be a cross section through the inferior alveolar canal. However, if the upper radiolucency on the left-hand side of the green line is the canal, there is less space for the implant, and if it is the lower radiolucency on the right side of the green line, there is more space for the implant. Using the scan, what could you do to make this determination?
1. Do you notice anything unusual in the alveolar bone in this area?
2. Is this a good implant site, and can the imaging guide be used as a surgical guide?

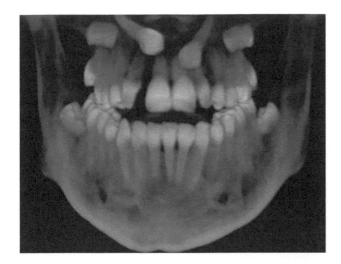

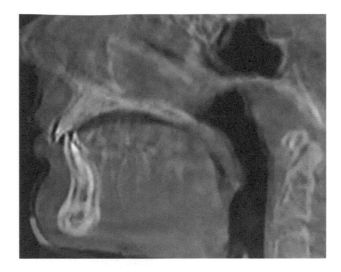

Figure **13-21**
1. What type of CBCT image is this?
2. What purpose does this type of image serve?

Figure **13-22**
1. What is wrong with this image?
2. How is it corrected?

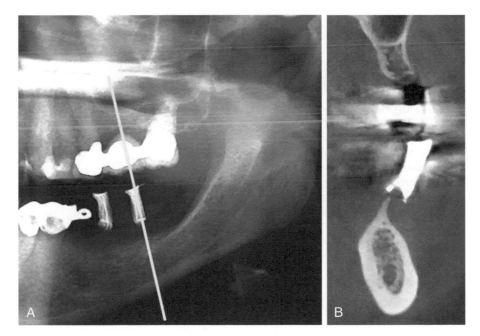

Figure **13-23** This patient was scheduled to receive implants because there was pain in the left mandible on chewing beneath her semi-precision partial denture. Because of this, the partial denture was removed, and the patient was worked up for implants.
1. What type of appliance was in the patient's mouth for both the panoramic and the CBCT images?
2. What view do we see in the CBCT image?
3. Name two artifacts present in the CBCT image.
4. What blackish, ovoid anatomic structure is at the very top of the CBCT image?
5. What is the source of the patient's pain?
6. Before implant placement, what treatment does this patient need at the implant site?

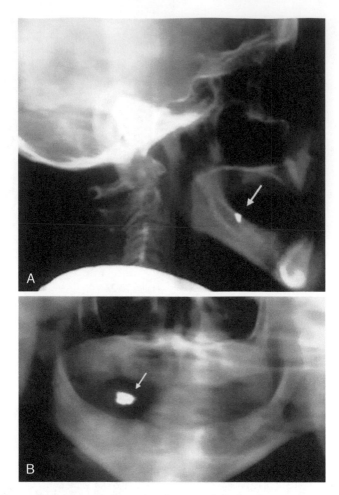

Figure **13-24**   This patient had two radiographs taken. On clinical examination, it was noted there was the presence of a purplish-blue macule (spot) in the right side of the mouth. The patient was asymptomatic.

1. What two types of radiographs do we see here?
2. What radiation safety measure was or was not taken?
3. Of what general type of material is the radiopacity, as indicated by the yellow arrow?
4. Approximately where is the radiopaque object? *Hint:* remember the panoramic projection geometry as seen earlier in this chapter.

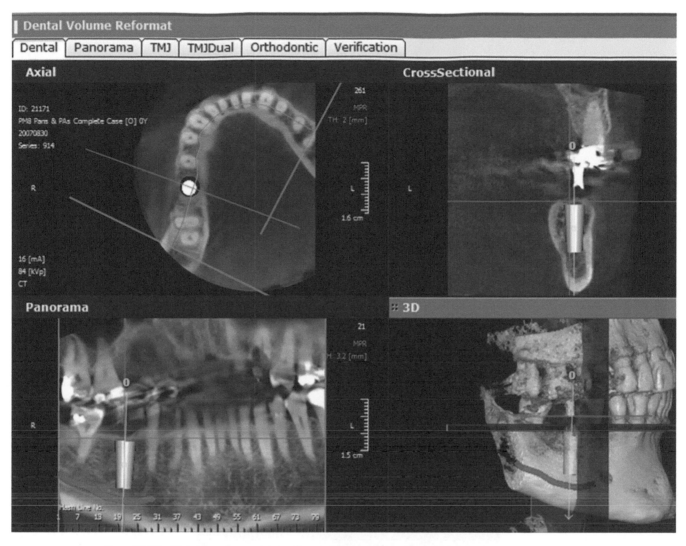

Figure **13-25**   This is a screen capture of a specific dental procedure.
1. What view do we see in the top left quadrant?
2. What view do we see in the top right quadrant?
3. What view do we see in the bottom left quadrant?
4. What view do we see in the bottom right quadrant?
5. What general type of software is being used?
6. In the top right quadrant, what specific imaging tool is the patient wearing in his mouth?
7. How does everything look with regard to proceeding with the next clinical procedure, which is being planned for the next dental appointment?

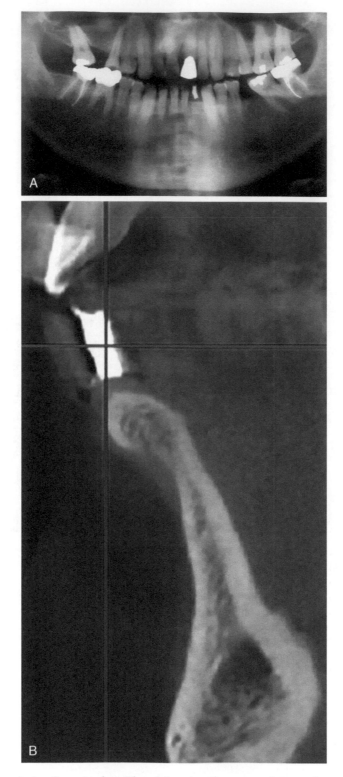

Figure **13-26**   This patient is being worked up for an implant. Though based on the panoramic image there was plenty of bone for the placement of an implant, the protocol called for a CBCT scan before proceeding to further treatment.

1.   What type of image do we see in A?
2.   Specifically what type of image and view do we see in B?
3.   What is the radiopaque object that we see in A in the edentulous space?
4.   What do you think about going ahead with the implant placement?

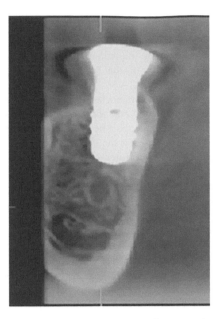

Figure **13-27** Please look at this image and answer the questions.
1. What type of image is this?
2. What is the view in this image?
3. What object do we see in the bone?
4. Comment on the efficacy of the treatment up to this point.

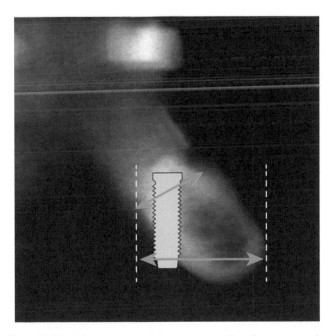

Figure **13-28** This is an image that was created to demonstrate the vertical orientation of an edentulous mandibular ridge and the possible resulting faulty implant placement.
1. What type of image is this?
2. Comment on the planned implant length.
3. What image could be taken to confirm the location of significant anatomic structures?
4. Comment on the vertical orientation of the mandible at the planned implant site.

MULTIPLE CHOICE QUESTIONS WITHOUT FIGURES

Instructions

Please select the best answer and check your selection with the correct answer in the Answer Key at the back of the book.

1. In implant planning, a periapical image may:
    A. Result in an implant that is too long
    B. Result in an implant that is shorter than necessary
    C. Result in an implant that projects outside of the bone
    D. All of the above
    E. Only A and B are correct

2. When a panoramic image is used to plan implant selection and placement in the posterior mandible, the location of the inferior alveolar canal in relation to the crest of the edentulous space:
    A. May appear shorter than it is if it is lingual to the ridge crest
    B. May appear longer than it is if it is buccal to the ridge crest
    C. May appear longer than it is if it is lingual to the ridge crest
    D. Is accurate, as panoramic imaging is a form of tomography
    E. Is accurate only if a magnification factor is calculated

3. When linear tomography is used for implant planning:
    A. Structural relationships are essentially accurate
    B. Several tomograms will be necessary to study the implant site in all three dimensions
    C. A magnification factor must be calculated
    D. All of the above
    E. Only A and C are correct

4. When planning an implant, an intraoral periapical image is sufficient as long as:
    A. The film or sensor is parallel to the bone at the implant site
    B. The x-ray beam is perpendicular to both the film/sensor and the bone at the implant site
    C. The bone at the implant site is oriented perfectly in the vertical dimension
    D. None of the above
    E. Only A and B are correct

5. When planning the placement of an implant, intraoral and panoramic imaging:
    A. Are never the best methods to assess an implant site
    B. Should be used in the initial evaluation of an implant site
    C. May be used only if an imaging guide is included in the image, for either imaging modality
    D. Should be used throughout the process as the x-ray doses are lower than other imaging modalities

6. Intraoral imaging is acceptable for the assessment of an implant site:
    A. As long as several periapical images are taken
    B. Only when an occlusal image is taken
    C. When periapical and occlusal images are used
    D. Choice C would be best
    E. None of the above are fully effective

7. In terms of planning an implant, cone beam computed tomography (CBCT):
   A. Involves higher doses than intraoral and/or panoramic imaging
   B. Involves lower doses than intraoral and/or panoramic radiology
   C. Involves selectable doses, depending on the image quality needed
   D. Should only be used in complex cases

8. The advantage(s) of CBCT for implant planning is/are that:
   A. The implant site may be studied in all three dimensions
   B. Linear and angular measurements are accurate
   C. The software allows for the placement of most brands of implants within the volume at the implant site
   D. All of the above are correct
   E. Only A and B are correct as only brand-specific software must be used for implant placement in the CBCT volume

9. Including an imaging guide with a CBCT volume allows the clinician to:
   A. Estimate the planned drilling angle, choose length and width of the implant, and assess the available bone and orientation of the bone to the planned drilling trajectory
   B. Mainly make the important accurate measurements in terms of the length and width of the available bone
   C. The imaging guide must be included in the scan as this is the best way to select the implant size and shape.
   D. Make accurate measurements

10. The most complete description of the available views of a CBCT scan are:
    A. Anterior, posterior, and cross-sectional
    B. Axial, coronal and sagittal
    C. Axial, coronal, sagittal, cross-sectional, and custom-created panoramic views
    D. Axial, coronal, sagittal, cross-sectional and custom-selected views

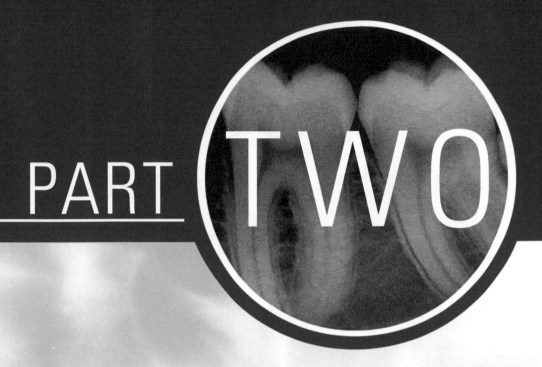

PART **TWO**

School, State, and National Board Examination Review

Section 1: Principles of Radiation Physics, Health, and Biology

Section 2: Radiographic Assessment and Interpretation

Section 1

Principles of Radiation Physics, Health, and Biology

MULTIPLE CHOICE QUESTIONS WITHOUT FIGURES

Instructions

Read the questions carefully. In some questions, the answer being sought relates to the "is not" phrasing of the question. The answer choices are based on the statement(s) in the question that, with rare exceptions, are factual. However, the answer sections also contain inaccurate or irrelevant but seemingly plausible selections, and the goal is to recognize the one most correct answer. Be wary of selecting the longest answer or the "C" choice. On the other hand, some of the correct answers *are* the longest or "C" choice. The same letter choice may occur as the correct answer several times in a row. Check your selections with the correct answers in the Answer Key at the back of the book.

1. An atom is said to be neutral when:
    A. It is ionized
    B. There are more electrons than protons
    C. The number of positive charges in the nucleus equals the number of negative charges of the orbital electrons
    D. It has a positive charge

2. X-rays interact with matter to produce:
    A. Ionization and desiccation
    B. Ionization and excitation
    C. Desiccation and excitation
    D. Ionization and replication

3. Which electron is bound most tightly to the nucleus?
    A. J-shell electron
    B. K-shell electron
    C. L-shell electron
    D. Q-shell electron

4. Electromagnetic radiation wavelengths are measured in:
    A. Kilometers
    B. Meters
    C. Angstrom units
    D. All of the above

5. Which of the following statements is true?
    A. X-rays have wavelengths, frequencies, and velocities
    B. X-rays can be reflected like light
    C. X-rays have mass and carry a positive electric charge
    D. X-rays do not travel in straight lines

6. Which of the following most adequately describes the radiation produced by high kilovoltages?
    A. Short wavelengths of low frequency
    B. Long wavelengths of high frequency
    C. Short wavelengths of high frequency
    D. High penetrating waves of low frequency

7. Secondary radiation is:
    A. Less when kVp is increased
    B. Most detrimental to the patient
    C. Less deeply penetrating than primary radiation
    D. Proportional to the square of the distance that the operator stands from the patient

8. Pocket dosimetry is an example of:
    A. Chemical dosimetry
    B. Photographic dosimetry
    C. Luminescent dosimetry
    D. Biologic dosimetry
    E. Air-ionization dosimetry

9. Which of the following is not applicable to thermoluminescent dosimetry?
    A. Ultraviolet light
    B. Heat
    C. Trapping centers
    D. Lithium fluoride
    E. Measurement of light

10. The long BID (cone) is recommended when using the paralleling technique because we can:
    A. Use the shorter time intervals allowable with an electronic timer
    B. Use a longer focal spot-film distance to compensate for a greater object-film distance to reduce magnification and distortion
    C. Hold the film closer to the tooth so there is less magnification and a better image
    D. Use a lower kVp
    E. B and C

11. The paralleling technique is recommended over the bisecting-angle technique because:
    A. Positioning the film is easier
    B. It uses slower film
    C. It gives a less-distorted picture of root length
    D. It shortens developing time
    E. A, B, and C

12. What is the main cause of foreshortening in the bisecting-angle technique?
    A. Improper placement of the film
    B. Improper horizontal angulation of the BID
    C. Vertical angulation of the BID is excessive
    D. Vertical angulation of the BID is insufficient

13. Which statement is the most correct?
    A. The long BID is used with the paralleling or the bisecting-angle technique
    B. The long BID is used with the paralleling technique only
    C. The short BID is used with either the paralleling or the bisecting-angle technique
    D. Film holders are not necessary with the paralleling technique

14. The intensity of x-radiation at any given distance from the source of radiation varies:
    A. Inversely with the square of the distance
    B. Directly with the square of the distance
    C. Inversely with the distance
    D. Directly with the distance

15. When an 8-inch target-film distance is changed to a 16-inch target-film distance (kVp and mA kept constant), the exposure time should be:
    A. Doubled
    B. Decreased by half
    C. Increased by half
    D. Quadrupled

16. In hand processing, if you place the film in the fixer first, this results in:
    A. A black film
    B. A clear film
    C. A mottled film
    D. No change

17. A tire track or other pattern throughout the image results from:
    A. Developer and fixer with different temperatures
    B. Bending the film
    C. Reversing the film to the beam
    D. Fluoride

18. Fluoride contamination of a film from the operator's fingers results in:
    A. White marks
    B. Black marks
    C. Generally increased density
    D. No change

19. The optimum time and temperature for hand development of film is:
    A. 3 to 4 minutes at 70° F
    B. 4.5 to 5 minutes at 83° F
    C. 4.5 to 5 minutes at 65° F
    D. 4.5 to 5 minutes at 68 to 70° F

20. To test for chemically fogged or age-fogged film:
    A. Develop the film without exposing it
    B. Develop the film after exposing it
    C. Hold the film up to a bright safelight
    D. Fix the film only
    E. C and D

21. In manual processing, the fixing time for films is usually:
    A. 5 minutes
    B. 10 minutes
    C. 15 minutes
    D. 20 minutes
    E. Dependent on the temperature

22. A radiographic film is underexposed. In manual processing, which of the following manipulations will produce diagnostically acceptable radiographs?
    A. Over-development
    B. Sight-development
    C. Treatment with Farmer's reducer
    D. None of the above

23. Which of the following are the components of Farmer's reducer that can be used to decrease the radiographic density (too dark) in a processed film?
    A. Sodium sulfite and hyposulfite
    B. Sodium sulfite and potassium ferricyanide
    C. Potassium bromide and potassium ferricyanide
    D. Sodium thiosulfate and potassium ferricyanide
    E. X-rays and duplicating film

24. Which is the hardening agent in film processing?
    A. Acetic acid
    B. Potassium bromide
    C. Potassium alum
    D. Potassium hydroxide

25. Which of the following tissues is most susceptible to radiation?
    A. Nerve tissue
    B. Muscle tissue
    C. Brain tissue
    D. Blood-forming tissue

26. Which of the following is the most radiosensitive?
    A. Young bone
    B. Nerve
    C. Muscle
    D. Reproductive organs

27. Which of the following is not a critical factor in the radiation response of cells?
    A. Cellular differentiation
    B. Size of cells
    C. Metabolic activity
    D. Mitotic rate

28. Which of the following effects can be associated with low-dose, whole-body radiation?
    A. Shock
    B. Epistaxis
    C. Epilation
    D. Leukemia

29. Relative to radiation biology, the latent period is that period between:
    A. Exposure of the film and development of the images
    B. Exposure to radiation and the appearance of clinical symptoms
    C. The states of cell rest and cell mitosis
    D. Subsequent doses of x-radiation

30. Which of the following effects is not considered to be dependent on dose rate?
    A. Death of the organism
    B. Local somatic effects
    C. Genetic effects
    D. Fetal somatic effects

31. Which of the following is the earliest clinical symptom for an individual exposed to a midlethal radiation dose sufficient to cause acute radiation syndrome?
    A. Nausea and vomiting
    B. Diarrhea
    C. Loss of hair
    D. General discomfort
    E. Fever

32. Which of the following is a unit of radiation absorbed dose expressed in joules per kilogram of irradiated tissue?
    A. Roentgen (R)
    B. Curie (Cu)
    C. Rem
    D. Gray (Gy)

33. The doubling dose is that dose:
    A. In which the LD-50 is doubled
    B. In which the rads delivered are doubled
    C. That causes a doubling of gene mutation
    D. That causes a doubling of interactions along the track of a high-speed electron

34. For dental radiography, the recommended collimation of the radiation beam of the BID at the patient's skin surface is:
    A. 2.65 inches
    B. 2.75 inches
    C. 3 inches
    D. 3.65 inches

35. A pregnant patient:
    A. Should be advised of her legal rights before being irradiated
    B. Should be warned about a possible miscarriage
    C. Should never be irradiated for dental radiographs
    D. May be irradiated for dental radiographs by taking the proper precautions

36. Which of the following reduces the radiation dose to the patient?
    A. Gonadal shields
    B. High-speed film
    C. Collimator
    D. Digital imaging
    E. All of the above

37. Which of the following is the most effective in reducing patient radiation dose?
    A. Fast films
    B. Proper collimation
    C. Higher kilovoltage
    D. Digital imaging

38. The electrons that revolve around the nucleus:
    A. Have a positive charge
    B. Have no charge; either positive or negative
    C. Have a negative charge
    D. Can be either positive or negative

39. Isotopes of an element have the same:
    A. Half-life
    B. A number
    C. Z number
    D. N number

40. The transformer used to heat the filament of the x-ray tube is:
    A. The autotransformer
    B. The step-up transformer
    C. The step-down transformer
    D. The rechargeable DC battery circuit

41. At diagnostic levels, what percentage of the electron energy is converted to x-radiation at the anode?
    A. Less than 1%
    B. 2%
    C. 10%
    D. About 98%

42. In a standard nonconstant potential machine, about 70% of the radiation in the x-ray tube is:
    A. Monochromatic
    B. Bremsstrahlung
    C. Characteristic
    D. Asynchronous

43. The substance that is the most resistant to the passage of x-rays is:
    A. Leaded glass
    B. Plastic
    C. Wood
    D. Rubber

44. X-rays are produced when:
    A. The anode is heated above 3000° C
    B. The filament becomes positively charged
    C. Electrons strike the cathode
    D. Electrons strike the anode

45. The x-ray beam of a standard nonconstant potential x-ray machine consists of photons of many different wavelengths, with the shortest wavelength photons determined by:
    A. Milliamperage (mA)
    B. Kilovoltage peak (kVp)
    C. Filtration
    D. Exposure time

46. The target material (in the anode) for dental x-ray tubes is:
    A. Copper
    B. Tungsten
    C. Lead
    D. Gadolinium

47. In a standard dental x-ray unit, the quality of x-radiation produced during the exposure is controlled primarily by:
    A. Exposure time
    B. Kilovoltage peak (kVp)
    C. Milliamperage (mA)
    D. Inherent filtration

48. In a standard AC-type x-ray machine, a 0.5 (½) second exposure would produce how many impulses of x-radiation?
    A. 5
    B. 15
    C. 30
    D. None of the above

49. To reduce the amount of heat given off during x-ray production, the source of x-ray energy is surrounded by:
    A. Copper
    B. Water
    C. Oil
    D. Lead
    E. Air

50. The number of electrons in a dental x-ray tube is determined by the:
    A. Kilovoltage used
    B. Distance between the filament and the target
    C. Step-up transformer
    D. Size of the focusing cup
    E. Low-voltage circuit

51. The efficiency of x-ray production in an x-ray generating tube (i.e., the percentage of electron kinetic energy converted to x-rays) is directly related to the:
    A. Z number of the target material
    B. Operational kVp
    C. Melting point of the target material
    D. A and B
    E. All of the above

52. Which of the following statements about radiation is true?
    A. General radiation is Bremsstrahlung radiation
    B. Bremsstrahlung radiation is the same as characteristic radiation
    C. All atoms have the same characteristic radiation
    D. Characteristic radiation is produced when cathode electrons collide with electrons of the outermost shell

53. To increase the penetrability of x-rays, their wavelength should be:
    A. Shortened by increasing the kVp
    B. Shortened by decreasing the kVp
    C. Lengthened by increasing the kVp
    D. Shortened by increasing the mA
    E. Lengthened by increasing the mA

54. In a constant potential (DC) x-ray machine, the x-ray beam is:
    A. A continuous beam of radiation
    B. A pulsating beam of radiation
    C. A pulsating divergent beam of radiation
    D. A continuous divergent beam of radiation

55. Which of the following statements is not correct?
    A. X-rays can penetrate opaque matter
    B. X-rays are differentially absorbed by matter
    C. X-rays cannot ionize gasses
    D. X-rays affect photographic film emulsion much like light

56. The number of oscillations or waves passing a point per second is known as the:
    A. Heat capacity of an x-ray photon
    B. Melting coefficient of an x-ray photon
    C. Tube capacity of the x-ray machine
    D. Frequency of an x-ray photon

57. The mean penetrability of an x-ray beam is not related to which of the following?
    A. kVp
    B. Filtration
    C. Wavelength
    D. Frequency
    E. mA

58. X-rays are a form of ionizing radiation. Ionization is:
A. The separation of the nucleus into positive and negative ions
B. Produced by photoelectric absorption only
C. Produced by the Compton effect and Bremsstrahlung only
D. Produced by photoelectric absorption and Compton scatter

59. The interaction in which the entire photon of x-radiation is removed from the beam by atomic interaction is known as:
A. The Thompson effect
B. The photoelectric effect
C. Compton scatter
D. Excitation

60. A recoil electron is produced during which of the following reactions?
A. The photoelectric effect
B. The Compton effect
C. Pair production
D. Photonuclear disintegration

61. The predominant mechanism of x-ray interaction with matter in the dental setting is:
A. Thompson (unmodified scatter)
B. Photoelectric effect
C. Compton scatter
D. Pair production

62. X-ray filters are usually made of:
A. Copper
B. Lead
C. Aluminum
D. Stainless steel

63. Collimators are usually made of:
A. Copper
B. Lead
C. Aluminum
D. Stainless steel

64. Dental x-ray machines that use 65 kVp are required to have a half-value layer (HVL) equivalent to at least:
A. 0.5 mm aluminum
B. 1.5 mm aluminum
C. 2.0 mm aluminum
D. 2.5 mm aluminum

65. The HVL is the amount of:
A. Lead necessary to absorb all of the radiation in the beam
B. Copper in the target needed to dissipate heat
C. Absorber necessary to attenuate the x-ray beam by one-half and is used to measure beam quality
D. Opening in the lead diaphragm needed to collimate the beam to its proper size
E. All of the above

66. The radiation weighting factor is used in the determination of which of the following radiation units?
A. R
B. Sv
C. Gy
D. Rad

67. The unit of x-radiation measurement that deals with the absorbed energy per kilogram of tissue is the:
A. R
B. Sv
C. Gy
D. Rem

68. A pocket dosimeter should be _____ before each use.
A. Checked for x-ray translucency
B. Sensitized with a standard radiation exposure
C. Loaded in the darkroom
D. Charged with the charging unit

69. Which of the following properties of x-rays is the basis for the rules of geometric projection?
A. X-rays travel at the speed of light
B. X-rays travel in diverging straight lines from a point source
C. The course of an x-ray photon can be diverted with an electromagnetic source
D. X-rays can form a latent image on photographic film

70. Regardless of the target-film distance, incorrect horizontal angulation will cause:
A. Elongation of the x-ray image
B. Foreshortening of the x-ray image
C. No significant change in the x-ray image
D. Overlapping of teeth in the x-ray image

71. The size of the focal spot in the x-ray tube influences radiographic:
A. Density
B. Contrast
C. Definition
D. Distortion

72. Which of the following does not control total magnification (includes penumbra) of the radiographed object?
A. Focal spot-film distance
B. Focal spot size
C. Object-film distance
D. Cathode size
E. None of the above

73. The optical density of an intraoral film indicates the:
A. Degree of darkness in an image
B. Difference between observers
C. Speed of the screens
D. Kilovoltage used
E. None of the above

74. Optical density is a function of:
    A. kVp
    B. mA
    C. mAs
    D. Exposure time
    E. All of the above

75. Subject contrast is primarily a function of:
    A. kVp
    B. kVp and mA
    C. mA
    D. kVp, mA, and exposure time

76. Fog affects the contrast of an intraoral film because it:
    A. Decreases film density
    B. Increases film density
    C. Produces white stains on the film
    D. Produces dark stains on the film

77. The primary advantage of the paralleling technique over the bisecting-angle technique is:
    A. The increased anatomic accuracy of the image
    B. The increased object-film distance
    C. The greater magnification of the image
    D. The easier handling of the long BID

78. Why is the long BID considered a necessary adjunct to the paralleling technique?
    A. To avoid magnification of the image
    B. To avoid shape distortion of the image
    C. To reduce secondary radiation
    D. To allow for easier handling
    E. To avoid superimposition of structures

79. The technique that shows the upper and lower crowns and associated alveolar bone on the same radiograph is called the:
    A. Retro-coronal technique
    B. Bitewing technique
    C. Bisecting-angle technique if a BID indicator is not used
    D. Paralleling technique if a BID indicator is used
    E. C and D

80. If a satisfactory radiograph was produced using a target-film distance of 8 inches and an exposure time of 5 impulses, what would be the correct exposure time for a target-film distance of 16 inches?
    A. 10 impulses
    B. 20 impulses
    C. ⅓ sec
    D. ½ sec
    E. B or C

81. In the bisecting-angle technique, the central ray of the beam is directed:
    A. Perpendicular to the long axis of the object
    B. Parallel to the long axis of the object
    C. Perpendicular to a line bisecting the angle formed by the object and the film packet
    D. Perpendicular to the film packet

82. Which of the following is a correct statement about intensifying screens?
    A. Thinner phosphor layers result in faster screens
    B. Thinner phosphor layers result in more unsharpness
    C. Thicker phosphor layers result in faster screens
    D. Thicker phosphor layers result in less unsharpness

83. BID (cone) cutting (partial image) on a radiograph is caused by:
    A. Underexposure
    B. Improper exposure technique
    C. A damaged BID
    D. Improper coverage of the film with the beam of radiation

84. A cassette:
    A. Emits light
    B. Is a container for films and screens
    C. Is an instrument to align the BID
    D. Records the patient's exposure

85. Intensifying screens are used with extraoral and panoramic films to:
    A. Increase the exposure time
    B. Improve image quality
    C. Decrease the radiation to the patient
    D. Increase the kVp

86. The efficiency with which film responds to x-ray exposure is known as film sensitivity or film speed. Which speed range is the best for reducing radiation to the patient?
    A. Speed B
    B. Speed D
    C. Speed E
    D. Speed F

87. A film is stripped from its packet and exposed to light. After processing it will:
    A. Be unaffected
    B. Turn clear
    C. Turn black
    D. Turn white

88. Which of the following films can be used intraorally and extraorally?
    A. Screen film
    B. Occlusal film
    C. Periapical film
    D. Bitewing film

89. Which of the following will not produce film fog?
    A. Unprotected films in the x-ray room or x-ray–equipped operatory
    B. Films stored for a long time in an unsafe place
    C. Light leaks in the darkroom
    D. Films stored in a refrigerator in the laboratory

90. Which of the following will produce film fog?
    A. Light leaks in the darkroom
    B. Films stored for a long time in an unsafe place
    C. Unprotected films in the x-ray room or x-ray—equipped operatory
    D. All of the above

91. The primary purpose of the lead foil in the back of the film packet is to:
    A. Eliminate penumbra
    B. Absorb remnant radiation after film exposure
    C. Identify film placed backward (back to front)
    D. Stiffen the x-ray packet

92. The base material used in dental films is:
    A. Sodium thiosulfate
    B. Metol
    C. Cellulose acetate
    D. Gelatin

93. Radiographic film emulsion is:
    A. Cellulose acetate
    B. Gelatin
    C. Gadolinium oxyphosphate
    D. Gelatin and silver bromide

94. Sensitization specks:
    A. Are defects in the gadolinium oxyphosphate crystals
    B. Are defects in the silver bromide crystals
    C. Act as electron traps
    D. A and C
    E. B and C

95. In hand processing, films should be washed in running water for at least:
    A. 10 minutes
    B. 20 minutes
    C. 30 minutes
    D. 40 minutes

96. What is the cause of yellow or brown stains appearing on films some time after processing?
    A. Aged film
    B. Improper exposure technique
    C. Films stored in a hot place
    D. Incomplete fixing and washing

97. The latent image consists of the accumulation of:
    A. Electrons in exposed silver bromide crystals
    B. Atomic silver at the sensitized specs
    C. Atomic silver in gelatin molecules
    D. Electrons in exposed silver bromide crystals and in gelatin molecules

98. The safety of a darkroom safelight depends on the:
    A. Distance of the safelight from the workbench
    B. Time the films are exposed to the safelight
    C. Wattage of the bulb in the safelight
    D. Speed of the film
    E. All of the above

99. Differences between manual and automatic processing include which of the following?
    A. Processing solution chemistry
    B. Solution temperature
    C. Solution concentration
    D. Time to completion of processing
    E. All of the above

100. During the processing of Insight "F"-speed film in the private dental office, which of the following is the most important source of film fog?
    A. Secondary radiation to the dental operatory
    B. Unsafe safelight
    C. Developing solutions that are too cold
    D. Use of an automatic processor

101. The theory that explains cellular damage by x-rays is the:
    A. Direct action poison chemical theory
    B. Indirect action poison chemical theory
    C. Bremsstrahlung theory
    D. Indirect nonionizing theory

102. Theoretically the biologic response to a given dose of radiation would be greater (more severe) with:
    A. The tissue being anoxic at the time of irradiation
    B. A higher dose rate
    C. A smaller area of tissue exposure
    D. Lower linear energy transfer (LET)

103. Which of the following x-ray photons (x-rays) are most apt to be absorbed by the skin?
    A. Central x-ray photons
    B. Filtered x-ray photons
    C. Long-wavelength x-ray photons
    D. Short-wavelength x-ray photons

104. The first clinically observable reaction to radiation overexposure is:
    A. Loss of hair
    B. Reddening of the skin (erythema)
    C. Cataract formation
    D. Agenesis of blood cells

105. In intraoral periapical radiography, which of the following is currently (2004) under consideration for abolition?
    A. Round, open-ended BIDs of any length
    B. ANSI "D"-speed film
    C. The protective apron for the patient
    D. None of the above
    E. All of the above

106. Ionization occurs:
    A. When atoms lose electrons; they become deficient in negative charges and therefore behave as positively charged atoms
    B. When atoms gain electrons; they become positively charged
    C. When an atom loses its nucleus
    D. Only when a K-orbit electron is ejected and replaced with an L-orbit electron

107. The structure that has a nucleus containing positive protons with surrounding orbits of one or more negative electrons is called:
    A. A molecule
    B. A neutron
    C. An atom
    D. A proton

108. Neutrons have:
    A. A negative charge
    B. A positive charge
    C. No charge
    D. A positive and a negative charge

109. The step-up transformer is used to:
    A. Step up the current to heat up the filament
    B. Allow the operator to vary the kVp
    C. Change low input voltage to high output voltage
    D. None of the above

110. If you wanted to increase the penetrating quality of the x-ray beam, what machine setting(s) would you change?
    A. Increase the mA
    B. Increase the kVp
    C. Increase the mA and the kVp
    D. Increase exposure time, mA, and kVp

111. Which of the following series indicates the correct progression of energy transformation in the production of x-ray photons?
    A. Kinetic energy, electrical energy, and radiation
    B. Kinetic energy, radiation, and electrical energy
    C. Electrical energy, kinetic energy, and radiation
    D. Electrical energy, radiation, and kinetic energy

112. Which of the following most adequately describes the radiation produced by high kilovoltage?
    A. Short wavelengths of low frequency
    B. Long wavelengths of high frequency
    C. Short wavelengths of high frequency
    D. High penetrating waves of low frequency

113. A dental hygienist wishes to change his mA from 10 to 15. If the original exposure time is 1.5 seconds, what must the new exposure time be to maintain the same density?
    A. 0.75 second
    B. 1.0 second
    C. 0.5 second
    D. 2 seconds

114. Thermionic emission is found at the:
    A. Positive anode
    B. Negative anode
    C. Positive cathode
    D. Negative cathode

115. The filament circuit in a dental x-ray tube:
    A. Requires a step-up transformer
    B. Is observed on a voltmeter
    C. Provides a cloud of electrons when the cathode is heated sufficiently
    D. Regulates the speed of the electrons

116. In a step-up transformer, the:
    A. Secondary coil has more wire turns than the primary coil
    B. Primary coil has the same number of wire turns as the secondary coil
    C. Primary coil has more wire turns than the secondary coil
    D. None of the above

117. The kilovoltage in an x-ray generating system regulates:
    A. The number of electrons produced
    B. Thermionic emission
    C. The velocity of the electrons traveling from the filament to the target
    D. The velocity of the x-ray photons produced

118. To increase the penetrability of x-ray photons, their wavelengths should be:
    A. Shortened by increasing the kVp
    B. Lengthened by increasing the kVp
    C. Shortened by increasing the mA
    D. Lengthened by increasing the mA

119. Which of the following statements about radiation is true?
    A. Electromagnetic radiation is the propagation of wavelike energy
    B. Light waves are electromagnetic radiation
    C. Radio waves are electromagnetic radiation
    D. A and C
    E. All of the above

120. Select the correct statement:
    A. X-rays cannot be focused to a point
    B. X-rays can be focused to a point
    C. X-rays cannot increase the electrical conductivity of a gas
    D. X-rays do not always travel in a straight line

121. Increased quantum energy of electromagnetic radiation is associated with increased:
    A. LET
    B. Velocity
    C. Frequency
    D. Wavelength

122. Bremsstrahlung production is:
    A. The primary source of x-ray photons in the dental x-ray tube
    B. The process by which x-ray energy is released as electrons rearrange themselves in the inner shells of an atom
    C. Important only in x-ray machines with rotating anodes
    D. Not important in the kilovoltage range below 69 kVp

123. Which of the following statements describes Compton scatter?
    A. The photon uses some of its energy to remove an electron from its orbit and then transfers the remaining energy to the electron in the form of kinetic energy that is capable of ionizing molecules
    B. The photon gives up some of its energy in ejecting an orbiting electron and is then deflected with a longer wavelength
    C. A high-energy photon passes close to a nucleus, releasing an electron and a positron. Some of the energy is used to give kinetic energy to the two particles
    D. None of the above

124. Diagnostic radiology is based on which of the following interactions of x-rays with matter?
    A. The Compton effect
    B. Coherent scatter
    C. The photoelectric effect
    D. All of the above

125. Radiopaque tissues:
    A. Absorb little of the x-rays
    B. Absorb x-rays more fully
    C. Are hollow regions
    D. Are cysts, granulomas, or abscesses
    E. None of the above

126. Which of the following statements is true regarding characteristic radiation?
    A. It is produced by the interaction of cathode electrons with target nuclei
    B. It is produced by the interaction of cathode electrons with target electrons
    C. It comprises the major component of the x-ray beam (more than 50%)
    D. A and B
    E. All of the above

127. Collimation of the beam refers to the:
    A. Selective removal of soft radiation from the beam
    B. Selective removal of hard radiation from the beam
    C. Reduction of the beam diameter
    D. Process of reducing the beam intensity by 50%

128. Filtration is used in dental x-ray machines to remove:
    A. Scatter radiation
    B. High-energy photons
    C. Long-wavelength photons
    D. Low-energy electrons

129. A lead diaphragm is used in dental x-ray machines to:
    A. Prevent Compton scatter
    B. Limit beam size
    C. Remove low-energy radiation
    D. Increase the photoelectric effect

130. Which of the following is true regarding the collimator?
    A. It is an aluminum disk with a hole in the center
    B. It has a smaller aperture for a long BID than for a short BID
    C. It removes soft radiation
    D. A and B
    E. All of the above

131. In the paralleling technique, an increased source-object distance:
    A. Prevents enlargement of the image
    B. Avoids overlapping
    C. Prevents shadows
    D. Causes blurring of the image outline
    E. None of the above

132. Which property of x-radiation must be utilized to control magnification of the radiographic image?
    A. X-rays travel in divergent paths from their source
    B. X-rays penetrate opaque objects
    C. X-rays cannot be focused
    D. X-rays cause secondary radiation when they strike the patient's face

133. An increase of which of the following factors causes an increase in subject contrast?
    A. Exposure time
    B. mA
    C. kVp
    D. None of the above

134. Increasing kVp results in:
    A. Low contrast (long scale contrast)
    B. High contrast (short scale contrast)
    C. Lighter film density (medium contrast)
    D. None of the above

135. How do you change from a low contrast to a high contrast image and still maintain density?
    A. Decrease the kVp and increase the mAs
    B. Decrease the kVp and mAs
    C. Increase the kVp and decrease the mAs
    D. Increase the kVp and the mAs

136. The localization rule whereby the lingual object follows the movement of the radiation source (tube head) is known as:
    A. Clark's rule
    B. Rapier's technique
    C. Miller's technique
    D. Richards' technique

137. The localization rule whereby the buccal object follows the movement of the tip of the BID is known as the buccal object rule, first described by _____ in 1952.
    A. Clark
    B. Rapier
    C. Miller
    D. Richards

138. The SLOB rule usually refers to _____ rule and stands for Same on Lingual; Opposite on Buccal.
A. Clark's
B. Rapier's
C. Miller's
D. Richards'

139. With the paralleling technique, it is important to use:
A. A short target film distance to avoid the loss of detail
B. A short BID to decrease magnification
C. A long target-film distance to increase magnification
D. A long target-film distance to decrease penumbra

140. In the paralleling technique, the most accurate image of a tooth is produced on the radiograph when the central ray is:
A. 30 degrees to the long axis of the tooth
B. 90 degrees to the film and the tooth
C. 90 degrees to the plane of the x-ray photon
D. 90 degrees to a plane bisecting the long axis of the tooth and the plane of the film

141. The focal spot—object distance is 8 inches, kVp is 65, mA is 10, exposure time is 12 impulses, and the resulting radiograph is acceptable. If we change the distance to 16 inches, what should the new exposure time be?
A. 3 impulses
B. 6 impulses
C. 24 impulses
D. 48 impulses

142. The "tire track" pattern appears in an image if it is:
A. Not processed properly
B. Given too much radiation
C. Not exposed to a sufficient amount of radiation
D. Placed in the oral cavity backward

143. A latent image is:
A. An image late in its formation
B. A very light image
C. Produced after exposure but before developing
D. A very dark image

144. What is the function of the raised dot embossed on intraoral film?
A. It identifies the side of the film facing the occlusal line
B. It identifies the side of the film facing the tongue
C. It identifies the side of the film facing the beam of radiation
D. It identifies the maxillary or mandibular teeth, depending on how the film is placed in the mouth

145. When the patient's lips are not kept closed during the panoramic exposure, what happens?
A. A radiolucent shadow obscures the anterior teeth
B. A radiolucent band obscures the apices of the maxillary teeth
C. A radiopaque band obscures the anterior teeth
D. No appreciable change is noted in the radiograph

146. In panoramic radiology, the collimator is:
A. A thin, narrow slit oriented in the vertical plane
B. A thin, narrow slit oriented in the horizontal plane
C. A small, rectangular aperture of the same proportions as the panoramic film
D. Similar to the rectangular collimator used with the rectangular BID

147. On a panoramic radiograph, the soft tissue of the nose appears as:
A. Bilateral radiopaque images
B. A midline radiopaque image
C. A midline real radiopaque image and bilateral ghost images
D. Bilateral real radiopaque images and a midline ghost image

148. On most newer panoramic machines, the tube head of the machine is:
A. Angled upward 4 to 7 degrees
B. Horizontal and directs the beam perpendicular to the film
C. Angled downward to avoid thick structures at the back of the head
D. Designed to adjust automatically for patient size

149. A dark shadow that obscures the apical region of the maxillary teeth in a panoramic image is usually caused by:
A. Positioning the patient too far forward
B. Positioning the patient too far back
C. The lips not being closed
D. Not having the tongue against the palate

150. In most panoramic machine designs, the one adjustment the operator can make for patient size is:
A. kVp
B. mA
C. Exposure time
D. mAs
E. Exposure cycle time

151. A single or series of dark, even, vertical radiolucent bands extending from the top to the bottom of the image is seen. This is usually caused by:
A. A cracked screen
B. A momentary obstruction of the machine by the patient
C. A defect on the rollers of the automatic processor
D. Static electricity

152. In current panoramic machines, special lights are fitted to:
A. Illuminate the patient
B. Assess proper patient exposure parameters
C. Ensure proper film density
D. Aid with patient positioning

153. Intraoral film speed is directly related to the:
A. Size of the AgBr crystals
B. Image exposure time
C. Exposure latitude
D. None of the above

154. In the darkroom, a cassette was opened to remove an exposed film. A piece of black paper was discovered on the surface of the intensifying screen. The paper would most likely produce:
    A. A white or light artifact
    B. A black artifact
    C. No artifact as the x-ray photons pass right through
    D. Black filament-like marks as is seen in intraoral films

155. Gelatin is a good radiographic film emulsion vehicle because it:
    A. Enhances contrast
    B. Is soluble in water at processing temperatures
    C. Is chemically inert
    D. All of the above

156. With the use of an automatic processor:
    A. Total darkness must be maintained in the darkroom
    B. Solutions should be kept as near to room temperature as possible
    C. Installation requires a properly designed darkroom
    D. Frequent solution replenishment is essential

157. Though rarely seen, reticulation is said to occur when the:
    A. Developer is too hot
    B. Fixer is too cold
    C. Developer and fixer temperatures differ too greatly
    D. Automatic processor needs cleaning

158. In the automatic processor:
    A. Unexposed silver salts are precipitated into the developer solution
    B. The latent image is activated by the action of the rollers in the fixer section
    C. Exposed silver salts are precipitated onto the film base
    D. Developer solution can be used for silver recovery
    E. A and D

159. In automatic processors, the daylight loader:
    A. Permits the loading of cassettes in daylight
    B. Can be contaminated by film wrappers
    C. Eliminates the need for a darkroom
    D. Requires filtration to protect film from fog
    E. All of the above

160. The normal cycle time for most automatic processing units is:
    A. 2 minutes
    B. 4 to 6 minutes
    C. About 10 minutes
    D. Significantly different for every machine

161. The rinse cycle in the water bath of automatic processors is to:
    A. Rid the film of chemicals
    B. Dissolve metallic silver
    C. Harden the emulsion
    D. There is no water bath in automatic processors

162. In manual processing, radiographs are rinsed in clean running water to:
    A. Rid the film of chemicals
    B. Dissolve metallic silver
    C. Shrink the emulsion
    D. Remove the latent image

163. The safety of safelight illumination does not depend on which of the following?
    A. Size of the darkroom
    B. Wattage of the light bulb
    C. Distance of the safelight from the work surface
    D. Duration of time the film is exposed to the safelight

164. When using the automatic processor, what is the most common cause of lost films?
    A. Mixing film up with wrappers
    B. Improper film identification
    C. Feeding bent films into the processor
    D. Combined use with intraoral and panoramic films

165. The perception of radiographic density varies inversely with the:
    A. Radiolucency of the object
    B. Quantity of silver in the radiograph
    C. Quantity of x-radiation exposing the radiograph
    D. Quantity of incident viewing light transmitted through the radiograph

166. When viewing a direct digital image on a monitor, the limiting factor in image perception is:
    A. Modified by reflected light in a dark room
    B. The quality of the original scanned radiograph
    C. The software
    D. The quality of the monitor

167. If resolution is measured in line pairs distinguishable by the eye within a millimeter of space (line pairs per millimeter, or lp/mm), what is considered as the outer limit of the eye?
    A. 6 lp/mm
    B. 10-12 lp/mm
    C. 14 lp/mm
    D. 22 lp/mm

168. In digital imaging exposure, dynamic range is best when using:
    A. Photostimulable phosphor plates (PSPs)
    B. Charge coupled device (CCD) sensors
    C. Complementary metal oxide (CMOS) sensors
    D. Film and then scanning it into the computer

169. The first "wireless" sensor in digital imaging was which one of the following?
    A. PSP
    B. CCD
    C. CMOS
    D. None of the above because all are "wired"

170. In digital radiology, "image processing" means:
    A. Using software to alter the original image
    B. Using processed film
    C. The process of capturing, storing, and archiving the image
    D. The conversion of the digital image to an analog image

171. The currently recognized official maximum permissible dose (MPD) of radiation to an occupationally exposed person is:
   A. 0.01 mSv/week
   B. 1 mSv/week
   C. 10 mSv/week
   D. 100 mSv/week

172. When a photon of x-radiation interacts with a molecule of water (H_2O) it results in the production of H^{1+} and OH^{1-}. Radiobiologically this is referred to as:
   A. Excitation
   B. Electrolyte formation
   C. Attenuation
   D. Free radical formation

173. On average, the dose rate from natural background radiation is:
   A. 0.005 mSv /year
   B. 0.05 mSv/year
   C. 0.6 mSv/year
   D. 1.3 mSv/year

174. Sievert (Sv) is a newer unit of radiation measurement. One Sv is equivalent to:
   A. 1 mrem
   B. 100 mrem
   C. 10 rem
   D. 100 rem
   E. None of the above; Svs are equivalent to rads

175. In terms of therapy, radiation is used to:
   A. Destroy tissue
   B. Increase mitotic activity
   C. Heat tissue
   D. Dehydrate tissue

176. A certain amount of radiation is needed before the clinical signs of damage to somatic cells appear. The amount of radiation after which damage can be produced is called the:
   A. Latent dose
   B. Threshold dose
   C. Maximum permissible dose (MPD)
   D. Background radiation dose
   E. Scattered radiation dose

177. As a radiation worker, you should not be exposed to more than 0.05 Sv (50 mSv) per year. But when you are a patient, you can easily receive 0.15 Sv (150 mSv) from certain types of dental radiographic procedures or an oral and maxillofacial CT scan. Which of the following statements best reconciles these contradictory statements?
   A. Any appropriate radiation dose may be given for diagnostic purposes
   B. A patient can be given any amount of radiation regardless of damage
   C. Documented exceptions recorded in the chart can be made
   D. Whole-body radiation is different from specific region radiation

178. The maximum permissible dose from diagnostic x-rays for a patient in 1 year is:
   A. 0.05 mSv
   B. 0.5 mSv
   C. 5 mSv
   D. 50 mSv
   E. Not specified

179. A dental assistant is using a radiation monitoring badge service. The service reports the badge was exposed to 0.05 mSv in the previous month. The assistant should:
   A. Stop taking x-ray films immediately
   B. Report to a radiation oncologist for a blood count
   C. Ignore the report because the reading is not significant
   D. Evaluate x-ray procedures and take steps to reduce unnecessary radiation

180. In normal dental radiographic procedures, the principal hazard to the operator is produced by:
   A. Gamma radiation
   B. Primary radiation
   C. Secondary radiation
   D. None of the above

181. Under no circumstances should the operator hold the:
   A. Film during exposure
   B. BID during exposure
   C. Patient during exposure
   D. All of the above

182. Traditionally, lead aprons are used _____, although pending federal guidelines may recommend discontinuance of their use. (This is true.)
   A. Only on women of childbearing age
   B. To reassure a pregnant patient
   C. To reduce radiation exposure to the operator
   D. On all patients

183. In a panoramic radiograph, the right premolars appear widened and are overlapped, whereas the left premolars appear narrowed with the contacts open. This indicates which positioning error?
   A. The patient was positioned too far forward.
   B. The patient's chin was tipped excessively downward.
   C. The patient's chin was tipped excessively upward.
   D. The patient's head was twisted or turned.

184. What is the most likely cause of a diffuse vertical radiopacity that obscures the center of the panoramic radiograph and gets progressively wider toward the bottom of the image?
   A. The ghost image of the spine that is not erect
   B. The ghost image of the hyoid bone
   C. The ghost image of the ramus of the mandible
   D. Movement of the patient

185. When the patient does not bite in the groove of the bite block, the most direct result would be that the patient is:
   A. Positioned in a rotated or twisted fashion
   B. Positioned with the chin too high or too low
   C. Positioned too far forward or too far back
   D. Slumped, thus producing a ghost image of the spine

186. If you are using a direct digital panoramic machine, which of the following statements is true?
    A. You can make all of the same positioning errors
    B. You cannot make darkroom errors
    C. You can immediately view the image on a monitor
    D. All of the above
    E. None of the above

187. A film-based panoramic machine may be converted to digital by:
    A. Installing a CCD sensor adaptor kit
    B. Replacing the old screen and film with a panoramic PSP in the cassette and a laser scanner
    C. A or B
    D. Neither A nor B because panoramic machines cannot be converted

188. Sensors such as the CCD and CMOS types are said to have a narrow degree of latitude with regard to radiation exposure. This means:
    A. The image size is narrower than the outside dimension of the sensor
    B. Image degradation occurs with very small increments of exposure above or below ideal
    C. Background and terrestrial sources of radiation can contaminate the image
    D. These sensors are subject to damage with excess exposure to radiation

189. "Blooming" is an undesirable image characteristic seen primarily with CCD and CMOS sensors. It results from:
    A. Sensor damage from infection control soaking
    B. Sensor protection with latex and polyethylene baggies for infection control
    C. Excessive wiping of the active side of the sensor with liquid infection control products
    D. All of the above
    E. None of the above

190. In digital imaging, "quantum noise" is:
    A. An undesirable characteristic produced by too little radiation
    B. A series of little black dots much like film fog
    C. A more significant feature of the CMOS sensor than the CCD type
    D. All of the above
    E. None of the above

191. In digital imaging, a laser scanner is needed for:
    A. PSP sensors
    B. CCD sensors
    C. CMOS sensors
    D. All of the above
    E. None of the above

192. In digital imaging, DICOM is:
    A. An abbreviation for bifunctional machines capable of standard and digital imaging
    B. A digital imaging system capable of simultaneous communication of the image to two different monitors or computers
    C. A contraction of the two Canadian codiscoverers of the CMOS sensor: Disette and Compeau
    D. A universal standard for digital imaging software

193. The intraoral digital sensor whose active portion most nearly approximates that of intraoral film is:
    A. PSP
    B. CMOS
    C. CCD
    D. None of the above
    E. All of the above

194. In a histogram stretch:
    A. The contrast histogram is shifted to the darker or lighter side of the scale
    B. The density histogram is shifted to the darker or lighter side of the scale
    C. The contrast histogram is expanded to include more shades of gray
    D. The density histogram is expanded to include more shades of gray

195. In a histogram shift:
    A. The contrast histogram is shifted to the darker or lighter side of the scale
    B. The density histogram is shifted to the darker or lighter side of the scale
    C. The contrast histogram is expanded to include more shades of gray
    D. The density histogram is expanded to include more shades of gray

196. The histogram stretch and shift are examples of:
    A. Digital image processing
    B. Ways of confusing the student
    C. Calibration tools needed for digital sensor adjustment
    D. A difference between panoramic and intraoral digital imaging

197. Which of the following statements is true?
    A. The K orbit is closest to the nucleus, and its binding energy is the lowest
    B. The M orbit is farther away from the nucleus, and its binding energy is greater than the K orbit
    C. The K orbit has the greatest binding energy
    D. The M orbit has the greatest binding energy

198. X-rays are produced at the:
    A. Filter
    B. End of the BID
    C. Cathode
    D. Anode

199. The workload, as related to structural shielding design, is a measure of the:
    A. Time during which a person to be protected is in the vicinity of the radiation source
    B. Radiation likely to be produced by an x-ray machine
    C. Time during which the radiation is directed at the barriers
    D. Parameters of the x-ray tube outside of which it will fail

200. Which of the following is not related to heat dissipation in an x-ray tube?
    A. Tube rating
    B. Duty cycle
    C. Copper block
    D. Oil around the tube
    E. Thermionic emission

201. In an x-ray generating system, turning the mA control adjusts the:
    A. Filament temperature
    B. Primary-to-secondary ratio of the step-down transformer
    C. Primary-to-secondary ratio of the step-up transformer
    D. Autotransformer

202. The instruction booklet accompanying an x-ray machine specifies that the unit should not be energized for more than 22 seconds at the maximum kVp and mA. This is referred to as:
    A. Tube rating
    B. Duty cycle
    C. Line-focus principle
    D. Workload

203. For CMOS and CCD intraoral digital radiography:
    A. Timer increments of 1/100 sec are desirable
    B. Constant potential–type x-ray machines are preferable
    C. Densitometer and sensitometer calibration are needed upon installation of the software
    D. A and B
    E. A, B, and C

204. Leakage radiation:
    A. Originates at the focal spot and leaves the tube head through the shielding
    B. Originates at the focal spot and leaves the tube head through the unleaded glass window
    C. Is the remaining radiation that passes through the patient
    D. Is the remaining radiation that passes through the walls of the x-ray room or operatory

205. In digital imaging, PSP and other sensor holders require infection control procedures because:
    A. Digital images do not require chemical processing
    B. The image can be immediately viewed on the operatory monitor
    C. The image characteristics are similar to those of film
    D. They become contaminated as part of the procedure

206. In the exposure phase of intraoral radiography, the following infection control procedures are recommended:
    A. Wrap the BID, tube head and yoke, and parts of the chair
    B. Wear gloves and use sterile BID indicators and bite blocks
    C. Isolate contaminated exposed films or PSPs to a defined area
    D. Wrap machine adjustment knobs and the exposure switch
    E. All of the above

207. In the transportation phase of the film to the darkroom or processor and of the PSP to the laser scanner, the following infection control procedures are recommended:
    A. Remove gloves and wash hands, or overglove
    B. Indicate the x-ray room is contaminated
    C. Place contaminated films inside daylight loader or bring them to processing area in the darkroom
    D. All of the above

208. In the processing phase, the films are developed or the PSPs are scanned. The following infection control procedures are recommended:
    A. Carefully shake out the films or PSPs onto a clean surface
    B. Dispose of contaminated wraps
    C. Remove contaminated gloves and wash hands
    D. Load films or PSPs into the machine
    E. All of the above

209. In the clean-up phase, the following procedures are recommended:
    A. Don gloves, throw away contaminated paper, and disinfect work area around machine
    B. Don overgloves to open darkroom door or to remove arms from daylight loader
    C. Repeat clean-up and dispose of contaminated wrap in the x-ray room
    D. Remove gloves and wash hands
    E. All of the above

210. X-rays behave a lot like light. However, they are also different in that they:
    A. Are electromagnetic radiation
    B. Have more energy
    C. Have a greater wavelength
    D. Are usually monochromatic

211. The characteristic that makes x-rays most useful in dentistry is that:
    A. They are affected by electric and magnetic fields
    B. They travel at the speed of light
    C. They penetrate opaque objects
    D. They are not differentially absorbed by matter
    E. They can be focused down to a small area

212. X-rays belong to that large group of radiations known as:
    A. Particulate radiations
    B. Hygroscopic radiations
    C. Alpha radiations
    D. Corpuscular radiations
    E. Electromagnetic radiations

213. Dense tissues:
    A. Permit the passage of x-ray photons and are radiolucent
    B. Resist the passage of x-ray photons and are radiolucent
    C. Resist the passage of x-ray photons and are radiopaque
    D. Permit the passage of x-ray photons and are radiopaque
    E. None of the above

214. The unit for measuring x-ray exposure is the:
    A. Coulomb per kilogram
    B. Rad
    C. Gray
    D. Rem
    E. None of the above

215. X-radiation is absorbed by different tissues during a diagnostic exposure. The effective dose is expressed in Sv (rems). Sieverts are calculated using:
    A. Roentgens × linear energy transfer (LET)
    B. Gy (rads) × radiation weighting factor × tissue weighting factor and summing over the tissues irradiated
    C. Gy (rads) × LET
    D. R × quality factor (QF)

216. Inside the x-ray tube, the anode is inclined at an approximately 17- to 20-degree angle to the vertical plane. This is referred to as the Benson line focus principle, which is used to:
    A. Increase the efficiency of x-ray production
    B. Serve as an x-ray focusing device
    C. Produce an effectively smaller focal spot
    D. Dissipate heat from energy conversion
    E. Immortalize Pete Benson, DDS, MS, OMF radiologist

217. In the processed radiographic image, contrast is defined as the:
    A. Differences between black and white areas of the film
    B. Overall blackening of the film
    C. Degree of overall grayness of the film
    D. Capacity to see soft tissues in the image

218. With reference to low kVp vs. high kVp, which of the following statements is true?
    A. 60 kVp produces short scale, high contrast with many shades of gray
    B. 60 kVp produces long scale, high contrast with few shades of gray
    C. 90 kVp produces long scale, low contrast with many shades of gray
    D. 90 kVp produces long scale, high contrast with few shades of gray

219. "Saturation" is an undesirable characteristic of a digital image and causes image details to "black out." Which of the following can produce "saturation"?
    A. Excessive exposure time, kVp, or mA, either singly or together
    B. Insufficient radiation exposure
    C. Software glitches
    D. Sensor exposure to water or saliva

220. In digital imaging, an 8-bit image would have how many shades of gray?
    A. 32
    B. 64
    C. 128
    D. 256
    E. 512

221. In digital imaging, some manufacturers are developing systems capable of producing 10- or 12-bit images. In normal clinical settings, what is considered the maximum number of shades of gray the eye can discern?
    A. 16
    B. 25
    C. 64
    D. 128
    E. 256

222. To view a digital image on a monitor, the software programs are designed to reject image bits that can be recognized as noncontributory, such as noise, and will display only the best _____ bits. In addition, most high-definition monitors used in dentistry are limited to displaying _____ bits.
    A. 6; 6
    B. 6; 8
    C. 8; 8
    D. 8; 6
    E. None of the above

223. To satisfy the need for accurate low increments of radiation for wired sensor digital imaging, the x-ray unit should have:
    A. Very low exposure times
    B. Exposure times in increments of 1/100 seconds
    C. A constant potential x-ray generator (constant flow of x-ray photons vs. 60 pulses/sec in traditional machines)
    D. B and C
    E. All of the above

224. The main reason for using faster films (currently speed F) in the dental office is to:
    A. Have exposures lower than digital imaging
    B. Improve image quality
    C. Decrease radiation dose to the patient
    D. Save time taking the radiographs

225. Films used with panoramic and cephalometric cassettes:
    A. Are more sensitive to x-rays than to light
    B. Are more sensitive to light than to x-rays
    C. Fluoresce by means of silver sulfide crystals
    D. Are gadolinium oxyphosphate crystals

226. In manual and automatic processing solutions, contrast in the radiographic image is enhanced by:
    A. Alum
    B. Hydroquinone
    C. Sodium acetate
    D. Sodium sulfate
    E. Sulfuric acid

227. In digital imaging, contrast may be enhanced by an image processing algorithm called:
    A. Histogram de-bit
    B. Image matrix intensification
    C. Histogram shift
    D. Histogram stretch

228. The gelatin coating on the film is softened in the developer solution by the addition of:
    A. Sodium sulfate
    B. Hydroquinone
    C. Acetic acid
    D. Potassium alum
    E. Sodium carbonate

229. When using automatic processors, a softening or swelling of the gelatin coating will cause it to stick to the rollers. Thus _____ is (are) added to the manual developer as (a) hardening agent(s) and to control swelling of the gelatin.
    A. Phosphates and sulfates
    B. Sodium carbonate and sodium sulfite
    C. Glutaraldehyde
    D. Glutamic acid and glutaraldehyde

230. In manual and automatic processing solutions, chemical fog is controlled in the developer solution by adding:
    A. Elon
    B. Acetic acid
    C. Sodium carbonate
    D. Potassium bromide
    E. Sodium sulfite

231. In manual and automatic processing, unexposed silver crystals are dissolved by _____ in the fixer solution.
    A. Acetic acid
    B. Sodium thiosulfate
    C. Sodium sulfate
    D. Potassium alum
    E. Sodium carbonate

232. In digital imaging, PSPs are manufactured with dark and pale sides. The pale side:
    A. Must be oriented toward the radiation
    B. Must be oriented toward the front of the cassette
    C. Must be oriented toward the laser beam in the scanner
    D. A and B
    E. All of the above

233. In manual and automatic processing, potassium bromide:
    A. Is an activator for reducing agents
    B. Is an activator for clearing agents
    C. Is a component of the developing solution
    D. Tends to increase chemical fog

234. In manual and automatic processing solutions, sodium sulfite is a component of the:
    A. Developing solution
    B. Fixing solution
    C. A and B
    D. None of the above

235. In manual and automatic processing solutions, which of the following requires an acid pH to function properly?
    A. Sodium thiosulfate
    B. Potassium alum
    C. Potassium bromide
    D. Sodium sulfite

236. Which of the following is a function of the rollers in an automatic processor?
    A. Transportation of film through the processor
    B. Massaging action for uniform distribution of chemicals on the film
    C. Squeegee action to remove chemicals from the film when changing baths
    D. Stirring action of solutions from roller motion
    E. All of the above

237. A panoramic radiograph on which there is an excessive "smile" line of the occlusion and streaking of the hyoid bone across the mandible indicates the:
    A. Patient was positioned too far back
    B. Patient was positioned too far forward
    C. Patient's chin was tipped excessively downward
    D. Patient's chin was tipped excessively upward

238. Infection control in panoramic radiology involves:
    A. Replacement or covering the bite block with a barrier; patient removes barrier or bite block after exposure
    B. Covering machine parts other than the bite block, and using gloves
    C. Using gloves for transporting and processing the radiograph
    D. Disinfecting contaminated machine parts after each use
    E. All of the above

239. Newer standard and digital panoramic machines can:
    A. Open the interproximal contacts like bitewings
    B. Improve resolution from the traditional 4-6 lp/mm to 9.5 lp/mm (bitewing film about 11-12 lp/mm)
    C. Project the panoramic x-ray photons perpendicular to the mandible
    D. Autocorrect for some operator errors
    E. All of the above

240. The acute radiation syndrome:
    A. Invariably results in the death of the exposed person
    B. Could be induced in a sensitive individual with a radiation dose of 50 Sv
    C. Occurs when the head and neck area is exposed to a radiation dose of 40 to 50 Sv
    D. None of the above

241. LD 50 (30d) stands for the:
    A. Dose of radiation that kills 30 experimental animals when 50 are irradiated
    B. Lethal dose to 25 out of 50 experimental animals within 30 days after an acute exposure
    C. Lethal dose to 50% of the experimental animals with the dose fractionated over 30 days
    D. Dose of radiation that results in 30 dead animals over a 50-day period

242. A radiation dose of 4 Sv (400 rem) given locally to the arm would most likely cause:
    A. Erythema
    B. Acute radiation syndrome
    C. Carcinoma of the skin
    D. Bone marrow death

243. The highest incidence of radiation-induced anomaly production occurs:
    A. Immediately after conception
    B. During organogenesis
    C. In disease-complicated aging
    D. When metabolism is reduced

244. When an x-ray photon interacts by the Compton effect, it sets in motion a high-speed electron. This reaction is called the:
    A. Target theory
    B. Threshold dose
    C. Primary interaction
    D. Recoil electron

245. In digital imaging, a computer is necessary to _____ the image.
    A. View
    B. Process
    C. Store
    D. Transmit
    E. All of the above

246. The delta ray is produced by:
    A. Interactions along a secondary track
    B. A fast-moving secondary electron moving away from the primary electron track
    C. The collision of a secondary electron with the primary track
    D. The collision of the incident photon with a secondary electron

247. The Bragg peak is an abrupt increase in the LET:
    A. Just before the fast-moving electron comes to a stop
    B. And involves a decrease in the energy transferred
    C. Measured at any point along the primary track
    D. And occurs at peak electron velocity

248. RNA differs from DNA in that it consists of a single sugar phosphate chain and that its base uracil replaces:
    A. Thymine
    B. Guanine
    C. Cytosine
    D. Adenine

249. The quality assurance procedure that checks for the integrity of the focal spot is the:
    A. Spinning top
    B. Line pair focal spot device
    C. Ionization chamber
    D. Sensitometer test
    E. Densitometer test

250. The quality assurance procedure that checks the beam to ensure it is collimated to the diameter of the open end of the BID is the:
    A. Specially designed fluorescent screen
    B. Line pair focal spot device
    C. Ionization chamber
    D. Sensitometer test
    E. Densitometer test

251. The quality assurance test that checks for the accuracy of the timer in an x-ray machine is the:
    A. Sensitometer test
    B. Densitometer test
    C. Coin test
    D. A and B
    E. None of the above

252. The acronym *ALARA* stands for:
    A. "ALArm: RAdiation" – type warning device
    B. "Alpha Long Ray Acquisition" – type tissue damage
    C. "All Low-let Radiologic Activity" resulting in tissue damage
    D. "Actual Low-dose Radiation Acceptability" for various tissue types
    E. None of the above

253. Which of the following statements is true?
    A. The spinning top can be used to check the timer accuracy of any intraoral machine
    B. Constant potential machine timers cannot be checked with a spinning top because there are no impulses.
    C. Traditional AC x-ray machines can have the timer checked with a pulse oximeter or a spinning top
    D. Constant potential machine timers are capable of small increments of pulsed radiation at intervals of 1/100 of a second

254. X-rays in the diagnostic range have a wavelength of approximately:
    A. 0.01 Å
    B. 0.10 Å
    C. 1.00 Å
    D. 10.00 Å

255. One of the easiest ways to check the integrity of the processing solutions either in manual tanks or the automatic processor is:
    A. To smell the vinegary odor of depleted solutions
    B. A daily check film
    C. To observe the accumulation of a surface scum and a soapy feeling
    D. To use one of the new electronic probes

256. Which of the following safelight filters is (are) recommended for best results with current intraoral and extraoral films?
    A. Kodak Morlite filter
    B. Kodak GBX filter
    C. Wratten 6B filter
    D. Kodak GBX II filter
    E. All of the above

257. The kVp can be measured with:
    A. An ionization chamber
    B. A pocket dosimeter
    C. A kVp meter or Wisconsin cassette
    D. A kVp meter
    E. Fluorescence of thermoluminescent dosimeters (TLDs)

258. A dosimetry badge:
    A. Is a plaque on the machine stating radiation dose specs per unit time (mR/sec)
    B. Is a wall plaque indicating x-ray doses for common examinations
    C. Is required on the machine and wall of any room with an x-ray machine
    D. Indicates operator exposure to ionizing radiation

259. The processor QA check should be done:
    A. Daily
    B. Weekly
    C. Monthly
    D. Yearly

260. Safelight integrity can be checked with:
    A. A check film
    B. The "coin" test
    C. A densitometer
    D. A colorimeter

261. The lead foil found in a typical size #2 film packet:
    A. Absorbs radiation after film exposure
    B. Adds needed weight to the film packet
    C. Is used mainly to make the film packet rigid
    D. Prevents film packet reversal
    E. All of the above

262. The smaller the focal spot or target area, the better is the radiographic:
    A. Intensity
    B. Density
    C. Contrast
    D. Detail

263. The waves of x-ray energy that are removed during filtration are characterized as:
    A. Short waves
    B. Long waves
    C. High-frequency waves
    D. Bremsstrahlung

264. Adumbration is another term for:
    A. Obscured roots
    B. The shadow usually referred to as penumbra
    C. Compton scatter effects
    D. Cervical burnout

265. Primary radiation originates from the:
    A. BID
    B. Cathode of the tube
    C. Autotransformer
    D. Anode of the tube

266. Another term for the small spot on the face of the anode where the x-rays originate is the:
    A. Focusing cup
    B. Filament
    C. Benson spot
    D. X-ray generator
    E. Focal spot

267. Limiting the size of the x-ray beam to that required to expose the film is achieved by:
    A. Collimation
    B. Filtration
    C. Absorption
    D. The BID positioning device

268. In digital imaging, a factor referring to image quality is termed spatial resolution. This factor is related to _____ and is measured in _____.
    A. Constant potential image acquisition; ergs/kg
    B. The shades of gray; bits
    C. Noise production; grays (Gy)
    D. The number of pixels in the image matrix; line pairs per millimeter (lp/mm)

269. In digital radiographic imaging, JPEG is a common term. JPEG is classified as a:
    A. Lossless compression technique
    B. Lossy compression technique
    C. Noncompressed image
    D. Type of image used in photography only

270. Image compression algorithms are used to:
    A. Improve image quality
    B. Reduce the size of the digital file
    C. Acquire the original image
    D. Create special effects like improved caries detection

271. Bridging software is often needed to:
    A. Integrate dental imaging into the paperless office
    B. Facilitate the recovery of specific image data from multiple sources such as intraoral and panoramic
    C. Render imaging sources from different manufacturers easily accessible after storage in the patient's electronic file
    D. All of the above
    E. None of the above

272. Apart from the master computer and monitors in each operatory, a server may make it possible to:
    A. Operate the wireless monitor network
    B. Operate the random access memory containing the image data
    C. Rapidly sort and recover stored image data
    D. Expand the personnel to operate the system

273. One of the differences between the CCD and CMOS sensors is:
    A. The low power requirement of the CMOS allows connection to a laptop via BUS
    B. The low power requirement of the CCD allows connection to a laptop via BUS
    C. The CCD is also known as an active pixel sensor (APS)
    D. The significantly lower noise production with the CMOS sensor

274. Digital images can be viewed for diagnostic information on:
    A. A high-resolution monitor
    B. Ink jet or laser printed photographic quality paper
    C. Dye subliminally printed acetate
    D. All of the above

275. In dental radiology, the longer the wavelength:
    A. The more penetrating are the x-ray photons
    B. The less penetrating are the x-ray photons
    C. The less absorbed are the x-ray photons
    D. The more useful is the x-ray beam

276. One geometric factor that will decrease the penumbra (increase sharpness) of the radiographic image is a:
    A. Short source-object distance
    B. Long object-film distance
    C. Short object-film distance
    D. Large focal spot

277. One geometric factor that will increase the penumbra (decrease sharpness) of the radiographic image is a:
    A. Short object-film distance
    B. Short source-object distance
    C. Long source-object distance
    D. Large focal spot

278. Using a short BID, the exposure time is 0.2 second. If the long BID is used, the exposure time becomes 0.8 second if mA and kVp are kept constant. In this scenario, the patient will receive:
    A. Less radiation dose with the short BID
    B. The same radiation dose with either BID
    C. More radiation dose with the long BID
    D. More radiation dose with the short BID

279. Which of the following demonstrates the indirect effect of x-rays on a biologic system?
    A. Chromosomal mutation
    B. Chromosomal break
    C. Enzyme inactivation
    D. Hydrogen peroxide production

280. When an exposed radiograph is placed in the developing solution:
    A. Developing time depends on the temperature
    B. The unexposed silver bromide is removed
    C. Developing time is decreased by cold solutions
    D. Developing time depends on the time needed for the image to appear

281. Which of the following film codes would you select for an adult bitewing radiograph?
    A. 1.1
    B. 1.2
    C. 2.0
    D. 2.2
    E. 3.4

282. In panoramic radiology, the usual adjustment you can make for a small person or child is to reduce the:
    A. Exposure time
    B. kVp
    C. mA
    D. All of the above

283. Traditional film-based panoramic radiographic images cannot achieve a resolution (image detail) much above 6 lp/mm. The film-based cassette capable of slightly more detail is:
    A. The soft plastic envelope
    B. The rigid metal cassette
    C. The digital cassette
    D. The soft plastic envelope with a fast screen

284. In all panoramic machines:
    A. Posterior interproximal contacts cannot be predictably opened
    B. The resolution is no better than 6 lp/mm
    C. The radiation dose is more than the full-mouth survey
    D. The exposure switch must be depressed throughout the exposure

285. In current digital panoramic radiology:
    A. The dose is about 10 times less than for the full-mouth survey
    B. Image detail approaches that of intraoral radiography (about 10 lp/mm)
    C. Few infection control procedures are needed
    D. The interproximal contacts can be opened predictably
    E. All of the above

286. In the year 2004, oral and maxillofacial radiology:
    A. Has been a recognized specialty for several years
    B. Will become a recognized specialty
    C. Will not become a recognized specialty in the near or distant future
    D. Will be merged with medical radiology by government decree

287. The most effective beam size—limiting device(s) is (are):
    A. The rectangular collimator
    B. A digital sensor
    C. A BID alignment ring
    D. Aluminum filtration
    E. All of the above

288. Proper replenishment of the solutions in the automatic processor can result in diminished patient exposure because it:
    A. Prevents overdevelopment of radiographs that are routinely overexposed
    B. Ensures a diagnostic image with minimum radiation exposure as weak developer results in light films
    C. Routinely develops films to a specific predetermined density regardless of exposure
    D. Minimizes film fog from scattered radiation

289. Which of the following factors will reduce the patient's somatic exposure by the greatest amount?
    A. Lead apron
    B. Short, pointed plastic cone
    C. Short, open-ended BID
    D. Long, round BID
    E. Long, rectangular BID

290. The amount of tissue damage after irradiation depends on:
    A.   The dose rate and intensity
    B.   The area or volume of tissue irradiated
    C.   The intensity of the exposure (chronic or acute)
    D.   The radiosensitivity of the tissue
    E.   All of the above

291. Which of the following is a major factor in reducing operator exposure?
    A.   Use high kVp because lower exposures can be used.
    B.   Use low kVp because these photons are less penetrating.
    C.   Throw away that old, pointed, plastic cone (BID).
    D.   Stand 6 feet away from the tube head and avoid the primary beam.
    E.   Have the patient wear a lead apron.

292. When x-ray photons are absorbed by silver halide crystals in the emulsion of the film:
    A.   Nothing happens to the crystal until processing
    B.   A large grain of metallic silver is formed
    C.   A minute speck of metallic silver is formed
    D.   A deposit of solid bromide initiates image formation

293. At the atomic level, x-ray photons from the dental x ray machine usually lose their energy through:
    A.   Collisions with the absorbing atom's nucleus
    B.   Collisions with other photons
    C.   The Compton effect
    D.   The photoelectric effect
    E.   The Bremsstrahlung effect

294. What is the greatest disadvantage of the bisecting angle technique?
    A.   Image distortion caused by film bending
    B.   Lack of definition in the image
    C.   Superimposition of the zygoma over the apices of the posterior maxillary teeth
    D.   Shape distortion of anatomic structures
    E.   Image magnification

295. Most genetic radiation exposure to human beings from human-made sources is the result of:
    A.   Emissions from nuclear reactors
    B.   Watching color television
    C.   Dental radiography
    D.   Medical radiography
    E.   Microwave ovens

296. In panoramic radiology, the focal trough is the:
    A.   Slit where excess radiation is filtered
    B.   Area where x-rays are generated
    C.   Zone of sharpest image detail
    D.   Area that is collimated

297. In digital imaging, the term *electron well* is used in association with:
    A.   PSP sensors
    B.   CCD sensors
    C.   CMOS sensors
    D.   The computer motherboard

298. The digital image matrix is based on a binary numbering system consisting of:
    A.   The numbers 0 and 1
    B.   Numbers to the power of 2
    C.   Rows and columns alphabetized binomially
    D.   Numbers divisible by 2

299. What is indirect digital imaging?
    A.   Image capture from a radiograph on a view box with a digital video camera
    B.   Image capture via scanner with a translucency adapter
    C.   Image capture from a film using a digital camera
    D.   None of the above
    E.   All of the above

300. What single dental x-ray system delivers the most diagnostic information to the doctor with the least patient dose, the least time and effort, the least infection control procedures, and the most patient comfort and acceptance and is available in a digital imaging format?
    A.   The constant potential intraoral x-ray unit
    B.   The constant potential intraoral unit combined with digital intraoral sensors
    C.   A multifunction, computer-operated panoramic machine
    D.   The Miles handheld, digital camera–like intraoral imaging system
    E.   You are dreaming; no such system exists!

301. In the x-ray tube, electrons are emitted from:
    A.   The target
    B.   The coil
    C.   The filament
    D.   Electrons are not involved

302. The focusing cup is usually made of:
    A.   Molybdenum
    B.   Tungsten
    C.   Hardened aluminum
    D.   Copper

303. X-rays, unlike light, do not travel very far. If you absolutely needed to stand right in front of the x-ray beam, at what distance are there no more x-rays?
    A.   3 feet
    B.   6 feet
    C.   9 feet
    D.   12 feet

304. Regarding the electrons in the x-ray tube:
    A.   Higher kilovolt settings increase the speed of the electrons striking the target
    B.   mA increases cause more electrons to boil off the filament
    C.   Increasing the exposure time causes more electrons to hit the target
    D.   All of the above
    E.   None of the above

305. Over time, and all other factors being equal, what part of the x-ray machine is the most responsible for the degradation of the image quality over time?
    A. Pitting on the focal spot
    B. Filament degradation
    C. Angular change in the target
    D. All of the above
    E. None of the above

306. Which of the following is not considered a critical organ?
    A. The brain and spinal cord
    B. Bone marrow
    C. The gonads
    D. The thyroid gland

307. A film badge:
    1. Is affected by ionizing radiation
    2. Is affected by other forms of radiant energy such as heat
    3. Should be worn by all occupationally exposed persons
    4. Was used to ID groups of films in the dark room
    A. 2 and 4
    B. 1 and 3
    C. 1, 2, and 3
    D. 1, 3, and 4
    E. All of the above

308. If you were asked what is the *one* thing that could have the greatest impact on diminishing the infection control procedures, materials, and time for dental radiology it would be:
    A. Obtain an omnifunctional pan machine capable of taking standard pans, bitewings, periapicals, and CBCT
    B. Go digital!
    C. Stick to electronic sensors as they capture directly into the computer with no need for scanning or darkroom processing
    D. Use disposable supplies and positioning instruments as they do not need disinfection

309. If a patient has routinely gagged on the bulky intraoral sensors and positioning device and has even thrown up several times, what would be the best procedure to obtain a current bitewing study?
    A. Don full protective gear with surface barriers to protect the equipment
    B. Sedate the patient
    C. Settle for only one bitewing image on each side instead of the usual two images
    D. Take a pan bitewing

310. Because all digital images are viewed in a computer screen or a monitor at a work station, the ability of the monitor to demonstrate all of the fine details in the digital image can be tested how?
    A. Purchase of a reliable brand of monitor
    B. Purchase of the most expensive brand of monitor
    C. Ask a colleague or dealer for a recommendation
    D. Test any computer screen or monitor with a specially designed SMPTE test pattern

311. When evaluating a computer screen or monitor for diagnostic quality, which of the following factors is the most important?
    A. Accuracy
    B. Contrast
    C. Detail
    D. All of the above
    E. None of the above; a special plug in the electronic device is required

312. What is the primary difference between the original USB cable connector and the USB 2 version?
    A. The newer type of plug involves less wear
    B. The USB 2 allows a faster (10×) transfer of digital data
    C. The USB 2 matches the plug design of newer computers
    D. There is no difference; it indicates newer stock

313. If a patient is positioned too far back in the machine, features of this error in the image consist of:
    A. The anterior teeth appear narrow, and the spine is superimposed on the ramus
    B. The anterior teeth are too wide, and the spine is not in the image
    C. The hard palate shadow is superimposed on the apices of the upper teeth, and the occlusal plane is flat
    D. This error is difficult to identify in the image

314. If a patient's head is twisted or turned to one side in the machine, features of this error in the image consist of:
    A. The condyles on one side are higher than the other
    B. The sinus becomes more apparent
    C. The turbinates are spread out horizontally in the sinus
    D. The teeth and ramus on one side are wider than the teeth and ramus on the other side

315. When we see a vertical radiopaque shadow in the midline of the image, the patient has been positioned:
    A. Too far forward, bringing the spine into the image
    B. With the neck in a "stooped" or nonvertical position
    C. With the chin too low, causing the neck to bend forward
    D. In the correct position, but there is severe arthritis in the cervical spine

316. If a digital panoramic image appears too dark overall:
    A. The exposure time is too high
    B. The exposure time is too low
    C. The mA is too high
    D. The mA is too low

317. When a patient is missing the upper or lower anterior teeth and does not have a prosthesis:
    A. The patient can be positioned too far forward
    B. The patient can be positioned too far back
    C. The patient can be positioned either too far back or too far forward
    D. The missing anterior teeth have no bearing on positioning

318. The single CBCT cut (slice) that can most often demonstrate the full length of the uvula is:
A. A sagittal cut
B. A coronal cut
C. An axial cut
D. Any of the above cuts

319. Turbinates are bilateral structures and they:
A. May differ in size due to location
B. May differ in size due to the "turbinate cycle"
C. May indicate an error in pan technique
D. All of the above

320. The clivus is:
A. Just beneath the pituitary fossa in a midline sagittal CBCT cut
B. A part of the cervical spine
C. Not a bone but consists of dense cartilage
D. A small bony protrusion on the heel of the foot sometimes associated with pain

321. The anterior arch is:
A. A part of the maxilla
B. A part of the mandible
C. Both A and/or B
D. A part of C1

322. It has been shown that calcifications at the carotid bifurcation can be seen in panoramic radiographs; they are most likely seen in:
A. Cases of injury to the cervical spine
B. Older patients
C. Patients with disorders of calcium metabolism
D. Patients in imminent danger of having a heart attack

323. Advantages of pan BWs:
A. They are excellent for patients with sensitive oral tissues
B. They are an option for gaggers
C. They involve fewer steps, less time, and more coverage
D. All of the above

324. If one were to compare a pan BW to a full-mouth survey, the problem(s) with the full-mouth survey is (are):
A. It may be less diagnostic as properly exposed electronic sensors do not routinely expose the tissues beyond the periapical regions
B. It is much more time consuming
C. It requires more infection control measures
D. It is much sharper, thus making it more diagnostic
E. A, B, and C only

325. If the dental office has a pan BW machine it may also be capable of:
A. Pan periapical or selected regional images
B. Cephalometric and cone beam CT imaging
C. A normal pan function but with the interproximal contacts open
D. A and B only
E. All of the above

326. The cadmium telluride photon counting (CdTePC) sensor:
A. Is a new type of intraoral sensor
B. Can be used on panoramic machines only
C. Is used for panoramic and CBCT imaging
D. In not currently used in dental imaging

327. The CdTePC sensor is capable of:
A. Lowering CBCT doses by 3 to 5 times
B. Producing both hard and soft tissue windows
C. Accurate bone density measurements
D. All of the above
E. None of the above

328. Which of the following statements is not true?
A. Large volume CBCT scans should not be used on children for orthodontic analysis
B. CBCT can be dangerous to patients with a lot of metallic restorations and appliances
C. CBCT is not generally recommended for routine endodontic procedures
D. CBCT is not affordable or advantageous for most types of dental practice
E. All of the above

329. Which of the following statements is true?
A. Some CBCT machines can be updated when new features are available
B. Sit down CBCT machines are better than those with the patient standing
C. A voxel size of 1 mm produces better images than a voxel size of 0.1 mm
D. The lowest priced CBCT machine is the best choice for most applications

330. In normal positioning for imaging the jaws, a CBCT volume of 8 mm × 8 mm × 8 mm will include in the volume:
A. Third molars in a small jaw
B. Third molars in all patient sizes
C. Third molars in most patients when they are not impacted
D. Not usually extend to the third molars

331. Beam hardening is:
A. A selectable beam quality improvement feature in CBCT
B. A low-density CBCT artifact
C. A characteristic that improves mainly detail and definition in most CBCT machines
D. A classic term associated with older CBCT machines

332. The Hounsfield number is:
A. A unit of density in CBCT and medical CT machines
B. A relative measurement in CBCT and a true value in medical CT
C. May be as accurate as medical CT only if a cadmium telluride photon counting (CdTePC) sensor is fitted on the CBCT machine
D. All of the above
E. Only A and B

333. If you are planning a CBCT scan to confirm a suspected cracked tooth you would:
    A. Select the highest resolution, even though this will increase the x-ray dose
    B. Select CBCT resolution, even though it does not affect dose but does increase scan time
    C. Select the smallest volume as this will increase the resolution
    D. Keep creating custom views through the suspected tooth until a crack can be seen

334. An important feature associated with localizing and confirming a cracked tooth is/are:
    A. A periapical radiolucency associated with the cracked tooth
    B. Evidence of trauma such as a chip in the crown
    C. Discomfort on mastication
    D. Erosion of the buccal and/or lingual alveolar cortex adjacent to the crack
    E. All of the above

335. In CBCT imaging "star" artifact is:
    A. The same as "beam hardening" artifact
    B. High density radiating lines in the CBCT volume
    C. The result of a software "glitch" in CBCT imaging
    D. Associated with older CBCT machines and the software

Radiographic Assessment and Interpretation

MULTIPLE CHOICE QUESTIONS WITH FIGURES

Instructions

Look at the illustration and read the questions carefully. The reader should be wary of selecting the longest answer or the "C" choice. On the other hand, some of the correct answers *are* the longest or "C" choice. The same letter choice may occur several times in a row. Check your selection with the correct answer in the Answer Key at the back of the book.

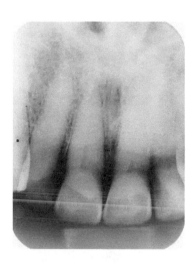

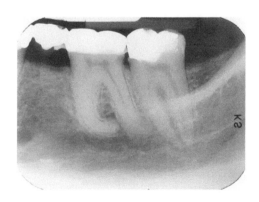

1. Select the most appropriate term for the anomaly associated with the 1st (most mesial) molar.
   A.   Diastema
   B.   Concrescence
   C.   Dilaceration
   D.   Dens invaginatus

2. This patient is a 60-year-old man with markedly shortened crowns. He does not work in an environment where particulate matter or acid-containing fumes can pollute the air. He has no known eating disorders and is healthy systemically. By what process have the crowns acquired this appearance?
   A.   Attrition
   B.   Abrasion
   C.   Erosion
   D.   Abfraction

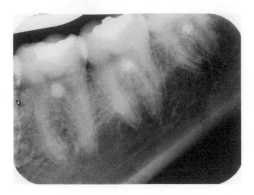

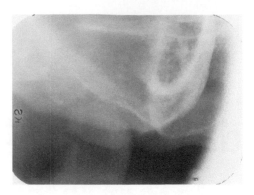

3. Observe the bifurcation area of these three molars. All have the same round, radiopaque, anomalous appearance. Note the overlap of the contacts. What term best describes this?
   A. Enamel pearl
   B. Pulp stone
   C. Buccal enamel defect
   D. "Faux" enamel pearl

5. At least two errors are in this edentulous maxillary posterior periapical view. Select the best choice.
   A. Improper horizontal and vertical angulation of the beam
   B. Excessive vertical angulation of the BID and round BID cone-cut
   C. Excessive vertical angulation of the BID and bent film in the processor
   D. Round BID cone-cut and excessive distal angulation of the BID

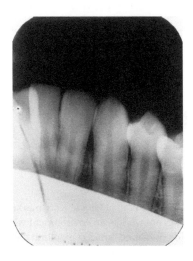

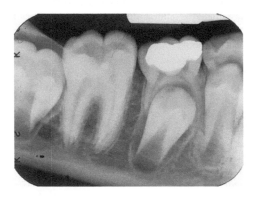

4. We can see at least two errors in this image. Which do you think they are?
   A. Rectangular BID cone-cut and film bending
   B. Rectangular BID cone-cut and static electricity
   C. Lead apron and static electricity
   D. Lead apron and film bending

6. One major error is in this radiograph. What is the cause?
   A. Foreshortening
   B. Elongation
   C. Improper horizontal angulation of the BID
   D. Excessive negative vertical angulation of the BID

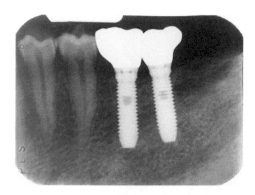

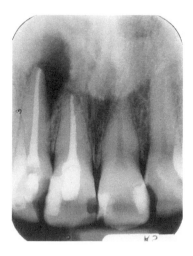

7. The correct term(s) that best describe(s) the radiopaque objects is (are):

A. Implants
B. Implants and appliances
C. Implants, appliances, and crowns
D. Screw-teeth

9. This patient first had the endodontic treatment done after a long period of abscess and fistula formation. Then the lateral incisor reabscessed and apicoectomy and curettage were done. Currently the patient is asymptomatic and clinically there is a scar, but the area appears well healed. What is your assessment of the periapical radiolucent area at the apex of the lateral incisor?

A. Recurrent abscess formation
B. Periapical cemental dysplasia
C. Surgical traumatic cyst
D. Apical scar

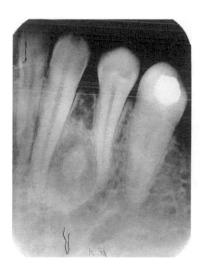

8. This patient is a 32-year-old white woman. This was the only lesion she had, and the adjacent teeth were vital. The condition we see here is:

A. Focal cemento-osseous dysplasia
B. Periapical cemento-osseous dysplasia
C. Florid cemento-osseous dysplasia
D. Ossifying fibroma

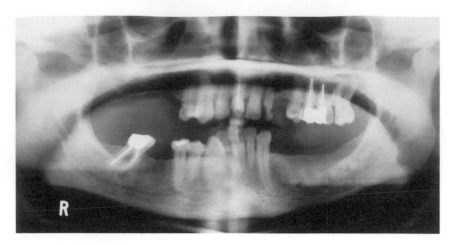

10. In this panoramic film, there are at least three positioning errors. They are:
    A. Chin too low, patient too far forward and slumped
    B. Chin too high, head twisted, and patient slumped
    C. Chin too high, patient too far back, and tongue not on palate
    D. Chin not on chin rest, head twisted, and tongue not on palate

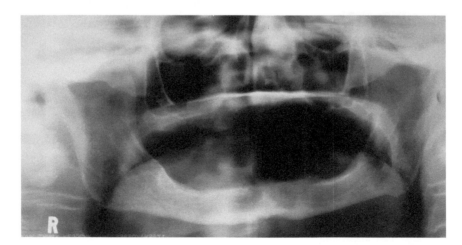

11. In this edentulous patient we can see a number of errors. The most complete and accurate list is:
    A. Chin too high, head tilted, tongue not on palate, movement, and film crimping
    B. Chin too low, head twisted, tongue not on palate, and film crimping
    C. Chin too high, head tilted, tongue not on palate, and film crimping
    D. Chin too high, head tilted and twisted, tongue not on palate, movement, and film crimping

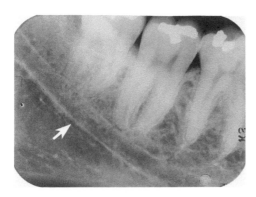

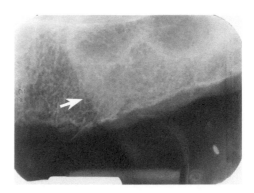

12. The arrow points to a normal anatomic structure. Which one is it?
    A. Inferior alveolar canal
    B. Posterior alveolar canal
    C. Lingual canal
    D. Mylohyoid line or ridge

14. In this edentulous patient we see an oblique shadow to which the arrow is pointing. This is:
    A. A ghost image of the ramus
    B. A bend in the film
    C. The nasolabial fold
    D. The lateral pterygoid muscle, anterior margin

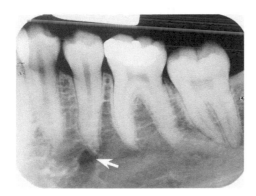

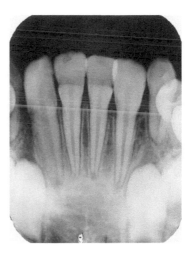

13. The 2nd premolar is vital and asymptomatic, and the patient is a black female. Identify the radiolucency to which the arrow is pointing.
    A. Periapical cemental dysplasia
    B. Periapical cyst or granuloma
    C. Mental foramen
    D. Lateral periapical cyst

15. We are interested in the central incisors of this 7-year-old boy who has had a lot of fevers during a certain period of his life. What condition affects the central incisors, and when during his life did this occur?
    A. Amelogenesis imperfecta; birth
    B. Enamel hypoplasia; first 2 years of life
    C. Dentinogenesis imperfecta; birth
    D. Amelogenesis imperfecta; first 6 months in utero

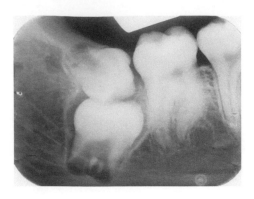

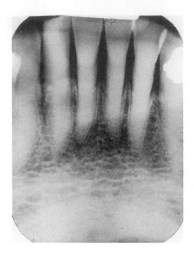

16. Here we see a very good radiograph of the 3rd molar region. List the anomalies seen in this radiograph.
  A. Impacted 2nd molar and microdontic 3rd molar
  B. Impacted 3rd molar and supernumerary 4th molar
  C. Impacted 2nd molar; microdontic, impacted 3rd molar; and dilacerated mesial root of the 2nd molar
  D. Impacted 3rd molar; impacted, supernumerary 4th molar; and dilacerated mesial root of the 2nd molar

18. This patient is a 72-year-old man. Notice that the pulp and root canal spaces are significantly diminished. What is the cause of this?
  A. Attrition and age
  B. Amelogenesis imperfecta
  C. Dentinogenesis imperfecta
  D. Dentin dysplasia type 1

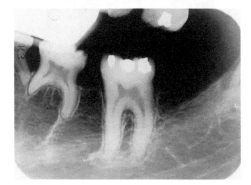

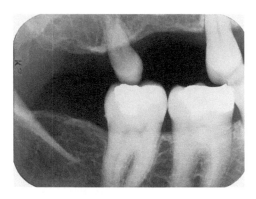

17. Notice that there are at least two, possibly three, missing permanent teeth with the retention of at least one or two primary teeth. Among the following list, what is the most likely diagnosis?
  A. Cleidocranial dysplasia
  B. Hypohidrotic ectodermal dysplasia
  C. Gardner's syndrome
  D. Cherubism

19. Observe the posterior maxillary tooth. What term(s) best describe(s) this tooth?
  A. Microdont
  B. Disto- or paramolar
  C. Macrodont
  D. A and B
  E. B and C

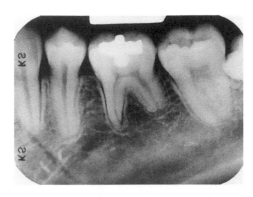

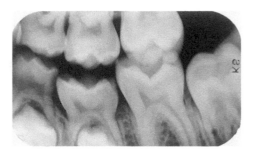

20. This young adult is missing her 1st premolars; there is also a technique error in this film. Which choice best represents this case?
    A. Bent film and foreshortening
    B. Static electricity and shovel-shaped incisor syndrome
    C. Nasolabial fold and taurodontism
    D. Bent film and orthodontic root resorption

22. Though the contacts are mostly open, what went wrong with this bitewing?
    A. Excessive positive vertical angulation
    B. Movement
    C. Excessive negative vertical angulation
    D. Nothing went wrong; it is okay

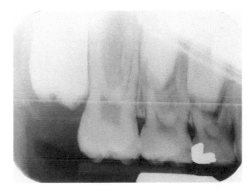

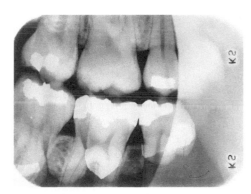

21. Two technique errors are visible in this image. Identify the cause of the two errors.
    A. Excessive positive vertical angulation and bent film
    B. Insufficient vertical film placement and rectangular BID cone-cut
    C. Insufficient positive vertical angulation and processor damage to bent film
    D. Elongation and partial image obscurity

23. Observe this radiograph. One of the other films in the series was blank. What went wrong here?
    A. Round BID cone-cut
    B. Fog
    C. Double exposure
    D. A and B
    E. A and C

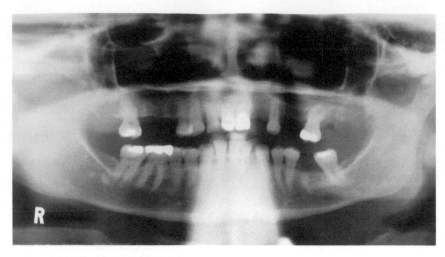

24. Note that the lips are slightly open and the tongue is not quite up against the palate; the lead apron may have ridden up very slightly on the shoulder. Several additional errors are in this panoramic radiograph. See if you can find them all.
    A. Chin too high and patient slumped
    B. Chin not on chin rest and head twisted (turned)
    C. Chin too high, patient too far back and slumped
    D. Chin too high, patient slumped, and head twisted (turned)

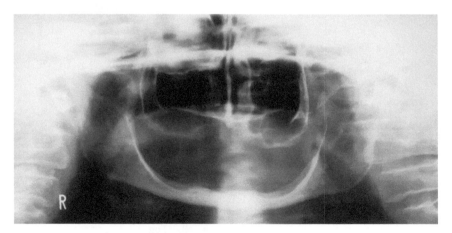

25. This patient's lips are closed (you can see them), and the tongue is against the palate. There are, however, several errors. What are they?
    A. Twisted (turned) and tilted
    B. Twisted (turned), tilted, and slumped
    C. Too far forward, tilted, and slumped
    D. Twisted (turned) and too far forward

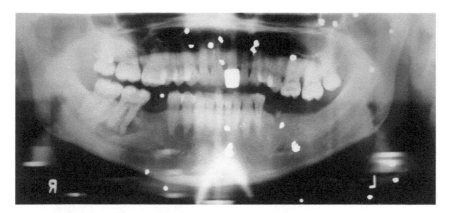

26. This patient survived a little run-in he had with Farmer Brown's shotgun. This is a bit tricky: Identify the metallic objects that have produced (a) ghost image(s).

A. Neck chain
B. Left/right markers
C. Shotgun pellets
D. All of the above

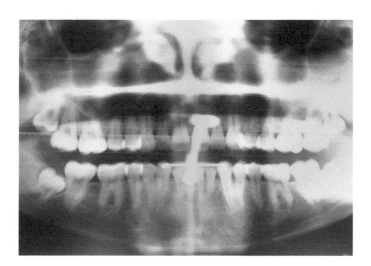

27. This radiograph has been cropped. Select the most accurate choice describing what we can see.

A. Tongue not on palate, barbell left in
B. Tongue not on palate, barbell left in, chin too high
C. Tongue not on palate, barbell left in, chin too high, patient too far back
D. Tongue not on palate, barbell left in, chin too high, patient too far back, lingual retainer

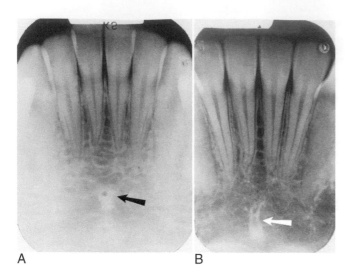

A　　　　　　　　　　　B

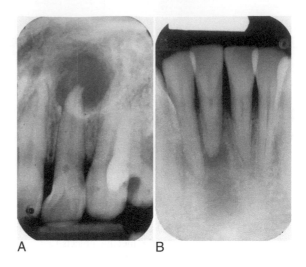

A　　　　　　　　　　　B

28. In part A, there is a black arrow, and in part B, a white arrow. Together they depict what anatomic structures?
   A. Variants of the genial tubercles
   B. Variants of the genial tubercles and the lingual foramen
   C. Lingual foramen and lingual canal
   D. All of the above

30. The maxillary lateral incisor (part A) and the mandibular central incisor (part B) both have periapical radiolucencies in this 59-year-old white man. Read the following question carefully: Select the best choice stating the nature of the periapical lesion and the one tooth with the visible cause identified.
   A. Periapical lesion of pulpal origin (abscess, cyst, granuloma) of both teeth; trauma to lower central incisor
   B. Periapical lesion of pulpal origin (abscess, cyst, granuloma) of both teeth; dens in dente maxillary lateral incisor
   C. Periapical lesion of pulpal origin (abscess, cyst, granuloma) of upper lateral; periapical cemento-osseous dysplasia of lower central incisor
   D. Periapical radiolucency of pulpal origin (abscess, cyst, granuloma) of both teeth; shovel-shaped incisor of upper lateral

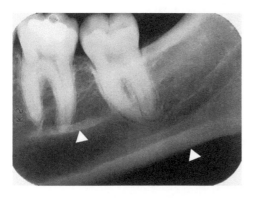

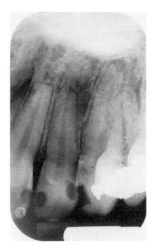

29. In this periapical radiograph, there are two white arrowheads. To what structures do they point?
   A. Inferior alveolar canal and inferior cortex
   B. Submandibular fossa and inferior cortex
   C. Inferior cortex and external oblique ridge
   D. Mylohyoid ridge and inferior cortex

31. Regarding this image, select the one most accurate choice listing what can be seen in this image.
   A. Orthodontic root resorption, radiolucent restorations, palatal torus
   B. Shovel-shaped incisor syndrome, class 3 caries, film bent and damaged in processor
   C. External root resorption, class 3 caries, palatal torus
   D. Orthodontic root resorption, radiolucent restorations, film bent and damaged in processor

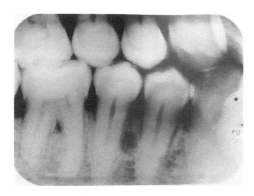

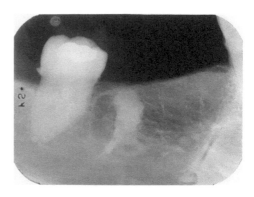

32. We are considering the radiolucent lesion between the lower premolars. Based on this radiograph, what would be your most likely clinical diagnosis before biopsy?
 A. Lateral (developmental) periodontal cyst
 B. Lateral (inflammatory) periodontal cyst
 C. Lateral radicular cyst
 D. Odontogenic keratocyst
 E. Botryoid odontogenic cyst

34. Okay, forget the bent film and chemical stains. What does the radiopaque lesion represent?
 A. Retained root tip
 B. Socket sclerosis
 C. Postextraction periapical cemento-osseous dysplasia
 D. Idiopathic osteosclerosis
 E. Parosteal osteoma

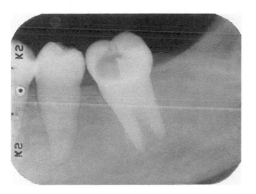

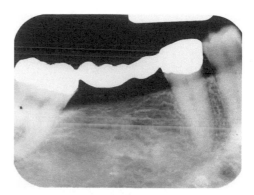

33. This patient is a 26-year-old woman with kidney disease. Note the ground-glass pattern of the alveolar bone and loss of the lamina dura. Select the most likely diagnosis.
 A. Fibrous dysplasia
 B. Primary hypoparathyroidism
 C. Secondary hyperparathyroidism
 D. Paget's disease of bone
 E. Nephrotic-induced osteoporosis

35. Observe the radiograph of this fixed 4 unit prosthesis (bridge). What material(s) is the prosthesis made of?
 A. All gold
 B. Gold with porcelain facings
 C. Gold with acrylic facings
 D. Acrylic temporary bridge

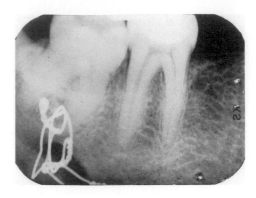

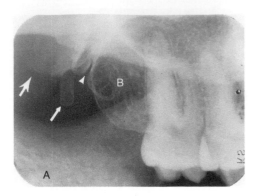

36. This patient has a history of a fractured mandible. What do you make of what we see at the apex of the 2nd (most posterior) molar?
   A. Ligature wire
   B. Ligature wire and fibrous scar
   C. Scratched film and abscessed tooth
   D. Some type of double exposure

38. First let's get oriented. Note the sigmoid notch and coronoid process of the mandible (black A) and the maxillary tuberosity (white B). Select the correct combination of answers listed from the most posterior (large arrow), the middle (small arrow), and the most anterior (arrowhead).
   A. Medial pterygoid plate, hamular process of the lateral pterygoid plate, hamular notch
   B. Lateral pterygoid plate, hamular process of the medial pterygoid plate, hamular notch
   C. Lateral pterygoid plate, hamular process of the medial pterygoid plate, pterygomaxillary fissure
   D. Lateral pterygoid plate, hamular process of the lateral pterygoid plate, pterygomaxillary fissure

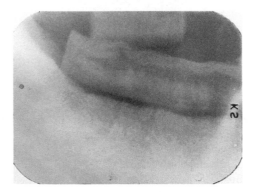

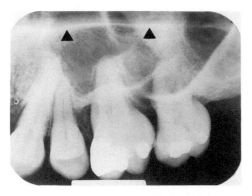

37. Name two materials associated with taking the radiograph.
   A. Bent film and fog
   B. Bite block and cotton roll
   C. Bent film and grainy image caused by depleted developer
   D. Bite block and acrylic stent for implant imaging

39. Note the many accessory canals in the lateral walls (anterolateral and posterolateral) of the maxillary sinus and the malar process of the maxilla superimposed on the 2nd molar. This question deals with only the structure indicated by the arrowheads. Select the best choice.
   A. Hard palate
   B. Floor of the nose
   C. Roof of the sinus
   D. A and B
   E. B and C

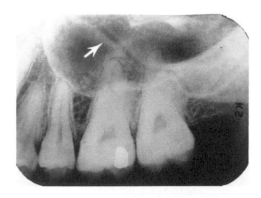

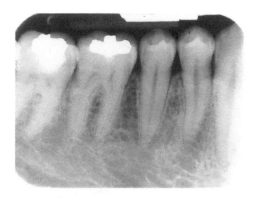

40. Look closely at the maxillary sinus. The arrow points to a radiolucent line bound by a more radiopaque line on each side that cuts diagonally across the maxillary sinus. This is:
A. The posterior superior alveolar canal
B. The roof of the sinus and floor of the nose
C. A septum of the sinus
D. A fractured sinus wall

42. For this radiograph, match the descriptive term that indicates the problem; after that, list the cause.
A. Shortened roots; orthodontics
B. Shortened roots; shovel-shaped incisor syndrome
C. Foreshortening of the roots; excessive negative vertical angulation of the BID
D. This is a problem without a cause because there is no problem or error

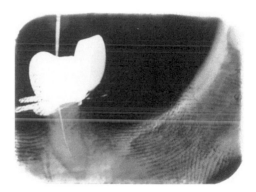

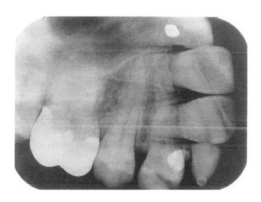

41. Because of the blackness of the fingerprints, what chemical do you think contaminated this film?
A. Fluoride
B. Developer
C. Fixer
D. Sodium thiosulfate
E. Water contaminated with developer and fixer

43. Okay, this is the one you have been waiting for. What happened?
A. Chemical stains
B. Grainy, fogged image
C. Class 4 partial denture with porcelain teeth that has become dislodged
D. Double exposure
E. None of the above

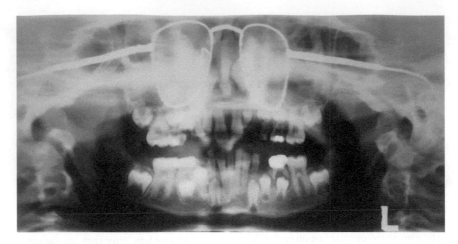

44. Oh yes, you can believe it! Stuff like this happens. Okay, select the most complete list of errors.
    A. Glasses left on
    B. Chin too high
    C. Tongue not on palate
    D. All of the above
    E. A and B

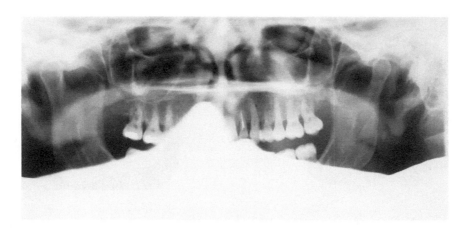

45. In spite of the fact that many of the teeth are obscured, three different errors can be noted:
    A. Apron shadow, head turned, patient too far back
    B. Large fixer stain, head tilted, patient too far back
    C. Paper in cassette, head turned, patient too far back
    D. Cassette light leak, head tilted, head turned

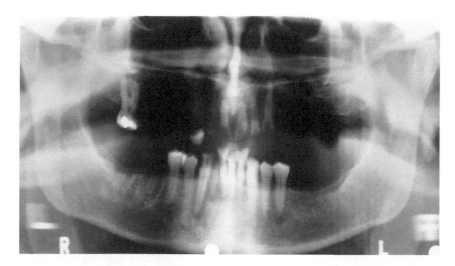

46. Read this one carefully. The patient is a middle-aged black woman. Match the radiographic findings with the associated disorder.
    A. Multiple anterior periapical radiolucencies; periapical cemento-osseous dysplasia
    B. Multiple anterior periapical radiolucencies and posterior radiopacities; florid cemento-osseous dysplasia
    C. Socket sclerosis; gastrointestinal or renal disease
    D. Multiple carious teeth; sialorrhea

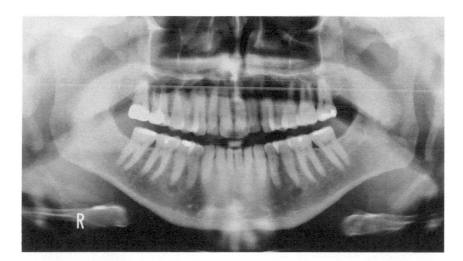

47. This patient had a tonsillectomy several years ago and has the following symptoms: a sensation like a fish bone stuck in the throat on swallowing and occasional lightheadedness when turning the head. The condition depicted here is caused by:
    A. Carotid artery calcifications
    B. Elongated styloid process and mineralized stylohyoid ligament
    C. A large bone stuck in the pharynx
    D. Falcon's syndrome
    E. Hawk's syndrome

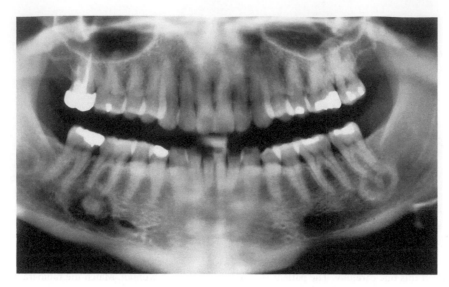

48. This patient is a 47-year-old black woman. There were some periapical radiopacities in the anterior region, which is obscured in this case. The diagnosis is:
    A. Focal cemento-osseous dysplasia
    B. Periapical cemento-osseous dysplasia
    C. Florid cemento-osseous dysplasia
    D. Chronic diffuse sclerosing osteomyelitis

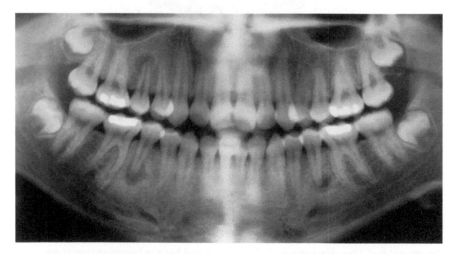

49. Amazingly, three of the four 2nd premolars were nonvital in this 14-year-old Asian teenager. All four 2nd premolars were affected by the same clinical finding. What could this be?
    A. Periapical cemento-osseous dysplasia
    B. Dentin dysplasia, type 1
    C. Deep occlusal caries
    D. Dens evaginatus

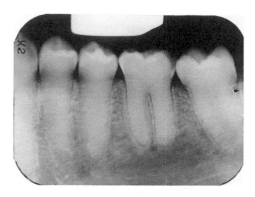

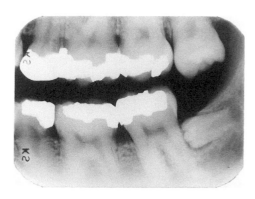

50. Observe these teeth carefully. What condition is present?
    A. Amelogenesis imperfecta
    B. Dentinogenesis imperfecta
    C. Dentin dysplasia, type 2
    D. Age-related pulp obliteration

52. Note the extruded maxillary 3rd molar. What term(s) best describe(s) the most distal mandibular tooth? Note that the 1st and 2nd molars are present and no teeth have been extracted.
    A. Distomolar
    B. Microdont
    C. Impacted
    D. All of the above

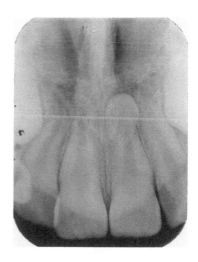

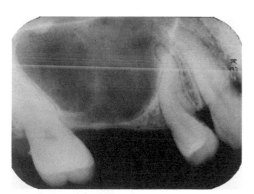

51. An anomaly is present in this patient. It is:
    A. Snow-capped tooth
    B. Periapical cemental dysplasia
    C. Rare double-crowned tooth
    D. Mesiodens

53. Note the dilacerated premolar root. The condition that affects this sinus is:
    A. Acute sinusitis
    B. Chronic sinusitis
    C. Sinus elongation
    D. Pneumatization

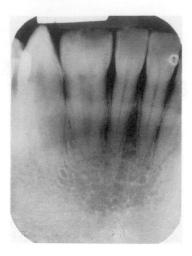

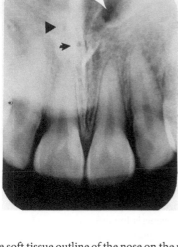

54. In this image you can see the two central incisors and a single lateral incisor. Clinically, there was a notch in the midincisal area. The problem here is:
A. Gemination
B. Fusion
C. Dilaceration
D. Twinning
E. Microdontia

56. Notice the soft tissue outline of the nose on the roots and lips at the incisal edge. We have three structures to identify here. The selections are listed from the left of the photo (large black arrowhead), middle (small black arrowhead), and right (white arrow).
A. Foramen of Scarpa, foramen of Stensen, nasal fossa
B. Foramen of Stensen, foramen of Scarpa, nasal fossa
C. Foramen of Stensen, foramen of Scarpa, superior foramen of the incisive canal
D. Foramen of Scarpa, foramen of Stensen, superior foramen of the incisive canal

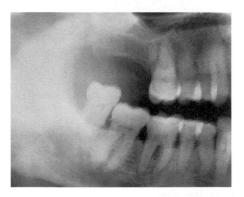

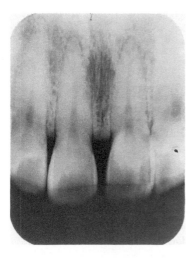

55. The maxillary 2nd and 3rd molars have been missing for several years. What has happened to the mandibular 3rd molar?
A. Partially extracted tooth
B. Dens evaginatus
C. Supraeruption (extrusion)
D. Eruption sequestrum
E. Floating tooth

57. Here we are looking at the radiolucent area between the central incisors. This is a:
A. Lateral (developmental) periodontal cyst
B. Incisive canal cyst (nasopalatine duct cyst)
C. Nasolabial cyst
D. Incisive foramen

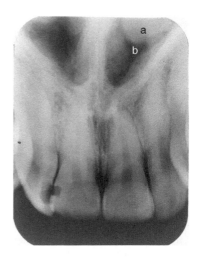

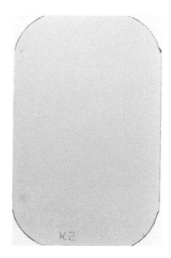

58. Here we want to identify the black letter *a* and the white letter *b*, in that order. Lastly, where are they located?
    A. Inferior turbinate, inferior meatus, nasal fossa
    B. Nasal polyp, air space, nasal fossa
    C. Palatal torus, air space, palatal and nasal fossae
    D. Soft tissue of the nose, air space, nasal fossa

60. This #1-size film was pretty well clear. What is (are) the possible cause(s) of this?
    A. Unexposed
    B. Left in fixer all weekend
    C. Fixed before developing
    D. All of the above
    E. None of the above; it is exposed to light

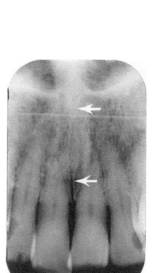

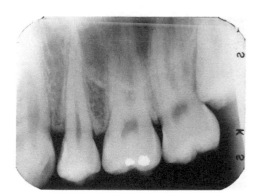

59. The top arrow points to a radiopaque structure; the bottom arrow points to a radiolucent line. The answer choices are listed from top to bottom.
    A. Anterior clinoid process; median maxillary cleft
    B. Vomer bone; median maxillary fracture
    C. Nasal bone; median maxillary cleft
    D. Anterior nasal spine; median maxillary suture

61. Here we certainly have a film placement problem, as the bottom of the film is not aligned with the occlusal plane. There is also something else that did not work out too well. What happened?
    A. Image distortion because of excessive digital pressure
    B. Inadequate positive vertical angulation of the beam
    C. Patient movement
    D. Processor damage to the image

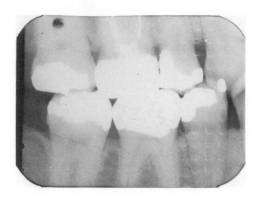

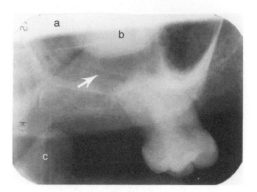

62. It was decided that this film should be retaken. Can you find the reason?
  A.   Somebody wrote on the film
  B.   Film packet was reversed
  C.   Excessive fog
  D.   Black, rectangular BID cone-cut

64. In this image, we need to identify four different entities. The choices are listed from top to bottom starting with (a), then (b), then the white arrow, and finally (c).
  A.   Bent film, turbinate, sinus septum, coronoid process
  B.   Rectangular BID cone-cut, sinus osteoma, sinus fracture, soft tissue osteoma
  C.   Rectangular BID cone-cut, palatal torus, posterior superior alveolar canal, coronoid process
  D.   Streaked fixer artifact, fingerprint with fixer, posterior superior alveolar canal, finger tip (phalangioma)

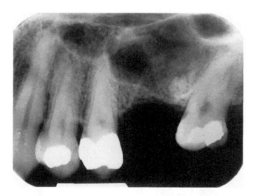

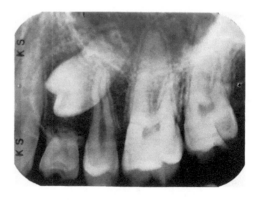

63. A small radiopaque object is in the maxillary sinus. Study the features carefully and see if you can select the correct diagnosis.
  A.   Antrolith
  B.   Antral exostosis
  C.   Retained root tip
  D.   Antral osteoma

65. The question was: "How come I have not lost my baby tooth?" Your answer:
  A.   Unerupted 1st premolar
  B.   Possible dentigerous cyst of 1st premolar
  C.   A and B
  D.   1st premolar is erupting; be patient

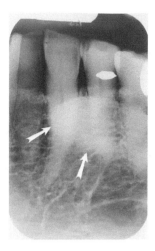

66. First, this patient's teeth are affected in a generalized way, and second, the arrows point to a good-sized radiopacity. Select the best choice.
A. Attrition, mandibular torus
B. Erosion, osteoma
C. Abrasion, large exostoses
D. Abfraction, idiopathic osteosclerosis

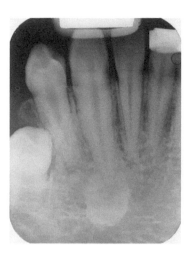

68. This patient is an 11-year-old boy; note the premolar is still erupting. What do you think the radiopacity at the apex of the canine represents?
A. Focal cemento-osseous dysplasia
B. Periapical cemento-osseous dysplasia
C. Condensing osteitis
D. Idiopathic osteosclerosis

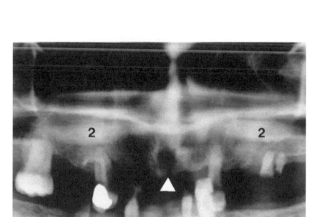

67. First, a white arrowhead is pointing to a radiolucent area in the maxilla; and second, the number 2 is seen within a radiopaque area bilaterally. Going from inferior to superior, what are the two entities?
A. Incisive foramen; ghost image of palate
B. Incisive canal cyst; palatal torus
C. Residual lateral periodontal cyst; bilateral buccal exostoses
D. Nasoalveolar cyst; bilateral mucus retention phenomena

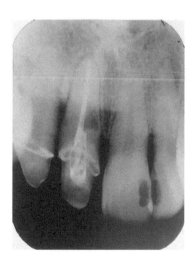

69. These teeth are restored with temporary acrylic crowns and radiolucent composite. There is a radiolucent area in the root of the lateral incisor. What does this represent?
A. Root caries
B. Internal root resorption
C. External root resorption
D. Internal/external root resorption

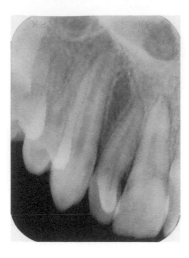

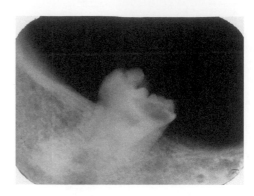

70. Study the lateral incisor. What features can you note regarding this tooth?
    A. Accessory lingual cusp
    B. Dens in dente
    C. Dilacerated crown
    D. Peg lateral
    E. All of the above

72. There's caries in this tooth; it's broken down, and you are contemplating extraction. Which one factor seen here is most likely to complicate the extraction?
    A. Ankylosis
    B. Large carious lesion
    C. Short crown length
    D. Apical osteosclerosis

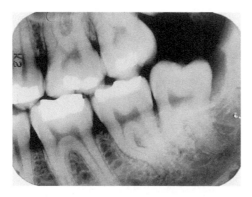

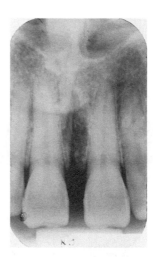

71. We are interested in the mandibular 3rd molar. Note the lesion at the distal aspect. This is consistent with a(n):
    A. Eruption cyst
    B. Inflammatory paradental cyst
    C. Periodontal pocket/abscess
    D. Normal follicular space

73. Note the anterior midline diastema. Can you identify a problem sometimes associated with the diastema?
    A. Fractured maxilla
    B. Anterior median maxillary suture
    C. Anterior median maxillary cleft
    D. Palatal orthodontic defect

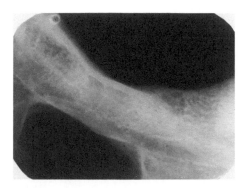

74. You are looking at the posterior mandibular region of a 67-year-old man. He is edentulous, and a full-mouth survey was done before making the new denture. He is asymptomatic and has no history of surgery. What is the problem?
    A. Deep submandibular fossa
    B. Submandibular salivary gland depression (Stafne defect)
    C. Large neuroma or neurilemmoma
    D. Large vascular lesion like an A-V malformation
    E. C and/or D

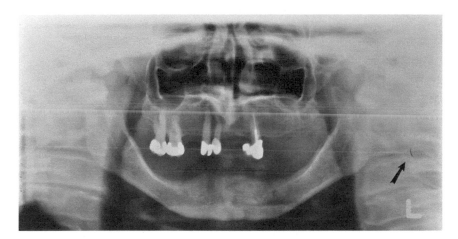

75. The black arrow points to a black, crescent-shaped radiolucent line. This is caused by:
    A. Long fingernails
    B. Static electricity
    C. Developer solution
    D. Crimping the film

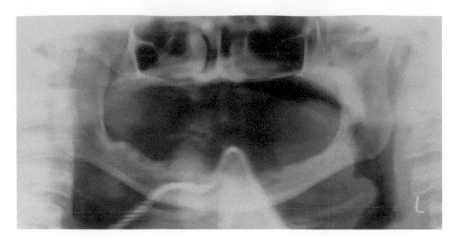

76. Okay. What was left on before taking the radiograph?
A. Napkin chain
B. Jewelry neck chain
C. A or B
D. None of the above; it was an antiswallow denture safety chain

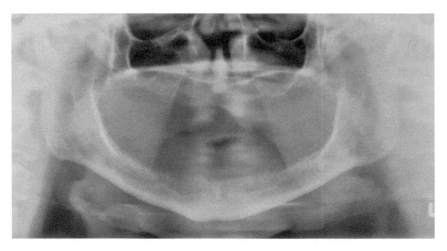

77. This film simply looks too light. The most common cause(s) of this is (are):
A. Inadequate kVp
B. Depleted developer solution
C. Failure of the autoprocessor heating element
D. All of the above

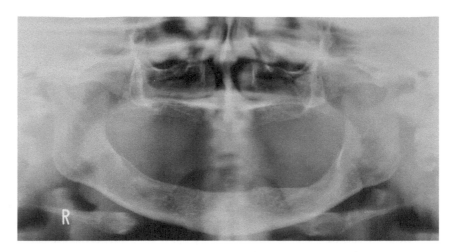

78. When you can see the turbinates spread bilaterally across the sinus and the shadow of the nose in the maxillary midline as we see here, the positioning error is:
    A. Too far forward
    B. Too far back
    C. Chin too low
    D. Slumped

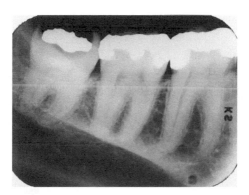

79. There is a dark shadow apical to these three molars. It is not unlike what we saw in Figure 74, yet this one is somehow different. What do you think?
    A. Submandibular salivary gland depression (Stafne defect)
    B. Submandibular fossa
    C. Corner of radiograph partially exposed to light
    D. Large periapical cyst as a result of carious 3rd molar

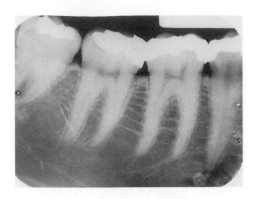

80. Although the stepladder trabecular pattern as seen here was once thought to be a sign of sickle cell anemia, this is no longer believed to be true. The trabecular pattern is, however, interesting. How would you classify this example?
A. Loose
B. Moderate
C. Heavy
D. Trabecular patterns are not classified

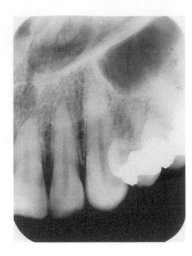

82. Here we see an anatomic landmark at the apex of the canine. It is the:
A. Maxillary sinus
B. Nasal fossa
C. Inverted "Y"
D. Ala of the nose

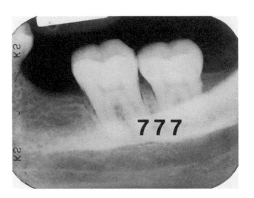

81. In this radiograph there is a large triangular radiopaque area labeled 777. (Why? …There was no "&" for the middle "7.") This area represents the radiographic confluence of two structures. Which ones are they?
A. Retromolar trigone and external oblique ridge
B. External oblique ridge and internal oblique ridge
C. Internal oblique ridge and the mylohyoid line
D. Internal oblique ridge and a deep submandibular fossa

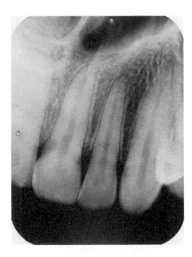

83. There is a prominent radiolucent area at the apex of the central incisor. What do you think this represents?
A. Nasal fossa
B. Superior foramen of the incisive canal
C. Periapical cyst
D. Unilateral high incisive canal cyst
E. Inferior meatus

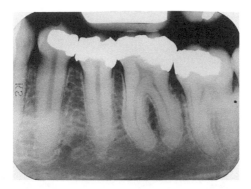

84. There are several interesting things to see in this radiograph. Notice how the root canal of the 1st premolar bifurcates and how bulbous the 1st molar roots are; but what do you see in association with the 2nd premolar?
    A. Bulbous root
    B. External resorption
    C. Hypercementosis
    D. Idiopathic osteosclerosis

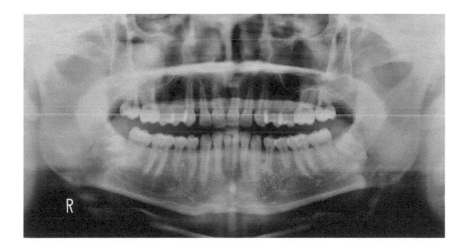

85. This panoramic radiograph is not perfect. Note how the chin is too high and the tongue not against the palate. Now take a look at the large round radiopaque area in the right maxillary sinus. WHOA!!! This is something we readily recognize in dental radiology. Do you know what it is?
    A. Mucous retention cyst (sinus mucocele, sinus pseudocyst)
    B. Periapical mucositis (odontogenic mucositis)
    C. Palatal torus (unilateral or hemisected)
    D. Osteoma (palatal or sinus)

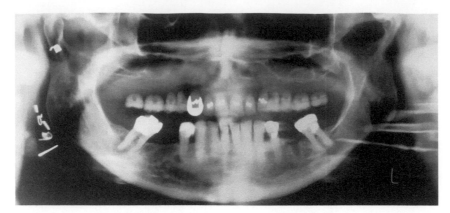

86. Jim has a scar on the right side of his neck. Here is an example of a perfectly acceptable procedure: Leave the denture in to assist positioning and to stabilize the patient. However, it looks like something else was left in or on. What is it?
    A. Some kind of earring on one ear
    B. Scratches on the film
    C. Scratched screen
    D. Vascular clamps

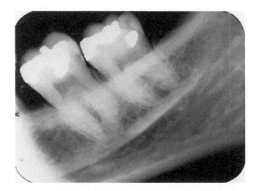

87. Yep… it's a round BID cone-cut! There are heavy radiopaque lines in this radiograph. The one at the cervical area is the external oblique ridge, and the lowest one is the inferior cortex. The opaque line crossing the apices of the molar is the:
    A. Internal oblique ridge
    B. Mylohyoid ridge
    C. A or B (terms are interchangeable)
    D. Submandibular fossa

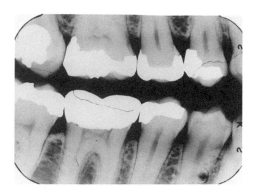

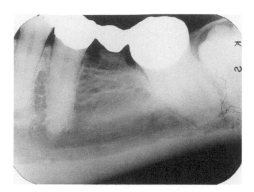

88. In this radiograph, you can see several thin, black lines on the maxillary 1st premolar and lower 1st molar. What are these?
    A. Static electricity
    B. Scratched film
    C. Fracture lines
    D. Lint contamination
    E. Fibers from the paper wrap

90. This patient has developed discomfort under the bridge. The soft tissues are red and swollen. What problem did you discover?
    A. Small osteoma
    B. Reactive subpontic exostosis
    C. Small wedged chicken bone
    D. Osteosarcoma

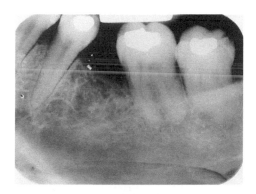

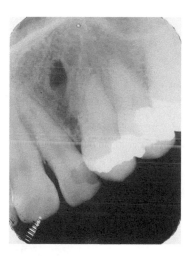

89. If you noticed the water contaminated with developer mark and the bent corner...you are catching on. If you were to look at this area of the patient's mouth clinically, what is the most significant thing you would look for?
    A. Space enough to make a bridge
    B. The angulation of the teeth regarding bridge design
    C. Whether there is caries on the 3rd molar
    D. Correlate pigmented lesion with amalgam fragments for amalgam tattoo

91. Notice the scratch made on the film by the mosquito forceps used for hand dipping. This 13-year-old female patient is asymptomatic; however, there is a scar in the region. Count the teeth. Now notice the radiolucent area distal to the lateral incisor. What do you think this is?
    A. Fibrous bone scar
    B. Globulomaxillary cyst
    C. Adenomatoid odontogenic tumor
    D. Residual cyst

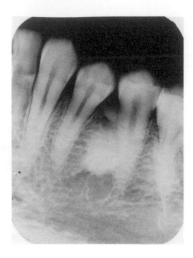

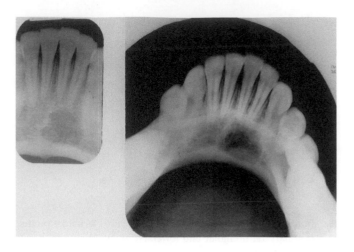

92. Here it is, plain and simple: What is the radiopacity between the premolars?
A. Osteoid osteoma
B. Osteoma
C. Mandibular torus
D. Idiopathic osteosclerosis
E. Osteosarcoma

94. This is an asymptomatic 14-year-old white female. The lesion was noted on a routine radiographic examination. All of the teeth were vital. What do you think the lesion is?
A. Developer solution artifact
B. Focal cemento-osseous dysplasia (radiolucent stage)
C. Simple bone cyst (traumatic cyst)
D. Adenomatoid odontogenic tumor
E. Primordial cyst of a supernumerary tooth

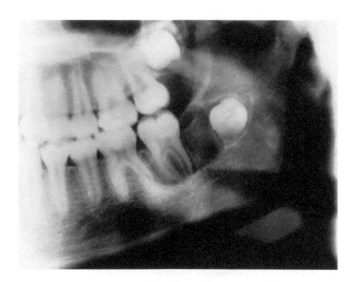

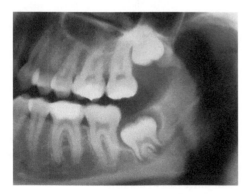

93. A deep periodontal defect was noted distal to the 2nd molar, and the lesion extended around to the buccal side. A buccal enamel spur was noted at the bifurcation of the 2nd molar. What condition do you think is present?
A. Lateral periodontal cyst
B. Botryoid odontogenic cyst
C. Inflammatory buccal cyst (inflammatory paradental cyst)
D. Eruption cyst of 2nd molar
E. Dentigerous cyst of 3rd molar

95. Look at the lower 3rd molar. We are interested in the radiolucent space around the crown. What do you think this is?
A. Normal follicular space
B. Eruption cyst
C. Dentigerous cyst
D. Inflammatory paradental cyst

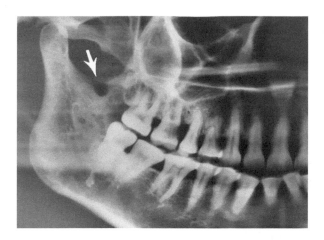

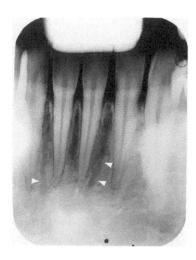

96. The arrow points to a radiolucency in the sigmoid notch area. This is:
    A. Fibrous bone scar
    B. Parotid salivary gland depression
    C. Foramen of the coronoid process
    D. Medial sigmoid depression

98. Note the prominent linear radiolucent areas indicated by the arrowheads. These are:
    A. Normal nutrient canals
    B. Abnormal nutrient canals
    C. A sign of susceptibility to destructive periodontal disease
    D. B and C
    E. Thinned radiolucent interseptal bone

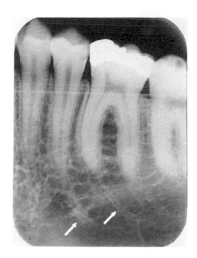

97. Yup! You can do vertical posterior periapicals, should the need arise. We are interested in the fine, thin, curved, parallel radiopaque structures indicated by the arrows. These are:
    A. A sign of a vascular lesion in the area
    B. Normal nutrient or accessory canals
    C. Abnormal nutrient or accessory canals
    D. The "wormian bone" sign

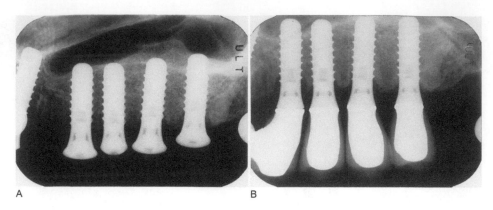

A   B

99. Parts A and B together represent an implant case. Select the most appropriate answer.
    A. Excellent osseous integration, sulcular bone breakdown
    B. Excellent osseous integration, sulcular bone normal for implants, poor crown contours
    C. Excellent osseous integration, sulcular bone normal for implants, sinus floor lift being repneumatized
    D. Excellent osseous integration, sulcular bone normal for implants, sinus floor lift being repneumatized, poor crown contours

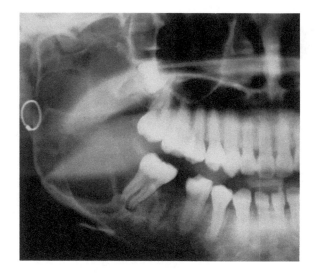

100. This is a 14-year-old female who presented with facial swelling on the right side. Select which group of three differential diagnoses would best suit this case.
     A. Ameloblastoma, mural ameloblastoma, odontogenic fibroma
     B. Ameloblastoma, central giant cell granuloma, odontogenic myxoma
     C. Mural ameloblastoma, odontogenic myxoma, odontogenic keratocyst
     D. Ameloblastoma, mural ameloblastoma, ameloblastic fibroma

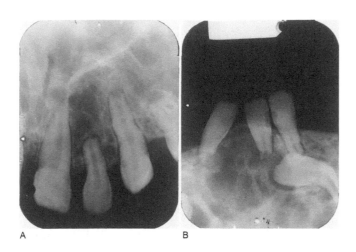

A   B

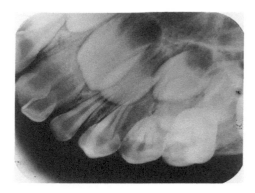

101. Parts A and B are from a 12-year-old female of Greek origin with a bilaterally swollen face. What do you think the problem is?
A. Fibrous dysplasia
B. Mediterranean anemia (thalassemia)
C. Cherubism
D. Greek restaurant syndrome
E. Maffucci's syndrome (multiple hemangiomas)

103. Assess the anterior region of this child. Select the best choice regarding the findings.
A. Supernumerary incisor
B. Possible fusion between central and supernumerary incisor
C. Lack of resorption of primary lateral apex indicates eruption problems and potential future crowding
D. A and B
E. All of the above

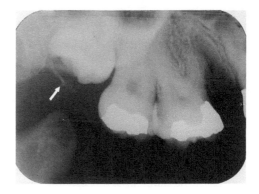

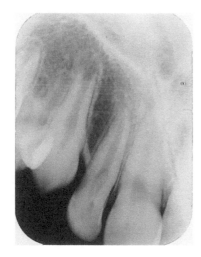

102. The arrow points to a small radiopaque bone fragment. This is:
A. A foreign body (chicken bone or similar)
B. An eruption sequestrum
C. An eruption cyst wall
D. Scratched film

104. Select the most complete answer regarding the lateral incisor.
A. Dens in dente
B. Dens in dente with enamel invagination
C. Dens in dente with enamel and dentin invagination
D. Dens in dente with enamel and dentin invagination, lingual pit
E. Dens in dente with enamel and dentin invagination, lingual pit, and possible lingual (palatal) groove

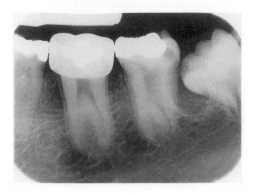

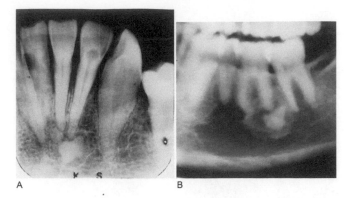

A   B

105. We are looking at the molars. Select the most complete description.
A. Taurodontism
B. Taurodontism, poorly adapted SS crown
C. Taurodontism, poorly adapted SS crown, caries
D. Taurodontism, poorly adapted SS crown, caries, lateral dentigerous cyst 3rd molar
E. Taurodontism, poorly adapted SS crown, caries, lateral dentigerous cyst 3rd molar, rule out genetic abnormality

107. Here are two areas from this 47-year-old black woman's mouth. The condition that is present is:
A. Focal cemento-osseous dysplasia
B. Periapical cemento-osseous dysplasia
C. Florid cemento-osseous dysplasia
D. Idiopathic osteosclerosis

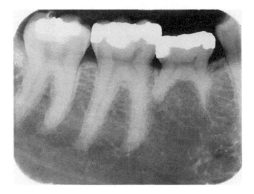

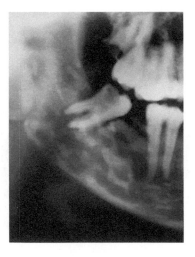

106. Assess this case regarding the retained primary molar.
A. Recognize the ankylosis and rebuild the occlusion
B. Chart the missing tooth
C. Assess the adjacent teeth for early root caries
D. All of the above
E. Leave it alone

108. This 60-year-old man is homeless and has an alcohol use disorder. He has come into the clinic with right facial swelling, pain, and several draining fistulas. The radiographic picture you see here is that of a "moth-eaten" pattern with several small bone sequestra and possibly a large radiopaque area of infarcted bone anterior to the molar. There is a faint periosteal reaction at the inferior cortex. The most likely diagnosis is:
A. Metastatic prostate carcinoma
B. Osteogenic sarcoma (lytic pattern)
C. Acute osteomyelitis
D. Chronic osteomyelitis
E. Garrè's osteomyelitis

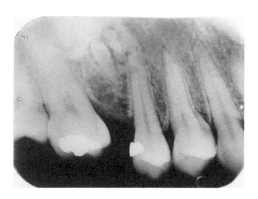

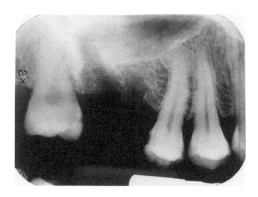

109. This patient has a finding at the apical region of the 2nd premolar. What is your assessment?
A. Compound odontoma
B. Complex odontoma
C. Idiopathic osteosclerosis
D. Dentinoma

111. What do we see at the apex of the 2nd premolar?
A. Condensing osteitis
B. Idiopathic osteosclerosis
C. Hypercementosis
D. Periapical cemental dysplasia

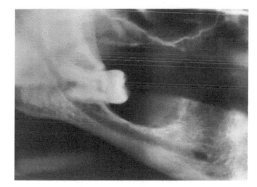

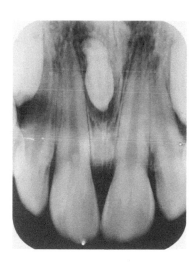

110. This patient came in stating she simply could not tolerate her old denture for another day and wanted to immediately have a new denture made. She never liked doctors or dentists and agreed to have the panoramic radiograph done only because it was "free" with the new denture. What did we discover?
A. Impacted 3rd molar
B. Impacted 3rd molar, dentigerous cyst
C. Impacted 3rd molar, infected dentigerous cyst
D. Impacted and partially ankylosed 3rd molar, infected dentigerous cyst
E. Impacted and partially ankylosed 3rd molar, infected dentigerous cyst, soft tissue swelling at crest of ridge

112. Pick out the one term that best describes the radiopacity between the roots of the maxillary central incisors.
A. Mesiodens
B. Hypodontia
C. Compound odontoma
D. Macrodont

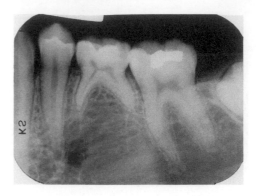

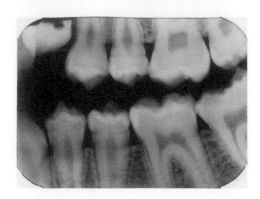

113. Assess this case regarding the retained primary molar.
   A. Recognize the ankylosis and rebuild the occlusion
   B. Chart the missing tooth
   C. Assess the adjacent teeth for early root caries
   D. All of the above
   E. Leave it alone

115. Note the occlusal anatomy of the occlusal surface of the mandibular 2nd molar that has just erupted. Now look at the maxillary 2nd premolar and the lower premolars. What is your assessment of these teeth?
   A. Enamel hypoplasia
   B. Amelogenesis imperfecta
   C. Dentin dysplasia, type 1
   D. Caries

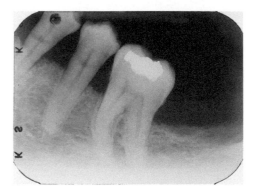

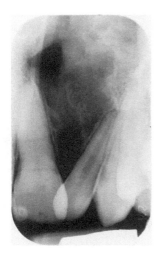

114. Note the linear horizontal radiolucent areas at the cervical aspect of the premolars. Though there is horizontal bone loss, these areas were slightly subgingival. What is your assessment?
   A. Toothbrush abrasion
   B. Abfraction
   C. Cervical caries
   D. Radiolucent cervical restorations

116. This 14-year-old patient is being worked up for orthodontic treatment. What is your assessment regarding this radiograph?
   A. Residual abscess or infection
   B. Fibrous bone scar
   C. Atypical globulomaxillary cyst
   D. Cleft palate

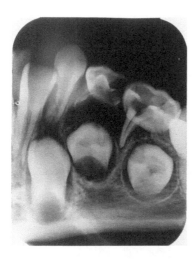

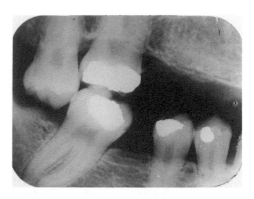

117. In your assessment of this case, you note that there is resorption of the mesial aspect of the primary canine in association with the eruption of the lateral incisor. This should be considered a sign of:

A. Normal eruption

B. Impending crowding of the permanent teeth

C. Macrodontia of the lateral incisor

D. Probable spacing between the permanent mandibular incisors

119. Okay, here it is. What is the source of this patient's pain on chewing?

A. Calculus associated periodontitis

B. Caries

C. Extrusion (supraeruption)

D. A problem not visible in this radiograph

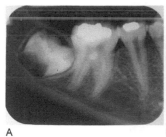
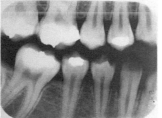

A   B

118. This is the "now you see it and now you don't" question. Notice the small round radiopacity in the furcal area of the molar in the periapical view (A). Now look at the bitewing (B) taken the same day. What is this?

A. A bitewing from another patient with similar restorations

B. A small drop of fixer in the periapical view (A)

C. The "faux enamel pearl" artifact

D. The bitewing (B) is the postoperative radiograph

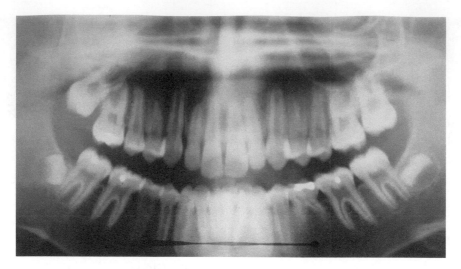

120. This 12-year-old boy has very large pulps and a systemic disorder. Select the best choice.
A.   Papillon-Lefèvre syndrome
B.   Renal osteodystrophy
C.   Vitamin D–resistant rickets
D.   Dentin dysplasia, type 2
E.   Wilson's disease

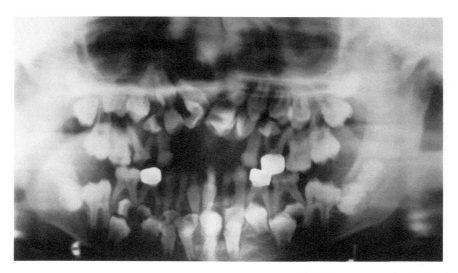

121. This is an 8-year-old girl with delayed eruption of the permanent teeth. She has other skeletal defects. What is your assessment of this case?
A.   Cherubism
B.   Cleidocranial dysplasia
C.   Gardner's syndrome
D.   Hypopituitarism

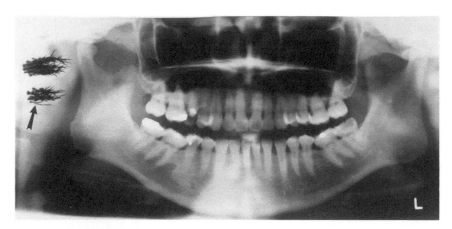

122. Note that the tongue is not against the palate, the patient is in a slumped position, and there are bilateral medial sigmoid depressions in the upper ramus. The arrow points to the area of interest. What is this?
    A. Static electricity
    B. Developer stain
    C. Light leak
    D. Scratched emulsion

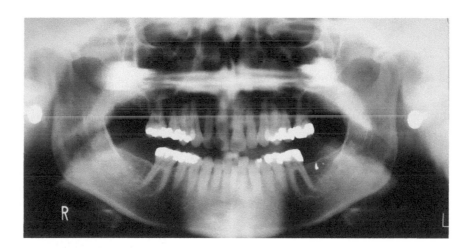

123. What was left on?
    A. Neck chain
    B. Bilateral hearing aids
    C. Bilateral earrings
    D. B and C

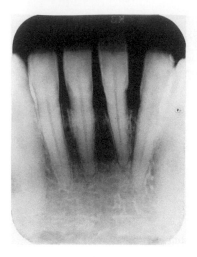

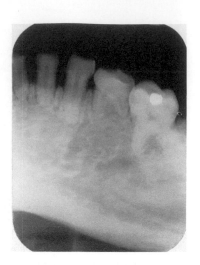

124. What error occurred in taking this radiograph?
A. Elongation
B. Lips open
C. Film on top of tongue
D. Using a #2 film in this area

125. This 18-year-old has a problem. Can you recognize what it is?
A. Microdontia
B. Hypopituitarism
C. Hypohidrotic ectodermal dysplasia
D. Agenesis of the permanent dentition

MULTIPLE CHOICE QUESTIONS WITHOUT FIGURES

Instructions

Select the correct choice and check your selection with the correct answer in the Answer Key at the back of the book.

126. Which are the most common microdontic teeth?
A. Third molars
B. Maxillary permanent lateral incisors
C. Maxillary 1st premolars
D. Primary canines

127. What is gemination?
A. The union between two separate tooth buds, usually by dentin and enamel
B. The union of the roots of two teeth by their cementum
C. The aborted attempt of a single tooth bud to divide into two teeth
D. The union of a permanent tooth bud with the roots of a primary tooth

128. What is fusion?
A. The union between two separate tooth buds, usually by dentin and enamel
B. The union of the roots of two teeth by their cementum
C. The aborted attempt of a single tooth bud to divide into two teeth
D. The union of a permanent tooth bud with the roots of a primary tooth

129. Dens in dente (dens invaginatus) is most often seen in:
A. Primary maxillary lateral incisors
B. Permanent maxillary lateral incisors
C. Permanent mandibular premolars
D. Primary mandibular molars

130. Dens evaginatus is most often seen in:
A. Primary maxillary lateral incisors
B. Permanent maxillary lateral incisors
C. Permanent mandibular premolars
D. Primary mandibular molars

131. In the hypomineralized type of amelogenesis imperfecta, an unerupted tooth may look radiographically normal. In the hypoplastic type of amelogenesis imperfecta, an unerupted tooth looks radiographically abnormal.
A. The first statement is true, but the second is false.
B. The first statement is false, but the second is true.
C. Both statements are false.
D. Both statements are true.

132. Dentinal dysplasia, type 1 has all of the following characteristics except:
A. Normal-sized crowns with normal enamel and dentin
B. Very short, blunted molar roots and short, tapered premolar and incisor roots
C. Thistle-tube pulp chambers and root canals
D. Susceptibility to early loosening, exfoliation, and idiopathic periapical radiolucencies

133. What is attrition?
A. The pathologic wearing away of tooth structure by a mechanical process
B. The physiologic wearing away of tooth structure as a result of normal mastication
C. Loss of tooth substance by a chemical process
D. Loss of tooth substance caused by hyperocclusion

134. What is abrasion?
    A. The pathologic wearing away of tooth structure by a mechanical process
    B. The physiologic wearing away of tooth structure as a result of normal mastication
    C. Loss of tooth substance by a chemical process
    D. Loss of tooth substance caused by hyperocclusion

135. What is erosion?
    A. The pathologic wearing away of tooth structure by a mechanical process
    B. The physiologic wearing away of tooth structure as a result of normal mastication
    C. Loss of tooth substance by a chemical process
    D. Loss of tooth substance caused by hyperocclusion

136. The most common supernumerary tooth is:
    A. Mesiodens
    B. Mandibular premolars
    C. Fourth molars
    D. Maxillary premolars

137. Which permanent tooth may demonstrate a wider follicular space than other teeth?
    A. Maxillary central incisor
    B. Maxillary 3rd molar
    C. Mandibular 3rd molar
    D. Maxillary canine

138. A variant of the dentigerous cyst (follicular cyst) characterized by a bluish, domelike bump on the gingiva over an erupting tooth is properly called a(n):
    A. Primordial cyst
    B. Traumatic cyst (simple bone cyst)
    C. Eruption cyst
    D. Mucous retention cyst

139. Abfraction is:
    A. The loss of tooth structure associated with traumatic occlusion
    B. The loss of tooth structure by a traumatic blow
    C. Minute craze lines seen in the enamel
    D. The root cause of the fractured tooth syndrome
    E. Abscess formation after tooth fracture

140. Hutchinson's incisors are associated with:
    A. Bertram's molars
    B. Congenital syphilis
    C. Infantile cortical hyperostosis
    D. Pyle's disease
    E. All of the above

141. The "phoenix" abscess:
    A. Arises from an asymptomatic chronic periapical infection like the mythical Egyptian phoenix arising from its own ashes in the desert every 500 years and then consuming itself in fire
    B. Was first described by a Dr. Miles Albert Phoenix, later known as a MAP lesion and eventually evolved to the term geographic abscess
    C. Was first seen among desert-dwelling Native Americans in Phoenix, Arizona
    D. Is a synonym for a Munro abscess
    E. Is probably as "mythical" as the above four choices (none of the above)

142. The most significant difference between the ameloblastic fibro-odontoma and the ameloblastic fibroma is that the ameloblastic fibro-odontoma:
    A. Occurs in an older age group
    B. Occurs in a younger age group
    C. May demonstrate radiopaque flecks
    D. Behaves more aggressively

143. What unusual feature most often characterizes the unerupted or impacted tooth associated with the calcifying epithelial odontogenic tumor?
    A. It is a 1st or 2nd permanent molar
    B. It is in an inverted position
    C. It is an anterior tooth associated with "driven snow"
    D. The crown of the tooth is partially resorbed

144. If you see a small cystlike radiolucency in the mandibular midline region of a panoramic film, what should you do next?
    A. Repeat the panoramic radiograph and see if the area can be duplicated
    B. Aspirate the area to check for vascular or cystic lesions
    C. Pulp-test all teeth in the area for vitality
    D. Take a periapical view of the area to see if the area can be duplicated
    E. A, B, and C above

145. A distinguishing characteristic of the calcification in the early-stage tooth crypt is the appearance of:
    A. Flecks, islands, or radiopacities
    B. Radiopacities resembling "driven snow"
    C. Inverted V-shaped ("circumflex" or ~-shaped) radiopacities
    D. Liesegang's rings
    E. None of the above

146. How long are postextraction sockets usually apparent on radiographs?
    A. 6 to 8 weeks
    B. 2 to 3 months
    C. 6 to 12 months
    D. 1 to 2 years

147. Focal osteoporotic bone marrow defect of the jaws occurs most often:
     A. Below the mandibular canal
     B. As an inherited trait in pale-complected females
     C. Secondary to hyperparathyroidism
     D. After tooth extraction

148. What is the radiographic appearance of the fibrous healing defect?
     A. An area of diffuse radiopacity
     B. A "punched out" or well-defined "see-through" radiolucency
     C. A radiolucency at first, gradually becoming radiopaque
     D. A radiolucency with internal trabeculations

149. A round or ovoid, well-corticated radiolucency located below the mandibular canal in the 2nd molar–ramus area is characteristic of a:
     A. Stafne defect (submandibular salivary gland depression)
     B. Residual cyst
     C. Simple bone cyst (traumatic cyst)
     D. Focal osteoporotic bone marrow defect

150. A developing tooth that undergoes cystic induction before calcification results in a(n):
     A. Dentigerous (follicular) cyst
     B. Odontogenic keratocyst
     C. Residual cyst
     D. Primordial cyst
     E. B and/or D

151. The lateral periodontal cyst tends to occur in the:
     A. Maxillary anterior area
     B. Maxillary 3rd molar area
     C. Mandibular premolar area
     D. Mandibular molar area

152. The most common developmental cyst is the:
     A. Incisive canal (nasopalatine duct) cyst
     B. Nasolabial cyst
     C. Globulomaxillary cyst
     D. Median mandibular cyst
     E. Primordial cyst

153. The simple bone cyst contains:
     A. A low, cuboidal, thin squamous epithelial lining
     B. Odontogenic epithelial lining
     C. Transitional epithelial lining
     D. No epithelial lining
     E. None of the above

154. The simple bone cyst usually affects the roots of teeth by:
     A. Causing resorption with the apices straddling the lesion
     B. Causing resorption with the apices protruding into the lesion
     C. Causing root divergence
     D. Forming a scalloped margin extending up between the roots

155. The simple bone cyst:
     A. May have a "cone" shape at its margin
     B. May have a very linear margin
     C. Has a wider dimension than the height
     D. May be seen with subtle signs of trauma
     E. All of the above

156. Which of the following conditions is considered pathognomonic?
     A. Ameloblastoma
     B. Cherubism
     C. Odontogenic keratocyst
     D. Dentigerous cyst
     E. All of the above

157. Socket sclerosis is a unique form of osteosclerosis:
     A. Seen in patients with current or past debilitating intestinal or kidney disease
     B. Where there is a lack of resorption of the lamina dura after tooth extraction
     C. That occupies only the socket area of a previously extracted tooth
     D. That is permanent once it develops
     E. All of the above

158. Stones and abdominal groans are associated with:
     A. Hypophosphatasia
     B. Hypoparathyroidism
     C. Hyperparathyroidism
     D. Fibrous dysplasia
     E. Myotonic dystrophy

159. The cyst that may be associated with a luminal radiopacity is:
     A. A residual cyst
     B. A calcifying odontogenic cyst (Gorlin cyst)
     C. A cystic odontoma
     D. B and C only
     E. All of the above

160. The radiologically evident "capsular space" is sometimes associated with:
     A. Adenomatoid odontogenic tumor
     B. Palatal pleomorphic adenoma with calcification
     C. Ameloblastoma
     D. Wall of the simple bone cyst

161. The lesion said to be attached to the root and that obliterates and/or resorbs the root(s) is the:
     A. Benign osteoblastoma
     B. Benign cementoblastoma
     C. Osteoid osteoma
     D. Aggressive ossifying fibroma

162. Myospherulosis:
     A. Is a developmental anomaly of marrow cells
     B. Is associated with the use of petrolatum jelly
     C. Is associated with the bone marrow effects of sickle cell anemia
     D. Is a type of fungal infection of bone most common in South America

163. Neuralgia-inducing cavitational osteopathosis (NICO) is a painful condition that may be associated with:
    A. A localized area of osteoporotic bone with vertically oriented lamina dura residues
    B. An area demonstrating radiolucent and radiopaque components
    C. A "bull's eye" lesion with a radiopaque center surrounded by a radiolucent ring and a radiopaque margin
    D. A "hot spot" with a technetium scan
    E. All of the above

164. The clinical impression of amalgam tattoo can be confirmed by:
    A. A lack of blanching on diascopy
    B. Noting a radiopaque metal fragment radiographically
    C. Biopsy
    D. B and C above
    E. All of the above

165. Taurodontism may be associated with:
    A. Amelogenesis imperfecta
    B. Down's syndrome
    C. Klinefelter's syndrome
    D. Osteoporosis
    E. All of the above

166. In ankylosis there is:
    A. A lack of a defined periodontal membrane space
    B. No lamina dura
    C. Regional sclerotic change resembling osteosclerosis
    D. A dull ringing sound in the ears
    E. Almost always external resorption

167. The term *antral pseudocyst* has now replaced the former appellation (mucous retention cyst) primarily because:
    A. Pathologists like to change the names of diseases from time to time
    B. The lesion contains a serous, not mucous, fluid beneath elevated sinus mucosa
    C. There is no epithelial lining
    D. Most lesions consist of solid soft tissue polyps

168. The lesion that is named after the "blown out" appearance of the bone is:
    A. A blow-out fracture
    B. Reactive proliferative periostitis (Garrè's osteomyelitis)
    C. Ameloblastoma
    D. Aneurysmal bone cyst

169. Which of the following cystic lesions is often multilocular radiologically and also multinodular grossly?
    A. Odontogenic keratocyst
    B. Botryoid odontogenic cyst
    C. Primordial cyst
    D. A and C
    E. None of the above

170. Cervical enamel extensions are associated with:
    A. The buccal bifurcation cyst
    B. Mainly primary molars
    C. Enamel pearls
    D. Amelogenesis imperfecta

171. Radiologically, a tooth in hyperocclusion may demonstrate:
    A. Hypercementosis
    B. Abfraction
    C. Widened periodontal membrane space
    D. Widened lamina dura
    E. All of the above

172. In Eagle's syndrome, the patient often has had a previous tonsillectomy and current pain on swallowing. Radiographically, we see:
    A. Nonspecific calcification in the carotid region
    B. Calcification in the tonsillar fossa
    C. Elongation of the styloid process
    D. Elongation of the styloid process and/or mineralization of the stylohyoid ligament complex
    E. All of the above

173. Histologically, which radiologic lesion has tissue very similar to brown tumor:
    A. Central giant cell granuloma
    B. Periapical granuloma
    C. Cherubism
    D. Aneurysmal bone cyst
    E. A and C

174. The lesion characterized as having a "tennis racket" or geometric pattern of bone destruction is:
    A. Multiple myeloma
    B. Fibrous dysplasia affecting the cranial vault
    C. Paget's disease affecting the cranial vault
    D. Odontogenic myxoma

175. In the nevoid basal cell carcinoma syndrome, the odontogenic keratocysts (OKCs):
    A. Recur with greater frequency than other OKCs
    B. Are greater in numbers but recur less frequently than other OKCs
    C. Are similar in number and behavior to other OKCs
    D. Are different in that the keratin is orthokeratinized
    E. Are greater in number but similar in behavior to other OKCs

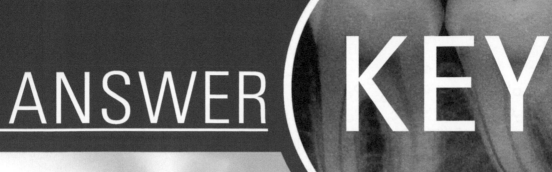

ANSWER KEY

PART 1
Chapter 1

MULTIPLE CHOICE QUESTIONS WITH FIGURES

FIGURE 1-1

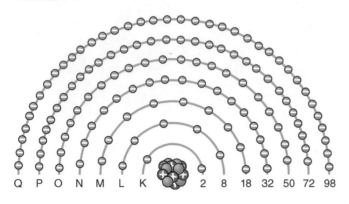

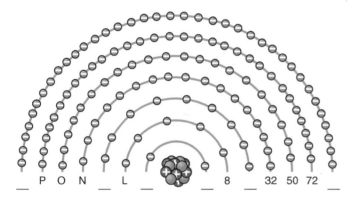

1. B. The Q shell is outermost and has 98 electrons
2. C. Protons and neutrons
3. C. Greatest for the K shell

FIGURE 1-2

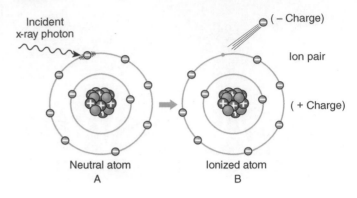

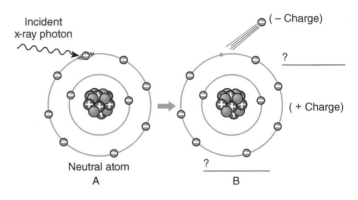

1. B. This reaction is called decay
2. D. The free electron and the positively charged atom

FIGURE 1-3

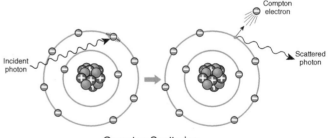

Compton Scattering

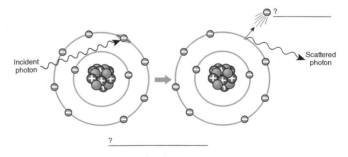

1. A. This reaction is called Compton scattering

FIGURE 1-4

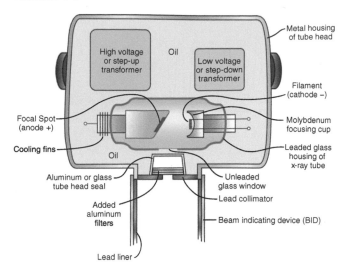

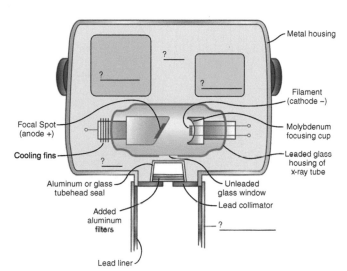

FIGURE 1-5

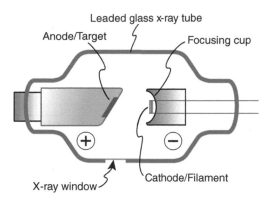

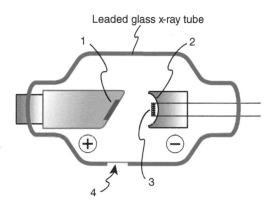

1. D. Anode/target, focusing cup, cathode/filament, window/aperture

1. D. Tube head
2. D. Step-up and step-down transformers, x-ray tube, and oil
3. D. All of the above

FIGURE 1-6

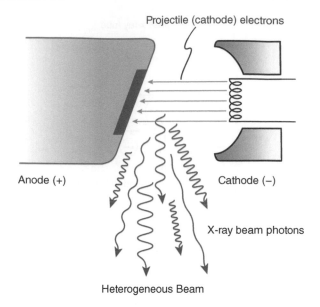

Projectile (cathode) electrons

Anode (+)

Cathode (−)

X-ray beam photons

Heterogeneous Beam

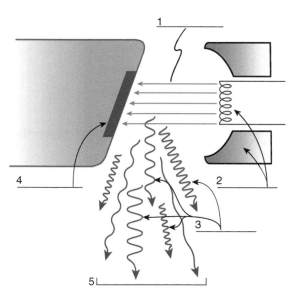

1. D. 1. Electrons, 2. focusing cup and cathode (−), 3. X-ray photons of different wavelengths, 4. Anode (+), 5. heterogeneous x-ray beam

FIGURE 1-7

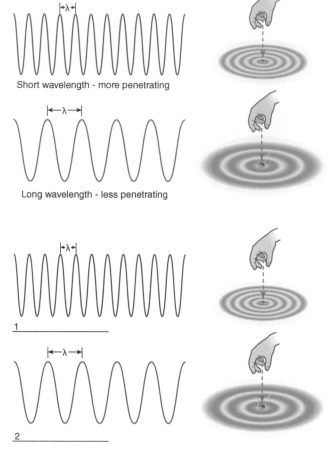

Short wavelength - more penetrating

Long wavelength - less penetrating

1. D. Lambda
2. A. The wavelength
3. D. All of the above
4. D. All of the above

FIGURE 1-8

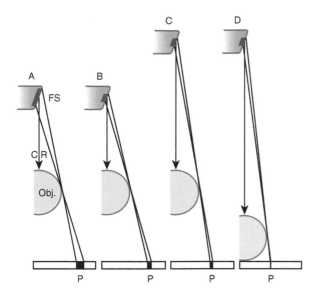

1. Penumbra
2. Focal spot size; the larger the focal spot, the greater is the penumbra
3. The distance between the object and the sensor/film; the longer the distance, the greater is the penumbra
4. The factors minimizing penumbra are:
    1. Small focal spot
    2. Longer distance between the focal spot and the sensor/film
    3. Shorter distance between the object and the sensor/film

FIGURE 1-9

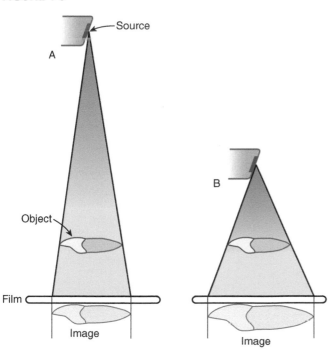

1. The variable is the focal-spot-to-object distance, which translates to cone length.
2. This variable causes magnification of the image, including the magnification of the objects themselves, e.g., the distance between objects or structures in the image.

FIGURE 1-10

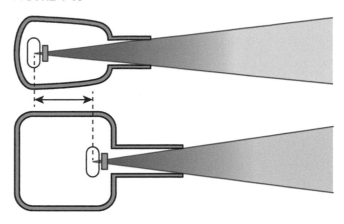

1. **Advantages of a long cone tube head:** Sharper images including less penumbra and less magnification. **Advantages of a short cone tube head:** The shorter arm is more stable and more maneuverable around the chair and patient, and the smaller operatory size saves space.

FIGURE 1-11

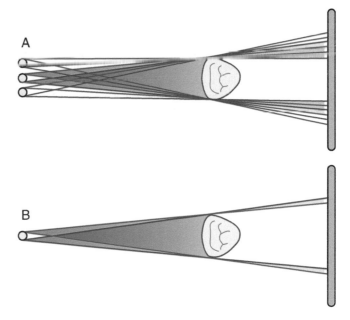

1. First, the more the tube head shakes or moves during the exposure, the greater will be the penumbra or fuzziness (unsharpness) of the image; however, the tomographic effect of the focal spot movement causes less magnification in the image; this effect is almost impossible to appreciate due to the fuzziness of the outline of the object caused by the penumbra. Second, in the case of the more stable tube head, the object is much sharper; however, it is also magnified. This problem can be sometimes greatly diminished by making certain the sensor/film is as close to the tooth as possible.

FIGURE 1-12

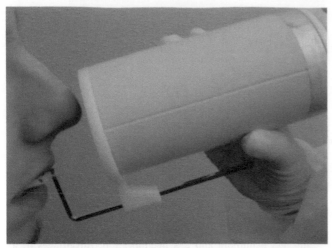

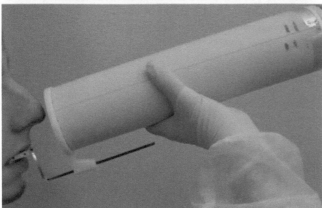

1. The first principle is magnification, and unsharpness will be greater with the short cone. The second is that parallel film/sensor positioning with a beam alignment device is exactly the same for a short cone vs. a long cone. Therefore from the aspect of image sharpness and detail and simplicity of technique, there is no advantage or reason to use a short cone. This is especially true when a machine with a long, recessed cone into the tube head is used, as was previously demonstrated.

FIGURE 1-13

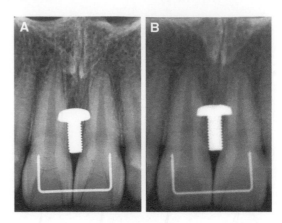

1. Image A is better than image B
2. The differences are as follows: Image A is sharper; note the cracks in the crowns, the lamina dura in the apical region, the trabecular pattern; the fine details of the screw in image A and the visible penumbra at the edge of the staple in image B. Finally image B is magnified as we see no nasal fossa and less of the lateral incisors.
3. The only difference is that image A was taken with a long, 16-inch cone while image B was taken with a short, 4-inch cone. While the short, round cone is not used anymore, it demonstrates more clearly the same effects that occur with an 8-inch cone, but to a lesser degree.

FIGURE 1-14

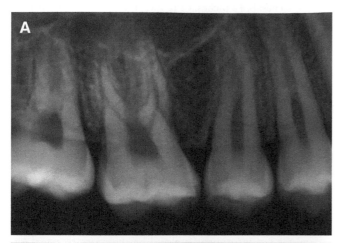

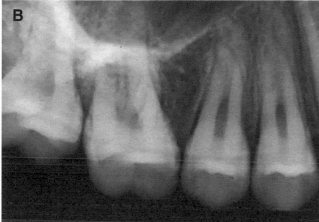

1. In image A: The buccal and lingual cusp tips are almost super-imposed; the interproximal alveolar bone level is seen; the palatal roots of the 1st molar are somewhat elongated, and the buccal roots are somewhat foreshortened; and the malar process of the zygoma does not obscure the apices of the 1st molar. In Image B: The buccal and lingual cusps are not super-imposed; the interproximal alveolar bone fills the interproximal space, and the palatal root of the 1st molar is elongated and the buccal roots are foreshortened; and the malar process of the zygoma is superimposed on the apices of the buccal roots of the 1st molar.
2. The best image is A. The reasons are as stated in answer #1.

FIGURE 1-15

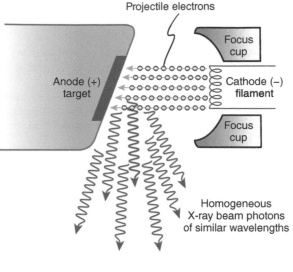

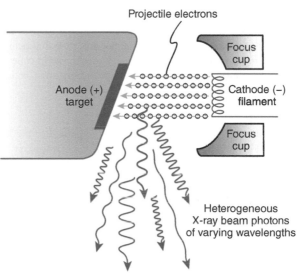

1. One machine has a heterogeneous beam; the other is homogeneous.
2. The heterogeneous type represents an AC (alternating current)-based machine. The homogeneous type represents a DC (direct current)-based machine
3. (a) The DC type will deliver about 20% to 22% less radiation resulting in a lower radiation dose. (b) The DC type will result in less noise in electronic sensors because weak long-wavelength photons of radiation produce unwanted noise in the digital images. (c) The DC type tube heads are much lighter and require no reinforcement of the wall for mounting. They can usually be mounted on any convenient stud.

MULTIPLE CHOICE QUESTIONS WITHOUT FIGURES

1.	A	9.	B
2.	D	10.	C
3.	D	11.	A
4.	B	12.	D
5.	D	13.	A
6.	B	14.	B
7.	A	15.	C
8.	D	16.	D

Chapter 2

SHORT ANSWER QUESTIONS WITH FIGURES

FIGURE 2-1

1. The pointed cone is being used. These are now illegal on new equipment; existing equipment should be retrofitted with open-ended BIDs.

   COMMENT: The pointed cone causes a wide area of the patient's tissues to be exposed to radiation. This wide area is much more than needed to expose the radiograph. They were nicknamed "scatter guns."

2. Pointed cones were usually 4 inches long.

FIGURE 2-2

1. BID diameter: 2.75 inches
2. Several of the rules of good technique (accurate image projection) are to have the film (sensor) parallel to the teeth, to have the film (sensor) as close to the teeth as possible to reduce magnification and penumbra, and to have the source (focal spot) as far away from the object and film (sensor) as possible (long BID or cone). For all of the maxilla, and to a lesser degree the mandibular anterior region, the film must be placed back away from the teeth to obtain parallelism. The magnification and penumbra are minimized with the long cone. Use of the short cone further contributes to magnification and penumbra and should be avoided in the paralleling technique.

FIGURE 2-3

1. No, the long, rectangular BID exposes the patient to the least amount of radiation. Within the next few years it is likely that round cones of any design will not be permitted for intraoral periapical radiography. Rectangular cones will be required. Long, round cones will be permitted for taking bitewings.
2. The long, round BID provides less exposure than the short BID because the beam is more highly collimated.

FIGURE 2-4

1. The collimator for the long, rectangular BID is smaller.
2. No, a cone-cut will not occur. There are slots in the round ring for the positioning of the rectangular BID. The ring slots correspond to the correct alignment with the film (sensor) if it is centered on the bite block.
3. To properly align the end of the rectangular BID with the slots in the ring, the rectangular BID can be rotated. Round BIDs cannot and need not be rotated because they are round.

FIGURE 2-5

1. The collimator is usually at the base of the BID, at the point of attachment to the machine.
2. Collimators are made of lead.
3. Refer back to the question. Note that all were said to be current. Therefore all of these collimators are legal.

4. Collimator D delivered the least radiation dose to the patient.
5. A: 8 inches; B: 12 inches; C: 16 inches; and D is also 16 inches.
6. D is the rectangular BID
7. There is no pointed cone because all are current.
8. C and D are both 16 inches long and have the same exposure times. D delivers less radiation to the patient because the collimator is considerably smaller than C, the long, round cone.

FIGURE 2-6

1. This is a quality assurance tool used to check the condition of the focal spot (target or anode) and "resolution." Resolution is the capacity of an x-ray machine to separate images that are very close together. These images are obtained by projecting the beam through standardized precut slits in the lead plate at the top of the test device.
2. The test is performed by placing an image receptor, such as an occlusal film or an occlusal or panoramic PSP, on the bench, and the test instrument is placed on the image receptor. An exposure is made that produces pairs of lines oriented both horizontally and vertically. The grid is on the top of the device so that the line pairs will only separate when a certain part of the x-ray machine is functioning properly.
3. Over time, the focal spot gets pitted, effectively making its surface area increase because of the pits. This increases the penumbra and decreases the resolution.
4. The slits that represent the resolution are measured and referred to as the ability to separate closely spaced pairs of lines in a 1-mm space. Thus they are called *line pairs per millimeter (lp/mm)*. In this case, the resolution will be at the labeled pair of lines that do not run together in either the vertical or the horizontal dimension. A resolution of 7 to 12 lp/mm is considered excellent to clinically acceptable and is typically seen with new machines. Five to 6 lp/mm is marginally acceptable if fine details are not needed; 1 to 4 lp/mm is considered unacceptable image quality. This old machine is resolving only 6 lp/mm, which in this case, is considered unacceptable for an intraoral machine.
5. This situation would indicate that the images being taken with this machine are unacceptable. Such images are said to be less diagnostic because of the blurring of fine details. Nondiagnostic radiographs are a waste of radiation to the patient. A new machine should be purchased. Thus this device can help to decide which machines need replacement including any handheld machines.
6. Some clinics and offices do have a variety of models and even sometimes a mixture of AC and DC machines. This device can help to decide which machines need replacement.

FIGURE 2-7

1. The collimator is being checked to ensure the radiation is limited to the diameter of the BID (beam indicating device or cone).
2. As you can see, there is no fluorescence beyond the open-ended BID.

FIGURE 2-8

ERROR #1: According to current National Council on Radiation Protection (NCRP) guidelines (2003), the protective apron is not needed. However here it is being put on the patient *backward*. Remember, it is the back of the patient that is potentially exposed to radiation in panoramic radiology.

ERROR #2: The (NCRP) Guidelines published on December 31, 2003, no longer require protective aprons for patients in dental radiography because of the low doses delivered with current technology. (New NCRP Guidelines are expected in the near future and are presently in draft form [2016]).

ERROR #3: Wearing gloves is not necessary in panoramic radiology unless the patient has a contagious skin condition or whose skin may be contaminated by secretions generated from the cold or flu virus.

FIGURE 2-9

1. The barrier material in the wall is lead. However, four layers (two layers on each side of the wall) of ⅝-inch sheet rock will also absorb any remnant radiation in dental radiographic procedures including intraoral, panoramic, cephalometric, and CBCT.
2. The glass is leaded, and no radiation passes through.

FIGURE 2-10

1. During exposure, the patient and machine should be observed by the operator. If there is any problem during the procedure, the exposure button can be released to immediately stop the machine. This minimizes unnecessary radiation exposure to the patient, protects the patient from injury by the moving parts of the machine, and can prevent damage to delicate parts of the machine such as the sensor.
2. As with intraoral radiography, the patient must remain under observation through a barrier window during the exposure.

FIGURE 2-11

1. The wavelengths are long and short, thus the beam is heterogeneous.
2. Aluminum
3. They are only the shorter, more penetrating and diagnostic wavelengths forming the image.
4. The filter removes long-wavelength photons, which are not diagnostic but which increase radiation dose.
5. A DC-powered machine has a homogeneous beam where all of the photons are of the same wavelength, thus reducing the dose by about 20% for the same AC-generated exposure.

FIGURE 2-12

1. Top exposure cone shape: rectangular
2. Bottom exposure cone shape: round
3. The round cone patient got more exposure.
4. Because more tissue was included in the x-ray beam when a round cone of any length (8, 12, or 16 inches) is used, and tissue area exposed decreases with round cone length.

FIGURE 2-13

1. Radiation protection or safety badge
2. The badge records any radiation the health care worker is exposed to while wearing the badge.
3. The ultimate goal is to identify individuals who become exposed to radiation levels that exceed guidelines and which may place such health care providers at risk for the acquisition of radiation-induced disease such as various types of cancers.
4. Most states require the wearing of such badges by personnel who operate x-ray equipment.

FIGURE 2-14

> The use of leaded aprons on patients *shall not* be required if all other recommendations in this Report are rigorously followed. However, if under exceptional circumstances any of these recommendations are not implemented in a specific case, then the leaded apron *should* be used.

The National Council on Radiation Protection (NCRP) report published on December 31, 2003, states the apron is not required. Pregnant patients may still request the apron, though it is not required in this situation. The thyroid collar has never been required for the panoramic image as it interferes with the beam. It is, however, required for intraoral images. New NCRP Guidelines are expected in the near future and are presently in draft form (2016).

Note: Please read the actual paragraph from the report.

FIGURE 2-15 No, the lead apron is not necessary. Pregnant patients may still request the apron, though it is not required.

FIGURE 2-16

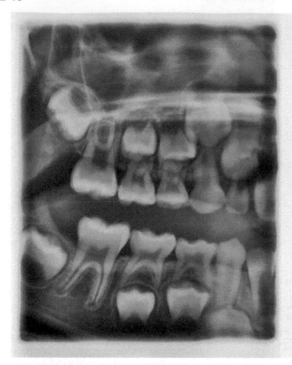 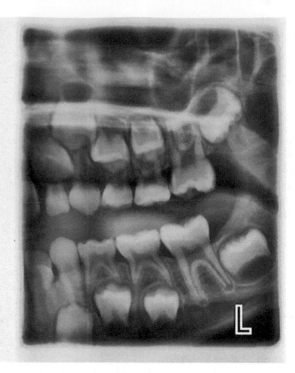

1. For children, the thyroid collar is still highly recommended for intraoral imaging because the thyroid gland, especially in children, is among the most sensitive organs to radiation-induced tumors.

> **3.1.9 Thyroid Collars**
>
> The thyroid gland, especially in children, is among the ***most sensitive*** organs to radiation-induced tumors, both benign, and malignant. Even with optimum techniques, the primary dental x-ray beam may still pass near and occasional through the gland.

2. Yes, take a panoramic bitewing as is seen here. This was a 5-year-old male. Note all of the interproximal contacts are open, and the developing permanent teeth can be seen as well as the periapical regions of the primary teeth. Thyroid collars are not required for any form of panoramic radiology as the beam is directed upward and does not expose the thyroid gland. The panoramic bitewing is more comfortable and is diagnostically the equivalent of a full-mouth survey with more apical coverage and the same dose as four intraoral bite wings. There is no thyroid gland exposure, and there is much greater comfort for the child. See Chapter 9 on caries detection and panoramic bitewings.

3. In general, patients should not hold the film, PSP, or electronic sensor. Films and PSPs can be distorted by digital pressure. Positioning devices achieve better paralleling, more stability, and more accurate positioning with respect to the desired area to be imaged.

FIGURE 2-17

1. This radiograph may not have been necessary under the circumstances as listed in Question 1.
2. It would appear that parts of the thyroid gland may be exposed under these circumstances.
3. Yes, a segmented panoramic image could have been taken. Segmentation allows the user to reduce the pan exposure to any selected area(s) of interest such as this with no risk of exposure

of the thyroid gland and possibly less radiation dose than the long cone periapical image.

4. In a space analysis, the mesiodistal measurements of the tooth widths would be magnified primarily because of the long distance between the image capture device, such as a PSP plate, and the tooth.
5. Totally accurate measurements can be made with a small-volume, low-resolution cone beam CT machine with doses no more elevated than with intraoral or panoramic images, and in many cases, with much greater comfort and less infection control procedures than with intraoral methods. Please refer to Chapter 12 on CBCT imaging.

FIGURE 2-18

1. The primary purpose of the cone or "beam indicating device" or simply "BID" is to collimate the beam of radiation to the narrowest width of the cone at the exit point.
2. The rectangular cone was the only cone that fully collimated the beam; however, in the experience of these authors, it is employed extensively in teaching programs and rarely used in dental practice.
3. Though the round cones both have the same exit diameter, you can see there is more area exposed with the short, round cone.
4. The pointed cone exposed the most tissue outside the area of interest and currently, manufacturers are prohibited from supplying pointed cones, though undoubtedly, a few old machines are still in use. It is also interesting to note that while the rectangular cone provides the greatest protection, it is the least used. It also seems that the 12-inch intermediate cone length between the 16-inch and 8-inch is in very popular use nowadays, even though it provides less protection than the 16-inch cone.

5. The longer the cone, the longer the arm must be and the more operatory space is needed. Presently, modern machines have the cone recessed into the tube head, thus requiring less maneuvering space around the chair.
6. The handheld intraoral machine is fully safe, requires the least space, can adapt to odd patient and/or chair positions, and can be transported from operatory to operatory. It may also be used in the field for public health and military applications.

FIGURE 2-19

1. None, zero, nada, and we have repeated this measurement in workshops many times with the same result.
2. No, lead lining of the walls is not necessary if two layers of ⅝-inch sheet rock are used on each side of the wall. Some state regulations require expensive lead lining of the walls, and there is no getting around this requirement, except to try to educate the legislators who make the sometimes unnecessary regulations.
3. If there is no barrier between a dental employee and the source of dental radiation, the safe distance is 6 feet right in front of the beam. In other words, the energy from the dental x-ray beam dissipates to zero after a distance of 6 feet.

FIGURE 2-20

1. The leading cause of decreased life expectancy in the United States is being an unmarried male.
2. Maybe you would respond being 30% overweight, but in fact. being a single female has more risk than the others mentioned in the question; undoubtedly being an unmarried female, 30% overweight, and with less than an eighth-grade education one might be just catching up with a single male at 3600 days. Conversely, medical x-rays may be responsible for 6 days' loss of life, and perhaps dental x-rays represent about 1% of medical x-rays, which is almost negligible. So if this is the case, the bigger worry is still being single for either sex while x rays probably have an almost negligible effect on our life expectancy. Also note that natural radiation and coffee drinking have about the same loss of life expectancy at 8 and 6 days, respectively.

FIGURE 2-21

1. The left machine (A) has a resolution of about 7 line pairs per millimeter (lp/mm) because you see a loss of separation between the lines at this point; the right machine (B) has a resolution of about 9 or 10 lp/mm. As a result, the left radiograph is much more blurred than the right image.
2. The most acceptable image is obviously on the right side.

MULTIPLE CHOICE QUESTIONS WITHOUT FIGURES

1. D
2. A
3. C
4. D
5. C
6. C
7. C
8. E
9. B
10. D
11. B
12. C
13. A

Chapter 3

SHORT ANSWER QUESTIONS WITH FIGURES

FIGURE 3-1 He is about to have a panoramic bitewing taken and significantly less infection control products and procedures compared with intraoral bitewings are required. Protection of the bite block or stick is the only barrier needed for the healthy patient with no infectious skin conditions. Additional infection control measures are not required.

FIGURE 3-2

1. These are intraoral x-ray film or PSP positioning instruments. Note the slots, which secure the film or PSP, are much too narrow to hold an electronic sensor.
2. The container is called a sterilization cassette.
3. The bag is a heat-resistant type.
4. Autoclave or chemiclave heat sterilization.
5. The film/PSP holder on the far left is for bitewings, and to the immediate right of this is the holder for the periapicals.
6. The round rings are BID (beam indicating device or cone)-positioning rings.
7. To be able to identify the contents in the bag after sterilization for storing and later retrieval.
8. The paperlike back is permeable to hot steam and or gasses used for sterilization.

FIGURE 3-3

1. The arrow is called an "indicator"; its purpose is to indicate that the time and/or temperature have resulted in sterility of the contents of the bag.
2. The EO stands for ethylene oxide gas.

FIGURE 3-4

1. "Air Techniques", it is the brand name of the barrier envelopes.
2. This type of barrier envelope is used to isolate a photostimulable phosphor plate (PSP) for infection control purposes.
3. These envelopes are used to isolate #1 and #2 PSP intraoral imaging plates.
4. The size difference is to accommodate #1-size PSPs on the top, and on the bottom, #2-size PSPs
5. The V-shaped notch allows the operator to tear the envelope open in a low-light area in order to allow the exposed PSP to fall to the countertop aseptically (after which it is dropped into the PSP scanner, which captures the image and sends it to the computer, and specifically, to the patient's chart).
6. The white strip is for labeling the patient ID with a marker pen.
7. None of the components are reusable.
8. The contents of the envelopes cannot usually be sterilized; they are already considered sterile.

FIGURE 3-5

1. This is an electronic sensor which may be of the CCD or CMOS types. (See Digital Imaging, Chapter 4)
2. The cost range is somewhere between $8000 and $14,000, each in 2016 U.S. dollars in the United States; however, the purchase price may be a little lower or higher, depending on whether there is more than one sensor being purchased and whether the purchase is being bundled with other equipment.
3. In general, it is better to use barrier materials rather than soaking the devices in a liquid disinfectant.

4. The reason this is not generally recommended is that the area of the connection between the wire and the sensor may allow leakage of the liquid or saliva into the sensor, which would ruin it. However, some manufacturers do recommend this type of disinfection for their sensors.

FIGURE 3-6

1. There are three people in this picture; the photographer was kibitzing with us during the photo session.
2. Infection control elements that are wrong:
   I: Because the operator is healthy, a mask is not needed for this procedure.
   II: The tube head and cone (BID) are not wrapped with barrier material.
   III: While the disposable gown may be worn all day in the office and need not be changed unless it becomes soaked with saliva and/or blood, it is not generally needed for the taking of radiographs.
3. The yellowish-orange container beside the sink is antiseptic liquid soap for handwashing.

FIGURE 3-7

1. This is an electronic sensor, and it may be of the CCD or CMOS types.
2. The sensor barriers: first a vinyl sleeve for the wire and second the latex finger cot for the sensor and retention of the vinyl sleeve; also remember the PPE (personal protective equipment) we see, consisting of disposable latex gloves, are required for this procedure.

FIGURE 3-8

1. Unwrapping exposed film from the supplied saliva-contaminated packets.
2. On the right, the cup is for the contaminated film packets; on the left, is a clean paper cup for the placement of the aseptically unwrapped film before loading it into the processor or placing the film on processing racks if hand processing is in use.
3. The operator is wearing disposable latex gloves.
4. Yes, it is the same pair of gloves used for the exposure phase with the patient; however, the clean vinyl overgloves were worn during the transportation phase and while inserting the hands into the daylight loader. The vinyl overgloves can be seen with the discarded contaminated film packets in the photo.

FIGURE 3-9

1. Left: electronic sensor of the charge coupled device (CCD) or complementary metal oxide sensor (CMOS); right: PSP sensors
2. First, the vinyl sleeve, about 12 inches long, is slipped over the sensor onto the wire with the last inch or 2 over the sensor; second, the latex finger cot is placed over the sensor and vinyl sleeve, which protects the sensor and anchors the vinyl sleeve on the first 10 or so inches of the wire.
3. On the right, there are two different brands of PSPs. The upper type is shown on the front-labeled side and the back phosphor layer, which captures the latent image and fluoresces when scanned with a laser light. The lower type can have a reusable rubber edge liner, which may in some anatomic locations, be more comfortable for the patient.
4. On the bottom, middle, and right photos we see two different brands of single-use PSP barrier envelopes.

5. The PSPs produce an image of the same size as the corresponding intraoral film; the electronic sensors are bulkier than PSPs, but the image is 25% to 30% smaller than the PSP image, making it difficult to get full periapical coverage with electronic sensors.

FIGURE 3-10

1. **A** Film
2. **A** Film
3. **D** Pair of latex gloves, pair of vinyl overgloves, receptor wrapping materials from the packet
4. **C** Daylight loader or darkroom

FIGURE 3-11

1. The operator is placing the intraoral film into one of the slots of the automatic processor.
2. For this part of the procedure it is appropriate not to wear gloves.
3. Continuing to wear contaminated gloves at this stage could contaminate the processing solutions or other internal parts of the processor and cause cross contamination of the processed film.
4. The image is reddish-yellow in color because work is being done in a daylight loader, and the colored Plexiglas cover both protects the film from being exposed to daylight or incandescent light in the area of the processor and also allows the operator to see what he or she is doing.

FIGURE 3-12

1. This part of the automatic processor is the daylight loader.
2. The cover is orange colored because it acts as a filter, similar to a safelight, to prevent exposure of the film yet lets enough light in so the operator can see what he or she is doing.
3. There are two paper cups; the top one is for the contaminated films; the bottom cup is to contain the unwrapped films as they cannot be aseptically loaded into the processor with contaminated gloves on, and the film packets cannot be unwrapped without gloves.
4. The operator has a clean vinyl overglove on his hand. This is done in order to cover the contaminated gloves while transporting the films from the x-ray machine to the processor; doors, parts of the processor, and other items on the way cannot be touched with the contaminated gloves, and the contaminated film packets can be unwrapped once in the daylight loader or in the darkroom with the same contaminated gloves after taking off the overglove.
5. Barrier envelopes are not necessary when using intraoral film because the packets themselves act as a barrier; however, barrier envelopes are necessary for PSPs.

FIGURE 3-13

1. The sensor is electronic, of the CCD or CMOS variants.
2. The apparatus attached to the sensor is a sensor holder and aiming device.
3. The apparatus holds the sensor in place once it has been properly positioned in the mouth.
4. The regions to be imaged are probably the upper right premolar or molar regions.
5. The infection control error is that the finger cot was not placed over the vinyl sleeve; the vinyl sleeve protects the wire but is not considered to be the most appropriate barrier for the sensor.

FIGURE 3-14 There is absolutely nothing wrong with this image. The yoke, tube head, and cone have been covered with a barrier, and the operator is wearing gloves. The disposable gown is not necessary but is okay and can continue to be worn for other patients, unless it becomes soaked through with water, saliva, or blood from other procedures because these fluids may carry other contaminants through onto the skin and clothing underneath.

From a radiation protection standpoint, it is appropriate to use a thyroid collar and a lead apron as seen here. However, according to NCRP (National Council on Radiation Protection) #145, the use of the lead apron is no longer a requirement.

FIGURE 3-15 Once again, there is nothing wrong with handling panoramic film in the darkroom with bare hands. Unlike intraoral imaging where the film, PSP, or electronic sensor barriers are contaminated after use, panoramic cassettes and films and panoramic PSPs do not normally become contaminated. Handling has no infection control components other than that the loading of cassettes should not be in an area in the darkroom that may be contaminated by recent unwrapping of intraoral films.

The problem we do see is that the safelight is much too close to the film loading area of the processor (about 2 to 3 feet). Most safelight manufacturers recommend a 15-watt bulb for direct safelighting and 25 watts for indirect reflected light from the ceiling and a minimum distance of 4 feet from the countertop or work area for direct lighting. The inverse square law in safelight illumination is that if we have × intensity at 4 feet, we will have 4× intensity at 2 feet and ¼ × intensity at 8 feet.

FIGURE 3-16 We can see that the cone, tube head, and one-armed vertical yoke have not been covered with barrier material. Note also that this picture was taken before scrubs and disposable gowns were in common use. Today scrubs and disposable gowns are in regular use by faculty and students working in the radiology clinic.

FIGURE 3-17 Infection control problems:
1. The tube head and yoke have not been covered by barrier material.
2. The cone is only partially covered with a barrier, and the operator actually seems to be touching the machine at the unprotected part of the cone as well as the tube head with her contaminated gloves.

FIGURE 3-18
1. This is a foot-operated exposure switch.
2. The simple answer is that the foot does not enter into the path of the spread of infection unless of course, as sometimes happens: "Once again, I put my foot in my mouth!" meaning I have said something I should not have said.

FIGURE 3-19
1. Here we see the x-ray film being aseptically removed from the black paper wrap and dropped into a clean paper cup.
2. The shiny material consists of the barrier envelopes used to transport the contaminated film packets to the automatic processor or to the darkroom and the barrier envelopes. Once we are ready to unwrap the film packets, the bulky, poorly fitting vinyl overgloves are removed and the film packets are unwrapped aseptically with the same contaminated gloves used during the image acquisition phase.
3. Yes, gloves are necessary; however, in this case the film packets could be removed from the barrier envelopes aseptically and

from there the gloves could be removed. However it is best to continue with the gloves on as there is a lot of discarded contaminated material in this small space.
4. If using PSPs, these imaging plates are much like film from an infection control standpoint and must also be removed aseptically from the barrier envelopes into a clean paper cup or onto a clean paper napkin while wearing gloves in a low-light area. After discarding the contaminated gloves and doing a hand wash, the PSPs are subsequently loaded into the laser scanner.
5. When using electronic sensors, the image is exported immediately after the exposure to the computer, thus saving time, space, and materials, which are necessary with film or PSP plates. The short answer: No, this procedural step is not necessary with electronic sensors.

FIGURE 3-20
1. With electronic sensors, this step is not necessary.
2. He has contaminated latex disposable gloves and clean vinyl overgloves on his hands in order to avoid contaminating the office items he must touch such as door handles or light switches on the way to the processing area.
3. In his left hand, he is actually holding two paper cups. The lower paper cup will be used to contain the unwrapped film before running it through the processor.
4. Dr. Langlais has worn a copper band on his wrist for many years for the relief of arthritis. Does it work? Who knows!

FIGURE 3-21 A mask is not necessary for the taking of intraoral radiographs if the operator and patient are healthy and are not subject to coughing or sneezing. If, however, the operator has a cold, it would be wise to wear a mask.

FIGURE 3-22
1. It is a photostimulable phosphor plate (PSP) laser scanner.
2. Its function is to cause the image on the PSP to fluoresce under a laser light.
3. The computer captures and stores the image for initial viewing for technique errors and ultimately exports the image to the patient's electronic chart.

FIGURE 3-23
1. This is the RVG (RadioVisioGraphie) original electronic sensor from France invented by Dr. Francis Mouyen and was (to our knowledge) the first electronic sensor introduced to the dental market in North America. It was small and bulky and was barely large enough to capture an image of a single molar. It was, however, an incredible step forward in the development of digital x-ray imaging.
2. The infection control error is as follows: usually a vinyl sleeve is first placed over the sensor and about 1 foot of the wire is connected to the sensor to protect the wire from spatter or other contaminants; then the latex finger cot is placed over the sensor and vinyl sleeve to both protect the sensor which may not be impermeable to fluids and to retain the vinyl sleeve in place over the wire.

FIGURE 3-24
1. He is looking at an RVG image of his molar taken with the sensor we saw in the previous question. It was among the first of the early electronic intraoral x-ray images taken in America.

FIGURE 3-25

1. Disposable protective gown; barrier protection for the tube head and cone, and operator protective gloves
2. The disposable protective gown is not necessary for radiology procedures, although it need not be removed during the radiology procedure.

FIGURE 3-26 Disposable latex gloves; surface barrier wrap for the yoke, tube head, long, rectangular cone, x-ray chair armrests and headrest; the non-disposable protective gown is not necessary, unless spatter is anticipated; however, it need not be removed once donned in the office for the clinical session. If ever the protective gown becomes soaked through, it must be removed immediately and properly disposed of. One does not anticipate this type of contamination for most radiology procedures. Although gagging is possible, vomiting is not usually anticipated. If the patient has been known to vomit, the panoramic bitewing and anterior periapical views of the upper and lower incisors offer a viable substitute to the full-mouth survey, including the bitewings.

FIGURE 3-27 In this clinical scenario the image is being captured onto a laptop computer. It is possible the images are a part of a study not involving a patient but simulating clinical conditions. Examples of such a study might be the testing of several sensors or to determine the best machine settings to obtain the best image with the lowest radiation dose. Alternately, the digital image can be captured onto a laptop computer, especially if a wired or wireless network is not available. After the procedure the images can easily be exported into the main office computer and into the patient's electronic chart.

FIGURE 3-28 This would be a setup for an electronic sensor. Therefore our primary infection control need with regard to the wording of the question is a vinyl sleeve to protect the wire attached to the sensor and a finger cot to protect the electronic sensor. Secondarily, the operator would need to wear gloves, and the cone, tube head, yoke, exposure setting controls, and the exposure switch of the x-ray machine would need to be barrier wrapped. The headrest, armrests, and position switches of the chair should be barrier wrapped.

FIGURE 3-29

The arms of the chair are not barrier wrapped.

MULTIPLE CHOICE QUESTIONS WITHOUT FIGURES

1.	C	9.	D
2.	D	10.	D
3.	A	11.	C
4.	B	12.	D
5.	B	13.	D
6.	C	14.	E
7.	B	15.	D
8.	D		

Chapter 4

SHORT ANSWER QUESTIONS WITH FIGURES

FIGURE 4-1B

1. It is controlled by the computer to which it is connected.
2. The device is called a scanner.
3. It must be equipped with a transparency adapter, which is not present on normal scanners.
4. The transparency adapter is on the top, which is thicker than a normal scanner or copier top with a scanning function.
5. To scan a radiograph no reduced light is needed.

FIGURE 4-2

1. The device is called a server.
2. It is needed because the office computer itself does not have enough memory to store all of the digital patient information, documents, pictures, and radiographs; there also may be several work stations where others such as office staff, the hygienist, and associate dentists will need to access the patient information at other locations within the practice.
3. This particular model contains the capability of adding six hard drives with each added hard drive being plugged in as the practice grows.

FIGURE 4-3

1. The most obvious missing item would be a digital sensor, which would also be plugged into the laptop computer.
2. Infection control: Parts of the laptop such as the screen area may be touched with contaminated gloves and should be covered with barrier material. The table is also being touched by the gloved right hand and may also be touched by contaminated gloves or sensors and therefore should be covered with a surface barrier or be surface disinfected after completion of the procedure; in the photograph, the cone of the x-ray machine may not be covered by a barrier.

FIGURE 4-4

1. Bit depth (binary digit) is determined by the number of bits used to define each pixel. The greater the bit depth, the greater the number of tones (gray scale) that can be represented.
2. Top image: 3 bits $(2^3) = 8$ shades of gray
   Bottom image: 4 bits $(2^4) = 16$ shades of gray
3. Theoretically, the 4-bit image is more diagnostic; however 8-bit or 256 shades of gray and sometimes 10-bit are standard for digital imaging while 12- to 15-bit depths are used in cone beam computed tomography.
4. The greater the bit depth, the larger the file size; the bottom image has the largest file size.

FIGURE 4-5

1. There are four shades of gray in this image; that is to say 2^2:

$$2 \times 1 = 2 \times 2 = 4 \text{ shades of gray}$$

FIGURE 4-6

1. The 4-bit image does not fully display the trabecular pattern of the alveolar bone and the crestal bone. The 4-bit image also appears to be slightly speckled overall with darker grayish dots referred to as noise, which is undesirable.

FIGURE 4-7 The most important difference between the two images is a much larger file size for figure B.

COMMENT: Figure A is an 8-bit image with 256 shades of gray; figure B is a 24-bit image with 16.7 million shades of gray. Figure B is not considered any more diagnostic than figure A; however, the file size for figure A is 459 kB (kilobytes) while figure B is 9120 kB. To sum up: the increased bit depth is not worth the extra file size.

FIGURE 4-8
1. The correct term for this appearance is "grainy."
2. The cause of this appearance on the image is not enough radiation, usually meaning insufficient exposure time.

FIGURE 4-9
1. The correct term for this appearance is "blooming."
2. The cause of this appearance on the image is too much radiation, usually meaning excessive exposure time.

FIGURE 4-10
1. Advantages of a DC-type x-ray machine:
   1. Approximately 20% less dose for the same exposure
   2. Less noise on images when using digital sensors
   3. Recessed tube allows a shorter cone to be used which makes it easier to manipulate and position the cone.
   4. Much lower weight negates the need for added wall support and allows simple installation to a wall stud.
2. The arrows point to a dot or other small symbol on the tube head indicating the position of the focal spot. In illustration B the focal spot is said to be "recessed," thus allowing for a shorter external cone.

FIGURE 4-11
1. DC involves less dose and therefore shorter exposure times because the kV rises to the peak (kVp) and stays there resulting in a constant production of radiation throughout the set exposure time.
2. The alternating current (AC) in AC-type machines produces 60 pulses of radiation per second in most of North America because the AC current cycles on and off 60 times per second. Thus, DC machines produce a homogeneous beam consisting of high energy short-wavelength photons, most of which will contribute to "image" formation; the heterogeneous A/C beam contains photons of radiation that have short penetrating wavelengths and longer, less, and non penetrating wavelengths. These lower energy photons do not contribute to the "image" as they appear as undesirable "noise," often looking like little black dots which obscure the clarity of the digital image. In digital imaging, the "image" is what you want to see like a tooth; noise does not contribute any information to the image of the tooth but does obscure the image of the tooth. Noise may mask critical details such as a fine crack in the tooth.

FIGURE 4-12
1. These two images demonstrate that the AC unit delivers the radiation in pulses as indicated by the dots; the DC unit delivers radiation continuously throughout the exposure as indicated by the curved black line.
2. The AC unit is not functioning properly as the first three pulses (black dots) are weak, nondiagnostic, and noise producing. These findings require this machine be repaired or replaced.

Note: In digital imaging, the weak pulses cause noise in the image.

FIGURE 4-13
1. Older AC-type machines
2. Adult; bitewings
3. This AC machine cannot be set at 8 mA.
4. A. Using these settings, the DC machine would deliver the most dose and is the reason why exposures are about 20% less for DC machines.
   B. The AC machine due to the heterogeneous beam containing long wavelength x-ray photons.

FIGURE 4-14
1. In general terms there are many interproximal caries on the sensor image and none on the pan BW image.
2. The reason for the lack of findings on the pan bitewing is that the image was subjected to several filters such as sharpen, sharpen edges, and remove noise. These filters also removed the interproximal caries from the image. Additionally, some of the existing noise, which did not interfere with the original image as captured, has been enhanced. Also a common artifact is the appearance of a dark line under metallic restorations resembling redecay when such filters are used. Bottom line: Filters should not be used to enhance caries detection; brightness and contrast, however, may be used to the viewer's advantage.

FIGURE 4-15
1. These three factors are:
   1. Dynamic range
   2. Contrast detail
   3. Spatial resolution

FIGURE 4-16
1. At the outset the most ideal situation is to have the same model of direct current x-ray machine and the same model of sensor throughout the office. However, any combination of sensor and x-ray machine can be used most effectively if a quality assurance device, such as the one pictured in the question, is employed to calibrate the machines and sensors to minimize exposure and maximize image quality. This quality assurance device is called the Dental Digital Quality Assurance Phantom (DDQAP) as illustrated in Figure 4-16 A and B. In Figure 4-16 B, the phantom consists of a top third, which consists of two rows of wells in a lead plate; in the upper row the wells are all of the same diameter but are of different depths; in the lower row the wells are all of the same depth but are of different diameters. When the sensor is exposed, the two rows of wells measure the *dynamic range* with the shallowest depths and the smallest diameter being the best values. The *contrast detail* is best when the most steps can be seen in the image of the aluminum step wedge on the bottom row. The *spatial resolution or detail* is measured in separable line pairs per millimeter (lp/mm), and the middle row is used for this. A value of 9 to 10 lp/mm would be an excellent result. Satisfactory image detail would be in the range of about 6 to 8 lp/mm.

FIGURE 4-17
1. Using the DDQAP quality assurance tool, each x-ray machine and sensor combination can be calibrated to deliver the highest quality image at the lowest dose. In the example here the image on the right was obtained from lower exposure factors than those suggested by the x-ray machine and sensor manufacturers by using the DDQAP quality assurance tool.

FIGURE 4-18

1. The monitor quality can be evaluated using a test pattern. This pattern is stretched out so that it covers the whole monitor screen from corner to corner. These patterns (SMPTE test pattern) test the ability of the monitor to display fine details, primarily evaluating three important features in radiographs:
    - Accuracy: First, straight lines throughout the test pattern need to be seen as straight, parallel, and undistorted or curved.
    - Contrast: Looking at the test pattern, subtle changes in the shades of gray should be seen in both darker and lighter shades of gray.
    - Detail: Fine details can be tested by looking in the corners of the pattern to see if the monitor can separate closely spaced thick and fine lines in both the horizontal and vertical dimensions as well as blurred lines toward the edge of the test pattern and monitor screen.

Note: Monitor specs for acceptable monitor quality are as follows: DPI (dots per inch), 96; dot pitch, 0.294 inches, or HD (high definition) 1080 p.

FIGURE 4-19

1. This is a type of digital assembly used for a film-based panoramic machine. Other than possible setting changes in the mA and kV, nothing else is needed to convert a film-based pan machine to a digital pan machine.
2. The device is a photostimulable phosphor plate, also referred to as a PSP.
3. The PSP must be scanned by a laser scanner connected to a computer before the image can be viewed in the computer monitor.
4. Before being reused, the PSP must be erased.

FIGURE 4-20

1. The type of panoramic digital imaging is called "indirect digital imaging" because the PSP plate must first be scanned by a laser scanner before the image can be viewed. In "direct digital imaging" electronic sensors are used instead of the PSP plate-cassette assembly, and the image can be viewed instantly. The advantage of the PSP plates is that they can be used to convert film-based pan machines to digital. Electronic sensors are only available on new digital pan machines and are not available for the conversion of film-based machines to digital.
2. The procedure is the erasure of the PSP image with a bright light. After this step the PSP plate can be reused hundreds of times but must be scanned and erased after each exposure.

FIGURE 4-21

1. This is a #2-size intraoral image.
2. This image was acquired with the use of a #2-size intraoral PSP plate wrapped in a barrier envelope and then exposed to acquire the "latent image" and then scanned with a laser scanner connected to a computer to view the image.
3. In this clinic, an out-of-service date is written on the PSP plate so that it may not be accidentally reused. In this case the PSP plate was reused after placing the "out-of-use" date on the PSP plate.
4. All of the above were done to this PSP plate for two reasons:
    a. There are scratches on the imaging surface of the plate.
    b. The so-called "emulsion" becomes partially removed from mishandling recently scanned PSP plates by slightly pressing on the scanned PSP plate on the smooth, flat countertop to bring it to the edge so that it may be easily picked up for further reuse.

FIGURE 4-22

1. This is a photostimulable phosphor plate indirect digital imaging system.
2. The PSP plate is being loaded onto a drum for scanning by a laser scanner, which is in the background and connected to a monitor; the image will then be viewable on the monitor, also in the background.

FIGURE 4-23

1. This is a portable handheld intraoral x-ray machine.
2. Even though the device is battery powered, many exposures can be taken on a single charge.
3. The machine is FDA approved for routine clinical use in dental practice, and in fact, some of the safety data that were supplied to the FDA during the approval process was acquired by the University of Texas Health Science Center Dental School at San Antonio, Texas.
4. The infection control set up is okay. What is incorrect is the placement of the orange barrier protective ring that fits on the cone; this ring should be placed at the end of the cone for the required protection of the operator.

Note: A newer, smaller, lighter model is currently available from this manufacturer.

FIGURE 4-24

1. Visually, the two images look the same diagnostically.
2. All of the factors were lower for the portable handheld machine, therefore the x-ray dose to the patient was lower.
3. The main advantage is that the machine is portable and can therefore be used anywhere in the dental office where x-ray images are normally taken. Second, the system is a DC type machine and theoretically less noise would occur because all of the photons would be of the same wavelength; conversely, the other machine was of the AC type and could produce more noise, although this author could not detect any more noise in the AC image. The final advantage involves maneuverability; because the machine is not anchored to the wall, the chair can be in a variety of positions during a procedure such as a root canal treatment whereby the operator can easily line up the machine to take an image without having to change the chair position.

Note: Because most operatories each have a wall-mounted machine, radiographs can be taken simultaneously as needed in any operatory by any practitioner or staff member while a single portable machine cannot supply this need.

FIGURE 4-25   Look at the radiograph. You can distinguish the white metal of the amalgam restoration from the black air nearby. You can also see the difference between the enamel, dentin, cortical bone, alveolar bone, and the soft tissue covering the maxillary tuberosity. These visible tissue densities in the image constitute the patient's "built-in step wedge," and when present, they indicate an adequately diagnostic image.

FIGURE 4-26   The answer to this problem is to use a USB connector adapter and attach this to the USB connector on the sensor wire. In this case it is the inexpensive USB adapter that wears out from connecting and disconnecting the sensor instead of the USB connector on the sensor wire. This is an inexpensive alternative to having sensors available in each operatory. However, even then, switching from larger to smaller sensor sizes will cause wear on the

USB connector on the sensor wire. Thus the USB connector adapter is a good solution to this problem.

FIGURE 4-27

1. This arrangement in a digital image is referred to as the "image matrix."
2. The squares on the left and right are referred to as "pixels."
3. The image matrix consists of pixels with different gray values arranged in horizontal "rows" and in vertical "columns."

FIGURE 4-28

1. The blue USB marking identifies this as a USB 2.0 type of plug. The USB 2.0 is said to transfer data many times faster than the ubiquitous original USB connector.
2. This part, attached to the sensor cabling, is a powered USB 2.0 router. Although the sensor may be powered by the sensor cable USB connection to the laptop capture computer in the operatory, to ensure adequate power, the sensor is plugged into the powered USB 2.0 router cable, which is in turn plugged into the operatory laptop computer. The USB 2.0 plug helps to ensure the fastest possible transfer of the acquired image data to the laptop computer. The laptop computer is plugged into the network to access and transfer the images to the patient's chart, which is in the office mainframe computer.

MULTIPLE CHOICE QUESTIONS WITHOUT FIGURES

1. A
2. C
3. B
4. B
5. C
6. D
7. C
8. A
9. A
10. C
11. A
12. D

Chapter 5

SHORT ANSWER QUESTIONS WITH FIGURES

FIGURE 5-1

1. thyroid collar
2. lead apron
3. round beam indicating device (BID) or round cone
4. focal spot location indicators
5. tube head
6. yoke
7. articulation of tube head with arm

FIGURE 5-2

1. This instrument is called a ring alignment device (also referred to as the XCP positioning instrument).
2. Taking bitewings.
3. The film is reversed. The bite block and ring are correct.

FIGURE 5-3

1. The maxillary central incisors are being radiographed.
2. A rectangular BID or cone.
3. BID not parallel to rod, with insufficient vertical angulation.
4. The teeth will be elongated.

FIGURE 5-4

1. A is the polysoft packet; B, the paper wrapper; C, the lead foil; and D, the film.
2. The film fits inside the paper wrapper; the lead foil is in back of the paper wrapper; these fit inside the polysoft envelope with the lead foil facing the back side of the packet.

FIGURE 5-5

1. The bite block is not centered in the ring.

FIGURE 5-6

1. A bitewing is being taken.
2. The rectangular BID (cone) is not properly centered on the ring.
3. There will be a rectangular cone-cut whereby some of the radiograph will not be exposed.

FIGURE 5-7

1. The kV setting: 63; the mA setting: 8; the timer setting: 0.160 sec.

FIGURE 5-8

1. The setup is for the upper right and lower left posterior quadrants.
2. This is #2-size film.
3. The corner of the film is bent.
4. A black line will be seen in this area of the processed image and a crimp mark will be seen on the corner of the image.
5. If the bent edge is fed into the automatic processor first (as the leading edge), there is a possibility the film will be flipped out of the roller assembly into the bottom of the tank and not emerge from the processor upon completion of processing. If films absolutely must be bent, they should be unbent and the bent portion should be the trailing edge in the processor.

FIGURE 5-9

1. The lower right posterior quadrant.
2. The BID is not parallel to the indicator rod.
3. The lower posterior teeth will be foreshortened, and the inferior border of the mandible (cortex) may appear in the image.
4. This should be avoided when making vertical measurements such as in endodontics.
5. This should be done on purpose if more periapical coverage is desired.

FIGURE 5-10

1. Paralleling technique.
2. The setup is for the upper right and lower left quadrants.
3. The film is not centered on the bite block, and someone has written the patient's name on the front of the film packet (with a ballpoint pen).
4. The film will be placed more anterior than desired; the patient's name will appear in the image as radiopaque writing.

FIGURE 5-11

- The Off button: This only turns the machine off.
- The 10-mA button: This turns the machine on when depressed and is backlit when the machine is on; it sets the mA at 10 milliamperes.

- The 15-mA button: This turns the machine on when depressed and is backlit when the machine is on; it sets the mA at 15 milliamperes. The 15-mA setting allows for shorter exposure times than the 10-mA setting; this is especially useful when using the long BID, which requires four times longer exposure times than the short BID if all other factors remain constant.

FIGURE 5-12

1. The rectangular BID is not parallel to the rod; excessive positive vertical angulation is being used.
2. The maxillary central incisors will be foreshortened.

FIGURE 5-13

1. A: #4; B: #2; C: #1.
2. Size #4 is used primarily for occlusal views; #2 is used for bitewings and posterior periapical views as well as anterior periapical views in some institutions and practices; #1 is used for anterior periapical views.

FIGURE 5-14

1. The patient's glasses have been left on.
2. The cone does not appear barrier wrapped.
3. If you said there is no apron please recall the apron is no longer required, though if a patient requests it, the apron can be used.

FIGURE 5-15

Errors in progress:

1. This setup is for imaging the maxillary and mandibular anterior teeth.
2. The film is placed backward on the bite block.
3. The image will be pale, and the lead foil pattern will be seen.
4. The film should be discarded because the dot will be reversed. Pathology may be interpreted on the wrong side of the patient. This view should be retaken.

FIGURE 5-16

Errors in progress:

1. The patient does not appear to be wearing the protective lead apron.
2. A cone cut with a long round BID (beam indicating device) is about to occur.
3. Note the BID is not barrier wrapped.

FIGURE 5-17

1. The rectangular BID is not parallel to the rod; a mesioangular horizontal angulation is being used.
2. Overlapping of the interproximal areas; possible cone-cut at the distal edge of the film; improper projection of the desired teeth on the film.
3. The BID is not barrier wrapped.

FIGURE 5-18   We are looking at the kVp meter, which can be adjusted with the kVp selector knob not seen here. Note, however, that the kVp varies with the two available mA settings. Thus the correct kVp scale must be used when adjusting the kVp according to the previously selected mA. If the wrong scale is used, the processed images may be too light or too dark.

FIGURE 5-19

1. The BID is not parallel to the rod; excessive positive vertical angulation is being used.
2. The maxillary premolars and 2nd molars will be foreshortened. The buccal roots of the maxillary 1st molar may be foreshortened and the palatal root elongated; this is known as

dimensional distortion and is most prone to occur with the bisecting-angle technique.

3. The cone is not barrier wrapped.

FIGURE 5-20

1. The lead foil backing.
2. To absorb remnant radiation after the film has been exposed; to indicate when the film has been placed in the mouth backward.
3. A: fish scale pattern; B: tire track pattern; C: table tennis ball geometric pattern. The so-called herringbone pattern has been retired.

FIGURE 5-21

1. The rectangular BID is not parallel to the rod; excessive distoangular horizontal angulation is being used.
2. The interproximal surfaces will be overlapped; there may be a cone-cut at the anterior edge of the film; the desired structures will not be properly projected on the radiograph.

FIGURE 5-22

1. The bite block is incorrectly placed on the rod; it should be rotated 180 degrees.
2. The profile of the bitewing bite block when placed correctly on the rod looks like the "tail of a jet plane."

FIGURE 5-23

Part 1

1. A long BID (cone) is specified; this is usually 16 inches, unless otherwise specified.
2. The mA setting is 15 mA.
3. Yes, the settings will be okay.
4. The film speed is "F" or Insight film.
5. The kVp is 70.
6. The exposure time for the maxillary anterior periapicals is 18 impulses.

Part 2

1. The exposure time would be 6 impulses. When you change from a 16-inch cone to an 8-inch cone, you can use ¼ of the exposure time if all other settings remain the same.
2. The molar exposure time would be about 30 impulses. (You can increase the exposure time by one increment for each 20 to 30 pounds.)
3. For the "D"-speed film, the exposure time would be about 30 impulses. ("D"-speed film requires about 50% to 60% more exposure time than "F"-speed film.)
4. For a 10-mA setting, the new exposure time would be 45 impulses. The mAs for the 15-mA setting is 15 mA × 30 impulses = 450 mAI. Therefore if we go to 10 mA, we will need 45 impulses to equal 450 mAI. Yep! That's how you do it!
5. If you switched to 85 kVp for the molar periapical, you could reduce the timer setting to 15 impulses. The rule of 15 kVp says that if you increase the kVp by 15, you can reduce the exposure time by approximately half; if you decrease the kVp by 15, you must increase the exposure time by about half.
6. No modifications are needed. "F"-speed film is the fastest available (2015).
7. The exposure chart specifies the values are the same for the two BID types.
8. The exposure time would be one increment less on the exposure chart; i.e., 24 impulses.
9. Thirty impulses is an exposure time of ½ or 0.5 second.
10. Three-quarters of a second (¾ sec) is 45 impulses.

FIGURE 5-24

1. The dot is not in the slot at the base of the bite block.
2. The dot can be superimposed on the apical region of the image and obscure important features.

FIGURE 5-25

1. The region is the maxillary premolar periapical area.
2. The exposure time would be 24 impulses.
3. The right image is an error.
4. The error is improper distoangular horizontal positioning of the BID. Note how the interproximals are overlapped and the contact areas are not properly seen in the photograph on the right.

FIGURE 5-26

1. It is a film mount for a full-mouth survey.
2. It is a film mount for two #2 films.
3. This full-mouth survey includes four bitewings using #2 film; eight posterior periapicals using #2 film; and eight anterior periapicals using #1 film. The complete survey consists of a 20-film survey. There are many other acceptable full-mouth survey configurations that use, for example, only #2 film.

FIGURE 5-27

1. The images were captured on an electronic sensor, the type attached to a wire.
2. These are digital images being viewed on a monitor; since some sensors have 25% to 30% less image size, it is possible this office was not getting a sufficient view of the alveolar bone when the sensors were placed in the standard horizontal position.
3. First, electronic sensors are expensive, in the range of $6000 to $14,000 each, depending on the brand, sale prices, and bundling with other equipment. Therefore it is possible this office is equipped with only #2-size sensors.

    Second, the bitewings appear to have been exposed in the vertical position instead of the normal horizontal position.
4. First, the mount has no indication of right and left sides; if these are digital images then there is not an embossed dot to correctly orient the image; therefore the mount should be labeled.

    Second, some images are mounted on top of other images, partially obscuring anatomic and possibly diagnostic information.

    Third, the bitewings on the right side of the photograph have been reversed; the premolar bitewing was taken too posteriorly, and the molar bitewing is angulated improperly, resulting in overlapping contacts.

FIGURE 5-28

1. This is a photostimulable phosphor plate (PSP) image.
2. These white spots represent scratches on the emulsion.
3. The radiopaque line is a fixed retainer following completed orthodontic treatment.
4. It is on the lingual side and makes flossing more challenging, although floss threaders work well.
5. It is the lingual foramen surrounded by the genial tubercles upon which the genioglossus and geniohyoid muscles insert.

FIGURE 5-29

1. First, electronic sensors are somewhat bulkier and larger than film or PSP plates, and the image in these sensors is up to 25% to 33% smaller than an image of the same area with film or a PSP plate. Therefore it is difficult to capture the alveolar bone beyond the apices.

    Second, in order to achieve this type of image, a negative projection angle of the beam is used. This results in an image of the periapical bone, but the teeth become foreshortened making endodontic measurements subject to inaccuracy (the roots and canals are foreshortened), possibly requiring a second image to be taken with the proper projection angle. However, this doubles the x-ray dose. Conversely, many dentists use apex locators that help to solve this problem. Vertical placement of electronic sensors in this circumstance is another solution. The best, most accurate and most comfortable endodontic imaging is with cone beam CT (CBCT) from which the canals can be measured accurately and other unapparent canals can also be located. CBCT is rapidly becoming the state of the art for even routine cases. CBCT is the subject of Chapter 13.
2. The endodontic filling of the distal canal appears to be short of the apex. The previously discussed foreshortening of the image and therefore short inaccurate measurements may have been responsible for this less desirable outcome. CBCT is highly recommended for endodontic procedures.

FIGURE 5-30

1. Bob's first and last names are written on the front of the plastic film packet before exposure. The ballpoint pen ink acted as a radiation barrier to produce the unwanted label. Students sometimes identify their films so as not to get their patient's film mixed up with someone else's.

FIGURE 5-31

1. This is the patient's finger. Some techniques call for using the patient's finger to retain the film.
2. Phalangioma

FIGURE 5-32

1. BID (beam indicating device) cut or cone-cut.

FIGURE 5-33

1. The two films were stuck together in the processor.
2. The answer is to not feed the films too quickly one after the other and to use alternating adjacent slots if available.

FIGURE 5-34

1. This indicates improper horizontal angulation of the beam in relation to these teeth. Note the interproximal overlap.
2. This error may be used to our advantage when trying to separate the two roots of this tooth.

FIGURE 5-35

1. Normally the periapical radiograph should include at least 5 mm to 1 cm of the periapical tissues.
2. To increase the area of apical coverage:
   - Ensure the film is placed as apically as possible.
   - This film seems to be well placed. However, inadequate negative vertical angulation of the beam was used.

FIGURE 5-36

1. A: An unexposed film was processed. Usually this means another film from the same patient will be double exposed.
2. B: An unwrapped, unexposed film was left on the darkroom countertop for 5 minutes and was fogged by an unsafe safelight. A 60-watt bulb was discovered in the safelight instead of the normal 7.5- to 15-watt bulb. If the film is left unprotected in the x-ray area, a similar appearance would be seen.
3. C: This film was exposed to light. The same appearance occurs if a film is exposed to a lot of radiation (60 impulses or 1 second).

FIGURE 5-37

1. The list of possible errors is:
   - Patient movement
   - Film movement
   - X-ray tube head movement

COMMENT: Here is how you can separate and identify the specific error:
   a. Patient movement often results in "double or triple edges" to objects in the image.
   b. Film movement occurs because the patient released biting pressure on the bite block, usually because of discomfort. Thus there would be increased distance between the teeth and the bite block, and the apical coverage would be diminished.
   c. Tube head movement effectively increases the focal spot size. This increases total magnification of the objects in the image with visible penumbra and unsharpness. Note the penumbra (shadow around the shadow or image) around the bottom part of the rubber dam clamp, the magnification, and the unsharpness (fuzziness) of this image. This error mimics the effect of an old, used-up, and pitted focal spot.

FINAL EXPLANATION: Tube head movement. (This is prone to occur in older, unstable machines and when the operator rushes the exposure because of patient discomfort.)

FIGURE 5-38

1. The appearance is "grainy," and normally this is supposedly caused by "clumping" of grains of silver if the developer is too warm and especially if exhausted.
2. In this case, the film that was found in the bottom of the processor still had the black wrapping paper on it. This caused it to flip out of the developer roller assembly. The recovered film was unwrapped and re-fed into the machine, and this is the result.

You missed that?...Anyone would have, unless you had seen this before, and even then, would you admit it?

FIGURE 5-39

1. Radiolucent stain: developer

2. Radiopaque stain: fixer

Yes, they were asked in the order used in processing!

COMMENT: To distinguish chemical stains, use the mnemonic "D-dark-developer." To learn the cause, remember that the fixer removes any unexposed or undeveloped silver grains. So if the film sits in a drop of fixer on the countertop (as happens all the time with "wet reading" manually processed films) before processing, parts of the image can be effaced. The same occurs with a drop of developer on the countertop, especially when the hand processing "quick developer" solutions are used for endodontics. This occurs to varying degrees as water droplets serve to dilute the droplets of developer and fixer on the countertop. The problems are avoided with neatness and tidiness in the darkroom.

FIGURE 5-40

1. Excessive curving of the anterior part of the film. This may be caused by:
   - Excessive finger pressure if the film is being held by the patient's finger
   - Excessive curving back of a bite block—retained film edge because of the curvature of the palate and the patient failing to complain about it. (Patients want to cooperate and sometimes do not report the discomfort that would signal an error.)

FIGURE 5-41

1. The error was caused by excessive vertical angulation of the x-ray beam:
   A: Excessive positive vertical beam angulation
   B: Excessive negative vertical beam angulation
2. The features identifying this error:
   A: Foreshortening of the roots. The molar has foreshortened buccal roots and an elongated palatal root; there is excess separation of the buccal and palatal cusp tips; several cusp tips of lower teeth can be seen.
   B: Foreshortening of the roots and excess separation of the buccal and lingual cusp tips
3. The advantage is increased apical coverage.

FIGURE 5-42

1. The chemicals are as follows:
   A: Fixer (Notice the developer stain as well.)
   B: Developer
   C: Stannous fluoride

COMMENT: The use of stannous fluoride is being rediscovered for patients with severe erosions or demineralized enamel that would be exacerbated by currently popular acidic fluoride solutions. Stannous fluoride does taste awful. The tin in the stannous fluoride causes excessive development of unexposed silver in the emulsion, producing very black marks.

FIGURE 5-43

1. Elongation
2. With the paralleling technique and the use of a BID positioning device, elongation results from inadequate positive vertical angulation resulting from the BID not being parallel to the positioning rod. In other situations, such as in endodontics, the bisecting-angle technique is used. Remember that the ala-tragus line or the occlusal plane must be parallel to the floor, and then the correct vertical angulation must be selected. Usually this is 45 degrees of positive vertical angulation; less will result in elongation.

FIGURE 5-44

1. Too light:
   - Insufficient exposure time
   - Insufficient milliamperage setting (if adjustable) for selected exposure time (mAs factor)
   - Insufficient kilovoltage (if adjustable)
   - Inadequate development (short time or cold temperature)
   - Weak or depleted developer solution
   - Expired or aged film
2. Too dark:
   - Excessive exposure time
   - High milliamperage setting (if adjustable) for selected exposure time (mAs factor)
   - High kilovoltage relative to selected exposure time
   - Light leak in darkroom

COMMENT: With an increase of 15 kVp, the exposure time can be reduced by 50% to maintain the same density (darkness). With a decrease of 15 kVp, the exposure time will need to be increased by 50% to maintain density. This works best between 60 and 75 kVp but is a good guide for any dental kVp setting.

If you maintain the same exposure time, you will need an increase or decrease of at least 5 kVp to be able to see a visible change in the density.

The most common cause of low-density (light) films is depleted developer solution in the automatic processor.

The most common cause of high-density (dark) films is too high an exposure time. The kVp controls contrast, which is the shades of gray in the image: low kVp gives high contrast (few shades of gray); high kVp results in low contrast (many shades of gray).

Fixer solution lasts twice as long as developer solution and thus needs replenishment only every second time. Remember the "6 and 6" rule for developer replenishment: most automatic processors will need 6 fl oz of fresh developer after processing six full-mouth surveys (about 120 intraoral films) or six panoramic radiographs. Also 6 fl oz of fixer for every second developer replenishment.

FIGURE 5-45

1. Double exposure

COMMENT: Remember, it is with this error that we usually find one unexposed film in the batch.

FIGURE 5-46

1. Errors:
   Roller mark (horizontal black line)
   Static electricity (V-shaped black lines on lower molar mesial root)
2. Error correction:
   Roller mark: Clean rollers weekly; pass a blank film through the processor daily first thing after warm-up.
   Static electricity: Humidify the darkroom with a humidifier or a large open container of water; do not pinch the packet or paper liner when removing the film for processing, and stand on an antistatic pad when processing.

FIGURE 5-47

1. Bitewing A was taken with a little too much positive vertical angulation; notice the lower cusp tips are not superimposed; the premolar-canine contacts are overlapped.
2. Bitewing B was taken with the incorrect horizontal angulation causing unacceptable overlapping of the interproximal surfaces of the teeth.

3. Both need to be retaken; in A we need to open up the canine-premolar contacts; in B we need to open all of the contacts.

FIGURE 5-48

1. The error is scratched emulsion from rough handling of the film, especially during processing when the emulsion is soft or a mosquito forceps is used to hand process the film.

FIGURE 5-49

1. The film packet was reversed with the back or printed side of the packet toward the beam of radiation. Thus the embossed lead foil backing filters out some of the radiation and the embossed pattern is recorded on the film. These patterns change from time to time with any film speed.
2. All should be retaken. Remember, the dot will be reversed so this film could be erroneously mounted on the wrong side of the film mount. This can produce a "good news–bad news" situation such as: "We treated the tooth well but we extracted the left molar instead of the right one"!
3. The film speeds are different:
   - A is "D"-speed or Ultraspeed film (KS embossed marking), which is about 50% faster than the old "radiatized" or "C"-speed film.
   - B is "E"-speed or Ektaspeed film (EKT embossed marking), which is about 40% faster than "D"-speed film.
   - C is "F"-speed or INSIGHT film (IN embossed marking), which is about 20% faster than "E" or "E+" speed film.

COMMENT: "E" and "E+"-films are the same speed. The "E+" uses a flat-shaped silver grain and has PLS embossed on the edge of the film. In 2015 "E"-speed film has generally been replaced with "F"-speed film.

FIGURE 5-50

1. The lower edge of the film was not placed parallel to the occlusal surfaces of the teeth. Actually, as often happens, the film was properly placed but was moved by the patient just before exposure.
2. The coronoid process of the mandible. You knew that!

FIGURE 5-51

1. Inadequate fixation. The film was not left in the fixer long enough after development, or the fixer solution needs replenishment.

COMMENT: The fixer removes all unexposed silver from the image and is said to "clear" the image. Remember: "There's silver in them thar hills!" Only in the dental office, it is in the fixer solution. Collection service companies will pay cash for fixer solution or supply a silver recovery unit.

FIGURE 5-52

1. Causes of film fog:
   Use of outdated film
   Film storage in a warm place
   Exposure of film to scatter radiation
   Light leaks in the darkroom
   Unsafe safelight:
   - Bulb brighter than 15 watts
   - Distance to countertop less than 4 feet
   - Incorrect safelight filter (Kodak GBX and GBX2 filters are safe for all dental films)
   - Two or more safelights with the above specs are all okay but too close to each other; the areas of light crossover will be too bright

FIGURE 5-53

1. In example A the complete upper denture was left in; in example B a cast removable partial denture was not removed.
2. Example A is acceptable in some situations because the denture helps to retain and stabilize the bite block holding the film. Denture acrylic is radiotransparent; i.e., it cannot be readily seen in the radiographs; not all plastics are radiotransparent. Example B is usually unacceptable because metallic parts may obscure structures or pathology, and the partial denture may not be needed to properly stabilize the bite block of the film holder.

FIGURE 5-54

1. The two errors in both examples A and B:
   Foreshortening caused by excessive vertical angulation
   Overlap of the canine-premolar contact, which should be open to best see the interproximal alveolar bone
2. These would not necessarily be retaken, depending on the purpose for which they were taken.
   COMMENT: Nowadays, even in training situations, students are not asked to repeat certain imperfect films if the areas of interest can be seen on other films in the series or if the less-than-perfect image suits the purpose. For example, these would not be good to measure root canal length (the crestal alveolar bone and periodontal membrane space are not perfect but perhaps adequate in the absence of disease); the apical regions are well imaged if periapical pathology is being sought.

FIGURE 5-55

1. This is known as consistency. In both instances the film was placed on top of the tongue, wedging it between the film and the mandible.
2. Look at the bottom left corner of the photo. This occurs in automatic processors. Bent film usually produces a radiolucent line. Apparently, when a slightly curved film edge is fed into the processor first the curved edge can somehow become entangled in the roller assembly. The ragged edge is actually torn and has lost emulsion. In this situation the film does not always come out of the processor.

FIGURE 5-56

1. The patient was probably uncomfortable or insufficiently instructed and let go of the bite block before the exposure was completed.

FIGURE 5-57

1. Two problems:
   Static electricity and how!
   "Fingernail" artifact, which is not from anyone's long fingernails but is from bending the film and causing it to crimp
   COMMENT: Take a piece of paper. Place it between your thumb on one side and your index and middle fingers on the other side (your index finger is the one you point with and your middle finger is the one…well…that you need to properly express yourself in some situations). As you bend back the piece of paper, watch the crimp mark appear.

FIGURE 5-58

1. The patient's glasses were left on.
2. Glasses material:
   Example A: A metal frame and a plastic (radiotransparent) lens
   Example B: A metal frame and a glass (porcelain-like density) lens

3. Film sizes:
   Example A: Size #1
   Example B: Size #2
   COMMENT: There are various techniques regarding film size in the full-mouth survey. In some cases the anterior teeth are imaged with #1 film and the posteriors and bitewings with #2; others use only #2-size film for the whole survey.

FIGURE 5-59

1. Error: cervical burnout (adumbration)
2. It could be root caries but…note that the horizontal angulation of the beam is incorrect. This is a very common location for cervical burnout.
3. Yes, if the clinical examination cannot confirm the absence of caries or if the interseptal alveolar bone needs to be seen.

FIGURE 5-60

1. Similar film-handling errors:
   Example A: Film crimping (crescent-shaped radiolucent line)
   Example B: Film bending (vertical black line)

FIGURE 5-61

1. Part of the image was exposed to light.

FIGURE 5-62

1. Increased apical coverage:
   Instruct the patient to keep biting on the bite block until the beeping sound (signaling x-rays being emitted) stops.
   Place the film more apically by positioning it more toward the midline of the palate.
   Increase the vertical angulation of the beam.
2. The dot is at the apex. Remember the "dot in the slot" rule. (The dot is darker than usual because it was inked in so you would not miss it.)

FIGURE 5-63

1. How to get 3rd molar apices:
   Example A: Increase the vertical angulation 10 to 15 degrees in excess of what the BID positioning device indicates, using the normal technique.
   Example B: There are two techniques:
   - Technique #1, mesioangular projection: Line the BID up correctly, then turn the cone tip about 10 to 15 degrees mesially, and then move the tube head and BID distally as one so that you do not cone-cut. This will project the coronal portion of the 3rd molar on the 2nd molar, but the apical region will be seen.
   - Technique #2, distal extension of film: Instead of placing the film centered on the bite block, move it distally from the centered position by about 1 or 2 cm. Place the film holder and BID indicating rod and ring as usual. Align the beam as usual, and then move the tube head and BID distally by the same amount you offset the film on the bite block.

FIGURE 5-64

1. Cone-cut

FIGURE 5-65

Errors:
1. Bent film
2. Film not placed sufficiently apically

FIGURE 5-66

1. Film too light as a result of factors causing insufficient radiation or depleted developer

FIGURE 5-67

1. Excess positive vertical angulation. This results in superimposition of the malar process and zygoma on the edentulous alveolar ridge.

FIGURE 5-68

1. Patient movement

FIGURE 5-69

1. Excess negative vertical angulation of the BID. Notice the shadow of the floor of the mouth crossing the inferior cortex. This is a newly recognized error by Weidman and Warman. The floor of the mouth rises up and gets wedged between the film and the mandible. This is distinguished from the tongue shadow by the straight linear nature of this shadow vs. the curved image of the tongue.

FIGURE 5-70

1. Insufficient apical coverage; probably because of pain, the child stopped biting on the bite block. Some film packets are made of paper; these can become soaked through with saliva and the black paper from the inner wrap sticks to the softened emulsion. With the polysoft film packets, this problem does not occur.

FIGURE 5-71

1. Excess biting pressure. Note the black marks at the occlusal aspect of the molar and incisal aspect of the canine. This is a pediatric partial occlusal technique taken with #2 film. This technique offers ease of film retention and comfort for the child.

MULTIPLE CHOICE QUESTIONS WITH FIGURES

FIGURE 5-72

1. A

FIGURE 5-73

1. D

FIGURE 5-74

1. C

FIGURE 5-75

1. A

FIGURE 5-76

1. C

FIGURE 5-77

1. D

FIGURE 5-78

1. B

FIGURE 5-79

1. B
2. A

FIGURE 5-80

1. C
2. A

FIGURE 5-81

1. A
2. B
3. C

FIGURE 5-82

1. E
2. C
3. D

FIGURE 5-83

1. B
2. D

FIGURE 5-84

1. A
2. D

Chapter 6

THE PARTS (ANATOMY) OF THE PAN-CEPH MACHINE

FIGURE 6-1

1. exit area of the radiation beam
2. CCD digital sensor
3. tube head
4. base for chin rest/bite block/side guide assembly; also housing for canine positioning light
5. hold-on handles for patient
6. platform for motorized machine adjustment knobs
7. touch screen for machine settings menu
8. primary vertical machine support column
9. support "C" arm for rotating tube head/CCD assembly

FIGURE 6-2

1. chin rest
2. bite block
3. side guides in closed position
4. base for chin rest/bite block/side guides
5. support arm
6. support housing for cephalometric assembly
7. center line nasion support/indicator
8. right and left ear rods

FIGURE 6-3

1. left ear rod
2. right ear rod
3. nasion support/indicator
4. CCD sensor
5. soft tissue filter
6. support housing for cephalometric assembly
7. ceph horizontal support arm

FIGURE 6-4

1. open/close side guides control
2. beam alignment controls for tomography

3. beam alignment control for tomography
4. raise and lower machine controls
5. support arm
6. housing for touch screen
7. touch screen machine function/settings menu
8. hold-on handles for patient
9. primary vertical machine support column

FIGURE 6-5A

1. base of support arm for special controls and rotating touch menu screen
2. housing for touch screen
3. panoramic program being selected on touch screen
4. touch screen
5. primary vertical machine support column

FIGURE 6-5B This picture represents an update of the control panel as seen in Figure 6–5A. It illustrates two things: 1. At any point in time, it is difficult for the authors to keep up with the progress that all manufacturers are constantly making. 2. This control panel is larger with easier to read graphics. The bottom line: Regardless of manufacturer or model, the panoramic anatomy and error identification principles remain the same.

QUESTIONS PART 1: IDENTIFICATION OF ERRORS IN CLINICAL TECHNIQUE

FIGURE 6-18 Error: The patient's head is turned or twisted.
Correction: Close the side guides; make sure the vertical midline positioning light is in the patient's midline.

FIGURE 6-19 Error: The patient is too far forward.
Correction: Use the bite block or bite stick; make sure the canine light is at the mesial aspect of the maxillary canine for this machine.

FIGURE 6-20 Error: The chin is positioned too high.
Correction: Tilt the chin down; make sure the positioning light is on the Frankfort plane (orbital rim to tragus of the ear).

FIGURE 6-21 Error: Glasses are left on.
Correction: Make certain all extraoral and intraoral items have been removed.

FIGURE 6-22 Error: Lips are open, and tongue is not against palate. (Note that side guides are also open and chin is a little high.)
Correction: Instruct patient to swallow or suck on his cheeks or suck on the bite block. This will usually cause the patient to close the lips and press the tongue against the palate. (Try this by biting on an object like a pencil eraser.)

FIGURE 6-23 Error: The patient is slumped. (The neck is not vertical because the patient is not standing up straight.)
Correction: Be sure the patient is standing upright so the neck is vertical with the feet advanced to the point where the patient must hold on to the handles. Some offices place two footprints on the floor for this purpose.

FIGURE 6-24 The most obvious error is that the patient's mouth is open, and in that circumstance, the tongue is usually not on the palate. The head appears somewhat tilted. The lead apron is no longer required.

FIGURE 6-25 Error: Chin is too low.
Correction: Make sure positioning light is on Frankfort plane. (Lower orbital rim to tragus of the ear, which is the little bump in front of the ear opening.)

FIGURE 6-26 Error: Chin is not on chin rest.
Correction: When you ask the patient to stand up straight, the chin often comes up off the chin rest. Be certain to bring the machine up to meet the chin when this happens.

FIGURE 6-27 Error: Head is tilted or tipped.
Correction: Close the side guides; ensure the vertical midface positioning light and the patient's midline happens.

FIGURE 6-28A Dad's errors:
1. Glasses are left on.
2. Earrings are left on.
3. Necklace is left on.
4. No protective apron is worn.
5. Positioned too far forward (canine light).
6. Head is turned (midline face light not on midline).
7. Chin is not on the chin rest (special edentulous chin rest has no bite block because the patient has no teeth).
8. Neck appears slumped.

FIGURE 6-28B The radiograph is of a different patient as can be seen by the missing earrings and glasses as well as possibly the necklace. The most obvious "error" is that the denture was left in; however, because acrylic is radiotransparent, leaving the denture in can help with positioning in some cases. Finally the patient was "slumped" when positioned in the machine, which produces a ghost image of the spine as a vertical, radiopaque band in the middle of the image.

FIGURE 6-29 The patient is "slumped" in the machine as the neck is not vertical; earrings and necklace are left on, mouth is open and tongue appears to be down from the palate; vertical stabilizers are not fully closed.

FIGURE 6-30A The patient appears to be positioned correctly.

FIGURE 6-30B This is a digital panoramic image of a well-positioned patient, except that the tongue was not against the palate causing a dark shadow across the apices of the maxillary teeth, and the lips were open causing a darkish shadow at the midline in the area of the crowns of the anterior teeth.

QUESTIONS PART 2: IDENTIFICATION OF ERRORS IN RADIOGRAPHS

FIGURE 6-43

1. Error:
   Chin is tipped too low.
2. Features:
   Excessively curved "smile line" of the teeth.
   Hyoid bone is projected as a horizontal, radiopaque band across the anterior mandible.

3. Correction:
    Raise chin up a little.
    Check Frankfort plane light is parallel to the ala-tragus line.

FIGURE 6-44

1. Error:
    Patient is "slumped" or "stooped."
2. Features:
    Lower anterior teeth are obscured.
    V-shaped radiopaque ghost image of the spine is seen in the midline.
3. Correction:
    Make sure patient is standing upright with back and neck straight.

FIGURE 6-45

1. First error:
    Patient is "turned" or "twisted" in the machine.
2. Features:
    Molars are wider on right than on left.
    Ramus is wider on right than on left.
3. Correction:
    Make sure patient is facing straight forward in the machine.
    Close side guides firmly against patient's head.
    Check anterior vertical midline light; make sure it is aligned with middle of nose and rest of face.
1. Second error:
    Patient is "slumped" or "stooped."
2. Features:
    Anterior left teeth are slightly obscured by radiopaque shadow.
    Ghost image of spine is seen on left midline, only as patient is turned in the machine.
3. Correction:
    Make sure patient is standing upright with back and neck straight.

FIGURE 6-46

1. First error:
    Patient is positioned too far forward in the machine.
2. Features:
    Excessively narrowed anterior teeth
    Spine is superimposed on ramus on both sides.
3. Correction:
    Make sure patient is biting in groove in bite block.
    Check that the canine light is aligned with middle of lower canine.
1. Second error:
    Patient is slightly twisted.
2. Features:
    Upper right molar is a little wider than upper left molar.
    Right ramus is a little wider than left ramus.
    Spine overlaps right ramus more than left ramus.
3. Correction:
    Close side guides firmly against patient's head.
    Check anterior midline light.

COMMENT: The lower anterior teeth are missing so the patient could not properly bite in the groove in the bite block, as indicated by the lack of an interocclusal space between the upper and lower teeth. Because the patient was not biting in the groove, he ended up too far forward and possibly contributed to the twisted position as well. A couple of cotton rolls in the edentulous space and careful attention to technique would have taken care of the problem.

FIGURE 6-47

1. Error:
    Insufficient kVp or depleted developer
2. Features:
    Image too light
3. Correction:
    Remember to adjust kVp to patient's size and build.
    Check processor with a pre-exposed radiograph; if it comes out light, replenish the solutions.

FIGURE 6-48

1. First error:
    Lower partial denture left in
2. Features:
    Partial denture seen in image
3. Correction:
    Be sure to ask patient if there is a denture or partial denture, barbell, etc.
1. Second error:
    Patient is slumped.
2. Features:
    Lower anterior teeth are obscured.
    Radiopaque ghost image of spine is seen in lower midline.
3. Correction:
    Make sure patient is standing upright with back and neck straight.

FIGURE 6-49

1. Error:
    Hoop and stud earrings were not removed on each side.
2. Features:
    Real and ghost images of earrings
3. Correction:
    Be sure to check for this in both men and women, especially those with long hair obscuring the ears.

FIGURE 6-50

1. First error:
    Tongue is not against palate.
2. Features:
    Dark shadow is obscuring apices of maxillary teeth.
3. Correction:
    Instruct patient to place tongue on palate; if this fails, ask patient to suck on his or her cheeks while still biting on the bite block.
1. Second error:
    Patient is positioned too far back.
2. Features:
    Normally we would expect to see widened teeth, but sometimes this feature is missing, as is the case here.
    Ghost image of the ramus on both sides. This is easy to see because a horizontal line is dividing the ramus from the body; above this line the ramus is excessively radiopaque, and below the line the body is of normal density. The radiopaque shadow is the ghost image of the ramus on the other side and happens only when the patient is too far back.
3. Correction:
    Make sure patient is biting in groove in bite block.
    Check canine light.

FIGURE 6-51

1. Error:
    Tongue is not on palate halfway through the exposure.

2. Features:
Black shadow representing air is superimposed on upper right maxilla and extending on to the ramus in the area of the coronoid process.

3. Correction:
Instruct the patient to suck gently on the bite block throughout the exposure.

Note: The medial sigmoid depression is seen bilaterally as a radiolucent area near the base of the coronoid process.

FIGURE 6-52

1. First error:
Chin is too high.

2. Features:
The occlusal plane is flat. Also when the chin is up, the head goes back causing a ghost image of the ramus on both sides.

3. Correction:
Make certain the ala-tragus positioning light on the side of the face is parallel with the floor and is in the middle of the ala of the nose and on the tragus of the ear; this will ensure the chin is at the correct down angle on the chin rest.

1. Second error:
Patient is slumped in the machine.

2. Features:
There is a light radiopaque shadow in the mandibular midline, and as a result of the slumping, the machine rubbed against the neck causing the patient to move slightly as seen by the wavy outline of the mandibular cortex in this area.

3. Correction:
Have the patient stand "tall" with the neck straight and vertical.

Note: The stylohyoid ligament is calcified and extremely large bilaterally. Such patients may have dizzy spells when turning the head as this movement causes pressure on the internal carotid artery.

FIGURE 6-53

1. First error:
Glasses are left on.

2. Features:
Foreign object is seen in the image (metal, glass lenses; space between metal and glass lens is a plastic rim).

3. Correction:
Remove all extraoral objects like glasses, jewelry, etc.

1. Second error:
Patient is positioned too far back.

2. Features:
Teeth are not widened again.
Ghost image of ramus is seen on both sides.

3. Correction:
Instruct patient to bite in groove of bite block.
Check cuspid light.

1. Third error:
Patient movement.

2. Features:
This is usually best noted by a "jiggly" or uneven image of a small portion of the inferior cortex of the mandible. Here we can clearly see this feature starting at the midline all the way to the right 1st premolar area. The movement sometimes causes vertical white streaks, as seen here in the midline.

3. Correction:
Instruct the patient to be still.
Explain what the machine will do so the patient is not startled.
Do a practice run, if necessary, with radiation turned off.

FIGURE 6-54

1. First error:
Chin is tilted too far upward.

2. Features:
"Flat" occlusal plane
Heavy, radiopaque horizontal line representing the hard palate obscures the apices of all the maxillary teeth. Inferior cortex of the mandible gives the mandible a "box-like" appearance.

3. Correction:
Tip the chin down 4 to 7 degrees.
Align the Frankfort plane light (ala-tragus line).

1. Second error:
Patient is "tilted" or "tipped" to one side.

2. Features:
Right condyle above left condyle

3. Correction:
Close side guides firmly against patient's head.
Check midline light.

1. Third error:
Patient is positioned too far back.

2. Features:
Widened anterior teeth are not seen (we expect to see widened anterior teeth, but this feature is not reliable).
Ghost images of the ramus on both sides (this time this feature is not so obvious but is there). The right-side radiopaque line is above the one on the left because the patient is tilted.
The radiopaque inferior turbinates are spread out across the maxillary sinus on both sides, immediately above the hard palate. (When present, this is another reliable feature of too-far-back positioning.)

3. Correction:
Make certain the patient is biting in bite block groove.
Check canine light.

1. Fourth error:
Patient is slumped in the machine.

2. Features:
Ghost image of spine is seen in anterior area.
Anterior teeth are slightly obscured by ghost image.

3. Correction:
Make sure patient stands upright with back and neck straight.

COMMENT: This can be facilitated by asking patients to take baby steps forward once in the machine until they must almost have to grasp the handles to avoid falling backward. You can also paste two footprints on the floor or base of the machine.

FIGURE 6-55

1. Errors:
First, the tongue is not against the palate and second, the lips are open.

2. Features:
There is a radiolucent shadow at the apices of the upper teeth. There is a dark oval shadow superimposed on the upper and lower anterior teeth.

3. Correction:
Ask the patient to suck gently on the bite stick to correct both errors.

FIGURE 6-56

1. First error:
The chin is too high.

2. Features:
The occlusal plane is flat, and in this case, both the real images and the ghost images of the hard palate are superimposed on

the apices of the upper teeth, thus obscuring the presence of any periapical lesions as can be seen in the mandible.

3. Correction:
Make certain the ala-tragus positioning light on the side of the face is parallel with the floor and is in the middle of the ala of the nose and on the tragus of the ear; this will assure the chin is at the correct down angle on the chin rest.

1. Second error:
The head is tilted down to the right.
2. Features:
The occlusal plane is canted upward toward the patient's left side; the left condyle is higher up in the image than the left condyle.
3. Correction:
Look at the patient face-on. The midline light will not pass through the midline of the face, and better still, align this light with the midline of the teeth as this is the most important from an imaging standpoint. The dental midline is not always aligned with the midline of the face or a structure on the face such as the nose.
1. Third error:
The lips are open.
2. Features:
There is a dark oval shadow superimposed on the upper and lower anterior teeth.
3. Correction:
Ask the patient to suck gently on the bite stick.

FIGURE 6-57

1. First error:
Neck chain is left on.
2. Features:
Ghost image of the neck chain in the mandibular midline.
Real image seen on right spine identifies the chain as jewelry vs. a napkin chain.
3. Correction:
Be sure to remove all extraoral items.
1. Second error:
Patient is too far forward.
2. Features:
Narrow anterior teeth
Shadow of spine overlaps the ramus on both sides.
3. Correction:
Make sure the patient is biting in bite block groove.
Check canine light.

FIGURE 6-58

1. First error:
Chin is too high.
2. Features:
The inferior border of the mandible is straight.
The mandible is box-like.
3. Correction:
Check ala-tragus light.
1. Second error:
Patient is too far back.
2. Features:
Ghosting of the ramus is seen bilaterally.
Turbinates are spread out across sinus bilaterally.
3. Correction:
Make sure patient is biting in bite block groove.
Check canine light.
COMMENT: This patient is slightly turned or twisted. See how the ramus is wider on the right, and we can only see the epiglottis below the angle of the left mandible.

FIGURE 6-59

1. First error:
Four necklaces are left on.
2. Features:
Note the four curved radiopaque images in the midline: one below the mandible, two superimposed on the lower centrals, and one on the maxillary centrals.
3. Correction:
Remove extraoral items.
1. Second error:
Earrings are left on.
2. Features:
Real and ghost images of earrings
3. Correction:
Remove extraoral items.
1. Third error:
Chin is too high.
2. Features:
Flat occlusal plane
Mandible is box-like.
3. Correction:
Check ala-tragus light.
1. Fourth error:
Lips are open.
2. Features:
Dark oval shadow partially obscuring the crowns of the upper and lower anterior teeth.
3. Correction:
Instruct the patient to close lips.
1. Fifth error:
Tongue is not on palate.
2. Features:
Dark shadow is obscuring apical region of maxillary teeth.
3. Correction:
Instruct patient to place tongue against palate or suck on cheeks or bite block.

FIGURE 6-60

1. First error:
Chin is not on chin rest.
2. Features:
Jaws are high up in image.
Wide space between chin rest just at lower middle edge of image and inferior border of mandible.
3. Correction:
When adjusting the chin, especially in tilting it up, or when asking the patient to stand up straight, the chin will come up off the chin rest. The machine must then be elevated so the patient's chin rests on the chin rest.
1. Second error:
Tongue is not on palate.
2. Features:
Dark shadow is seen above maxillary apices.
3. Correction:
Instruct patient to place tongue against palate.

FIGURE 6-61

1. First error:
The tongue is not against the palate and the lips are open.
2. Features:
There is a radiolucent shadow at the apices of the upper teeth.
There is a dark oval shadow superimposed on the upper and lower anterior teeth.

3. Correction:
    Ask the patient to suck gently on the bite stick

1. Second error:
    The chin is too high.
2. Features:
    The occlusal plane is flat, and in this case, both the real images and the ghost images of the hard palate are superimposed on the apices of the upper teeth thus obscuring the presence of any peri-apical lesions, as can be seen in the mandible.
3. Correction:
    Make certain the ala-tragus positioning light on the side of the face is parallel with the floor; this will ensure the chin is at the correct down angle on the chinrest.

1. Third error:
    The head is tilted down to the left.
2. Features:
    The occlusal plane is canted upward toward the patient's left side; the right condyle is higher up in the image than the left condyle.
3. Correction:
    Look at the patient face-on. The midline (midsagittal) light will not pass through the midline of the face. Better still, align this light with the midline of the teeth as the dental arch is the most important from an imaging standpoint. The dental midline is not always aligned with the midline of the face or a structure on the face such as the nose.

FIGURE 6-62

1. Error:
    Patient movement
2. Features:
    Wavy outline of inferior cortex of mandible
3. Correction:
    Instruct patient to hold still.
    Explain function of machine so patient will not be startled.

FIGURE 6-63

1. First error:
    The patient is too far forward in the machine.
2. Features:
    The main feature seen here is that the spine is superimposed on the ramus bilaterally.
3. Correction:
    Have the patient bite in the groove in the bite block and bring the canine light to the correct position. This is often in the middle of the canine or on the mesial aspect of the canine.
1. Second error:
    The tongue is not against the palate.
2. Features:
    There is a radiolucent shadow at the apices of the upper teeth.
3. Correction:
    Ask the patient to suck gently on the bite stick.

FIGURE 6-64

1. Error:
    Patient is positioned too far back.
2. Features:
    The only sign of this error is that the nasal turbinates are spread across the sinus above the hard palate on both sides.
3. Correction:
    Some machines have a special chin rest for edentulous patients. These usually have a bit of a cup-and-lip configuration so the chin can fit in there snugly.

Check the canine light; it should be somewhere near the corner of the mouth, depending on the machine.
COMMENT: In this case we can see the outline of the lips, which are closed around the bite block.

FIGURE 6-65

1. Error:
    Patient is twisted or turned in machine.
2. Features:
    Right ramus is much wider than left ramus.
3. Correction:
    Close side guides firmly against patient's head.
    Check midface vertical light.

FIGURE 6-66

1. Error:
    Patient is tilted or tipped in machine.
2. Features:
    One condyle is lower than the other.
3. Correction:
    Check midface vertical light.

FIGURE 6-67

1. First error:
    Patient movement
2. Features:
    Note bend, curve, or "chink" in mandibular outline and in tur-binate directly above.
3. Correction:
    Instruct patient to hold still.
    Explain machine function and movements.
1. Second error:
    Patient is positioned too far back.
2. Features:
    Turbinates of nose are spread out across sinuses.
3. Correction:
    Place chin properly in the special edentulous chin rest.
    Check canine positioning light at or near corner of the mouth.
1. Third error:
    Patient is twisted (turned).
2. Features:
    Left ramus wider than right ramus
3. Correction:
    Close side guides firmly against patient's head.
    Check midface positioning light.

FIGURE 6-68

1. First error:
    The patient is slumped in the machine.
2. Features:
    There is a light radiopaque shadow in the mandibular mid-line, and as a result of the slumping, the machine rubbed against the neck causing the patient to move slightly, as seen by the wavy outline of the mandibular cortex in this area. On the left side, there is a hint that the spine is not vertical.
3. Correction:
    Have the patient stand "tall" with the neck straight and vertical.
1. Second error:
    The chin is too high.
2. Features:
    The occlusal plane is flat.

3. Correction:
Make certain the ala-tragus positioning light on the side of the face is parallel with the floor; this will ensure the chin is at the correct down angle on the chin rest.
1. Third error:
The head is turned toward the left side of the midline.
2. Features:
The interproximal surfaces of the teeth on the left side are more "open" than on the right side, and the left ramus is narrower than the right ramus.
3. Correction:
Look at the patient face-on. The midline light will not pass through the midline of the face. The face will appear to be at an off angle relative to the midsagittal light.
1. Fourth error:
The head is tilted down to the left.
2. Features:
The occlusal plane is canted downward toward the patient's left side; the left condyle is lower down in the image than the left condyle.
3. Correction:
Look at the patient face-on. The midline (midsagittal) light will not pass through the midline of the face. Better still, align this light with the midline of the teeth as the teeth are the most important from an imaging standpoint. The dental midline is not always aligned with the midline of the face or a midline structure on the face such as the nose.

Note 1: This is a digital panoramic image which has been over-processed in functions such as sharpen, sharpen edges, despeckle, and remove noise. This causes a dark line to appear under metallic restorations, which can mimic recurrent caries. In the case of a panoramic bitewing, however, this is a significant error as these electronic filters will remove smaller interproximal caries.

Note 2: This is an older patient as can be seen by the receded pulp chambers. Look at the area of the "L" marker. This is carotid artery plaque, which may occlude the internal carotid artery when the patient turns his head, or if a piece of plaque breaks off it can cause a stroke.

FIGURE 6-69 When you look at this image you can say "wow" if you want because it is an example of what a really nice digital panoramic image can look like.
1. First error:
The chin is too high.
2. Features:
The occlusal plane is flat, and in this case, both the real images and the ghost images of the hard palate are not superimposed on the apices of the upper.
3. Correction:
Make certain the ala-tragus positioning light on the side of the face is parallel with the floor and lined up with the ala of the nose and the tragus of the ear. This will ensure the chin is at the correct down angle on the chin rest.
1. Second error:
There is a wavy outline of the inferior cortex of the mandible in the midline.
2. Features:
Although the spine is not vertical, it was not sufficiently canted to produce a ghost image. However, it was canted sufficiently to cause the tube head of the machine to rub against the back of the patient's neck, which caused the patient to move slightly.

3. Correction:
Have the patient stand "tall" with the neck straight and vertical.
Note: Look at the apex of the upper left lateral incisor. There is a radiolucent area at the apex and resorption of the tooth at the apex. This could be interpreted as pathology. However, the patient has had orthodontic treatment, which can be deduced by the fixed retainer at the lower midline. Excessive orthodontic forces can cause resorption of the apex of one or several teeth. The radiolucent area is the air within the left nostril with its twin on the right side.

FIGURE 6-70
1. First error:
Patient's chin is tipped too low.
2. Features:
Excessive smile line of occlusal plane
Apices of lower teeth out of image
Usually all of the hyoid bone is seen as a horizontal radiopaque shadow crossing the mandible; it is not in this case because of the next error.
3. Correction:
Check ala-tragus positioning light.
1. Second error:
Patient is twisted or turned.
2. Features:
Right ramus is narrower than left ramus and toward the buccal or film side of machine.
Hyoid is spread out only on left or wide side, which is toward the machine (wide side is lingual; machine or tube head is always lingual).
3. Correction:
Check vertical midline light.

FIGURE 6-71 If you are having trouble finding an error it is because there is nothing significantly wrong with image.
1. Error:
Slight movement.
2. Features:
There is slight waviness of the mandibular inferior cortex at the midline. The spine is not perfectly vertical, and the machine may have momentarily rubbed against the back of the neck.
3. Correction:
Have the patient stand "tall."
Note: Figures 6-39, 6-40, 6-43, 6-44, 6-49, 6-51, 6-56, 6-57, and 6-59 are all digital panoramic images. Please read the introduction regarding these images.

FIGURE 6-72
1. First error:
Nose ring is left on.
2. Features:
Observe item.
3. Correction:
Remove extraoral objects.
1. Second error:
Some sort of body-piercing object is seen in back of neck or metallic clip on clothing.
2. Features:
Observe item.
3. Correction:
Remove extraoral objects.
1. Third error:
Tongue is not on palate.

2. Features:
Palatoglossal air space (same dark shadow covering maxillary apices)
3. Correction:
Instruct patient to place tongue against palate.
1. Fourth error:
Patient is positioned too far back.
2. Features:
Bilateral ghosting of ramus
3. Correction:
Make certain patient bites in bite block groove.
Check canine positioning light.
PHEW!!! I guess that was hard work, although the cases were selected to be progressive with lots of repetition of the errors. Hope you are starting to catch on.

FIGURE 6-73

1. Dark stains are developer; whitish stains are fixer.

FIGURE 6-74

1. Fog

FIGURE 6-75

1. Scratched screen

FIGURE 6-76

1. Machine not started at home base
COMMENT: Many of the machines with soft cassettes fitting on a drum can have this error. The drum must be set at a certain starting point before starting the exposure. If this is not done, a sort of panoramic "cone-cut" occurs.

FIGURE 6-77

1. Film crimping while removing from box or from cassette
2. Pits in the screen; each white spot is a small damaged area of the screen.

FIGURE 6-78

1. Static electricity
2. The problem is from dry air. Humidify the darkroom, especially in winter.

FIGURE 6-79

1. The pattern of the white lines suggests they are physical damage to the emulsion. This can be confirmed when holding the film in your hand. Instead of looking directly at the radiograph, look at the reflected surface of each side of the film. If there are scratches, you will see them this way.
In the absence of finding damage to the film emulsion, you then look at the intensifying screen in the cassette. You will see the scratch marks, and every film taken with that cassette will have the same pattern.

FIGURE 6-80

1. Old plastic cassettes tend to split at the seams after a time. This was the case here, with the resulting light leak that produced the black mark.

FIGURE 6-81

1. Cracked screen; the operator would pull the screen and film about one third of the way out of the soft cassette and then flip back the top screen to remove and insert films. Over time, the screen became cracked. In such areas there is no image because it does not fluoresce in these areas.

FIGURE 6-82

1. In some machines (current models also), the cassette can be put into the machine back to front. The result is the same as for intraoral film, only this time things on the back of the cassette are in the image.
2. It is not recommended that it be kept. Having both L and R markings can lead to "good news–bad news" mistakes. These reversed images should be retaken.

FIGURE 6-83

1. First error:
Chin is too high.
2. Features:
The occlusal plane is flat, and in this case, both the real images and the ghost images of the hard palate are superimposed on the apices of the upper teeth.
3. Correction:
Make certain the ala-tragus positioning light on the side of the face is parallel with the floor and is in the middle of the ala of the nose and on the tragus of the ear; this will ensure the chin is at the correct down angle on the chin rest.
1. Second error:
The tongue is not against the palate and the lips are open.
2. Features:
There is a radiolucent shadow at the apices of the upper teeth. There is a dark oval shadow superimposed on the upper and lower anterior teeth.
3. Correction:
Ask the patient to suck gently on the bite stick.

FIGURE 6-84

1. First error:
The tongue is not against the palate, and the lips are open.
2. Features:
There is a thin, radiolucent shadow at the apices of the upper teeth.
3. Correction:
Ask the patient to suck gently on the bite stick.
1. Second error:
Chin is too high.
2. Features:
The occlusal plane is flat, and in this case, both the real images and the ghost images of the hard palate are superimposed on the apices of the upper teeth.
3. Correction:
Make certain the ala-tragus positioning light on the side of the face is parallel with the floor and is in the middle of the ala of the nose and on the tragus of the ear; this will ensure the chin is at the correct down angle on the chin rest.

FIGURE 6-85

1. First error:
Earrings are left on.
2. Features:
The real images are seen in the area of the earlobe but in the image seen at the anterior arch of C1 bilaterally. The ghost images are above and long and spread out, indicating they were

just behind the rotation center where the horizontal magnification factor goes to infinity.

3. Correction:
Remove earrings before the scan.

1. Second error:
Patient is positioned too far forward in the machine.

2. Features:
Narrow anterior teeth and the spine is prominent, almost touching the posterior border of the ramus and has a reverse curvature.

3. Correction:
Make certain the canine light is on the upper canine and have the patient stand "tall." In this case the patient was asked to bring the shoulders forward in an effort to prevent the tube head from rubbing against the back of the neck. Check the neck and shoulders, making certain the neck is straight vertically.

1. Third error:
The head is tilted slightly to the left.

2. Features:
The occlusal plane is canted upward toward the patient's left side; the right condyle is higher up in the image than the left condyle.

3. Correction:
Look at the patient face-on. The midline (midsagittal) light will not pass through the midline of the face. Better still, align this light with the midline of the teeth as the dental arch is the most important from an imaging standpoint. The dental midline is not always aligned with the midline of the face or a structure on the face such as the nose.

FIGURE 6-86

1. First error:
The patient is slumped in the machine.

2. Features:
There is a radiopaque shadow in the mandibular midline, and as a result of the slumping, the machine rubbed against the neck causing the patient to move slightly, as seen by the slightly wavy outline of the mandibular cortex in this area. On the edges of the image, the spine is not vertical.

3. Correction:
Have the patient stand "tall" with the neck straight and vertical.

1. Second error:
The tongue is not against the palate and the lips are open.

2. Features:
There is a radiolucent shadow just below the edentulous maxilla and above the radiopaque soft tissue shadow of the tongue. There is a dark horizontal shadow midway between the mandible and the maxilla centered on the midline.

3. Correction:
Ask the patient to suck gently on the bite stick.

Note: The radiopacities we see just medial to the cervical spine between C3 and C4 most likely represent calcifications at the bifurcation of the carotid artery. There is some risk of a stroke in these patients and heavy deep palpation in the area of the pulsing carotid artery should be avoided if possible.

FIGURE 6-87 (also Figure 6.30B) See if you can still recognize the slight problem with this image. Part B: This is a current digital pan image. It is pretty good. The dark shadow above the apices of the upper teeth indicates black air because the tongue was not against the palate. With that error, the lips are often open and close examination shows an ovoid shape of dark air in the area. However, these

problems are hard to see, and the software in digital pan images can help to minimize the effects of these errors on the image.

1. First error:
The tongue is not against the palate and the lips are open.

2. Features:
There is a radiolucent shadow at the apices of the upper teeth. There is a dark oval shadow superimposed on the upper and lower anterior teeth.

3. Correction:
Ask the patient to suck gently on the bite stick.

1. Second error:
The patient is too far forward.

2. Features:
Narrow upper and lower anterior teeth, and the spine approximates the posterior border of the ramus.

3. Correction:
Check the canine light and make certain it is not further posterior than the middle of the upper canine.

Note: This error is a result of trying to get the patient sufficiently forward in the machine so that the tube head will not rub against the back of the neck.

1. Third error:
Movement

2. Features:
On the patient's right side, the spine is not vertical, but it is vertical on the patient's left side.

3. Correction:
Make certain the neck is vertical and bulky clothing is not going to interfere with the rotation of the machine as it passes behind the neck.

Note: Modern digital pan machines are truly more forgiving of technique errors as, in spite of the errors in technique, this image is of excellent quality.

QUESTIONS PART 3: MATCHING THE CLINICAL ERROR WITH THE RADIOGRAPH

FIGURE 6-88 Matches 6–100

FIGURE 6-89 Matches 6–105

FIGURE 6-90 Matches 6–107

FIGURE 6-91 Matches 6–98

FIGURE 6-92 Matches 6–103

FIGURE 6-93 Matches 6–101

FIGURE 6-94 Matches 6–104

FIGURE 6-95 Matches 6–102

FIGURE 6-96 Matches 6–106

FIGURE 6-97 Matches 6–99

QUESTIONS PART 4: MULTIPLE CHOICE QUESTIONS WITHOUT FIGURES

1. D
2. B
3. B
4. A
5. A
6. D

7. C	12. A
8. D	13. C
9. D	14. D
10. C	15. A
11. C	

Chapter 7

SHORT ANSWER QUESTIONS WITH FIGURES

FIGURE 7-1

Part 1: The structures include the facial parts of the skull including the mandible, maxilla and orbits.
Part 2: The view is from the anterior straight on to the buccal
Part 3:
1. anterior nasal spine
2. interseptal bone
3. crestal alveolar bone
4. inferior turbinate (concha)
5. cartilaginous nasal septum
6. inferior process of the ethmoid bone
7. nasal fossa
8. infraorbital foramen
9. zygomatic process of the maxilla
10. mental ridge
11. mental foramen
12. external oblique ridge
13. retromolar trigone
14. zygomaticomaxillary suture
15. zygomatic bone
16. zygomaticotemporal suture
17. zygomatic process of the temporal bone
18. nasal bone
19. zygomaticofrontal suture

FIGURE 7-2

Part 1: The structure is the mandible
Part 2: The mandible is slightly tilted down and the view is from the right buccal/anterior aspect
Part 3:
1. mental ridge
2. mandibular symphysis
3. mental foramen
4. mandibular body
5. external oblique ridge
6. angle of the mandible
7. retromolar trigone
8. ramus
9. neck of the condyle
10. head of the condyle
11. sigmoid notch
12. coronoid process
13. medial sigmoid depression
14. mandibular foramen
15. lingula

FIGURE 7-3

Part 1: The structure is the mandible
Part 2: The mandible is slightly tilted down and the view is from the lingual/posterior aspect
Part 3:
1. coronoid process
2. sigmoid notch
3. head of the condyle
4. medial sigmoid depression
5. mandibular foramen
6. angle of the mandible
7. inferior cortex of the mandible
8. digastric fossa
9. submandibular (salivary gland) fossa
10. mylohyoid (internal oblique) ridge
11. inferior genial tubercle of the geniohyoid muscle
12. superior genial tubercle of the genioglossus muscle
13. accessory lingual foramen for lingual vessels (lingual foramen)

FIGURE 7-4

Part 1: The anterior mandible
Part 2: The view is from the posterior looking forward (anteriorly).
Part 3:
1. accessory foramen
2. superior genial tubercle
3. accessory lingual foramen for lingual vessels (lingual foramen)
4. inferior genial tubercle
5. digastric fossa (digastric muscle attachment)

FIGURE 7-5

Part 1: The overall structure is a cut away of the left maxilla, the nose, and several adjacent sinus cavities and second, a view of the maxilla including the pterygoid complex. Third, the foraminae of the canals within the incisive canal as they are seen on the floor of the nose are pictured.
Part 2: The top diagram is a lateral view of a medial cut away; the view of the maxilla is from the palatal or inferior side. The superior foraminae in the floor of the nose are from the top (superior) view look downward (inferiorly).
Part 3:
1. hard palate
2. infundibulum
3. ostium of the nasolacrimal canal
4. inferior turbinate
5. middle turbinate
6. nasal bone
7. nasolacrimal canal
8. frontal sinus
9. sphenoid sinus
10. pituitary fossa
11. medial pterygoid plate
12. lateral pterygoid plate
13. hamular process of the medial pterygoid plate (hamulus)
14. maxillary tuberosity

15. incisive foramen
16. median maxillary suture
17. palatal process of the maxilla
18. palatomaxillary suture
19. shadow of the nasolacrimal duct
20. palatine bone
21. greater palatine foramen
22. lesser palatine foramen
23. posterior nares
24. foramen of Stensen
25. incisive canal
26. foramen of Scarpa

FIGURE 7-6

Part 1: The overall structure is a cut away of the maxilla including the lower parts of the maxillary sinus
Part 2: The view is from the anterior-superior aspect
Part 3:
1. interdental groove
2. maxilla
3. vertical process of the maxilla
4. floor of the nasal fossa
5. vomer bone
6. palatomaxillary suture
7. palatal bone
8. posterior nasal spine
9. sinus recess
10. maxillary sinus (antrum of Highmore)
11. bony septum of the maxillary sinus
12. anterior nasal spine

FIGURE 7-7

Part 1: The overall structure is a diagram of the branches of the carotid artery which supply the mandible and maxilla
Part 2: The view is from the lateral
Part 3:
1. common carotid artery
2. external carotid artery
3. internal carotid artery
4. facial artery
5. inferior alveolar artery
6. internal maxillary artery
7. posterior superior alveolar arteries
8. infraorbital artery
9. labial artery
10. incisive artery

FIGURE 7-8A

Part 1: Body of the mandible
Part 2: Lingual view
Part 3:
1. mylohyoid (internal oblique) ridge
2. submandibular fossa
3. inferior cortex or border of the mandible
4. mylohyoid (artery) groove
5. enamel
6. cementum
7. cemento-enamel junction
8. retromolar trigone (fossa)

FIGURE 7-8B

Part 1: Part of the body, angle, and ramus of the mandible
Part 2: Lingual view
Part 3:
1. mylohyoid (internal oblique) ridge
2. submandibular fossa
3. mandibular foramen
4. lingula
5. angle of the mandible
6. inferior cortex

FIGURE 7-8C

Part 1: Mandible
Part 2: Buccal view of the left body and ramus and lingual view of the upper part of the right ramus
Part 3:
1. external oblique ridge
2. retromolar trigone
3. mental foramen
4a. coronoid process, lateral view
4b. coronoid process, medial view
5a. mandibular condyle, lateral view
5b. mandibular condyle, medial view
6. body of the mandible
7. ramus
8. angle of the mandible
9a. sigmoid notch, lateral view
9b. sigmoid notch, medial view
10. medial sigmoid depression

FIGURE 7-9A

Part 1: Mandible (anterior midline area)
Part 2: Lingual view
Part 3:
1. accessory foramina
2. genial tubercles; (normally four tubercles serving as the attachments of the genioglossus [upper tubercles] or geniohyoid [lower tubercles] muscle)
3. accessory lingual foramen
4. digastric fossae (attachment of the digastric muscles)
5. fenestration; loss of bone covering the root without marginal involvement

FIGURE 7-9B

Part 1: Maxilla
Part 2: Buccal or lateral view
Part 3:
1. anterior nasal spine
2. fenestration (with involvement of the bone at crestal margin; condition is termed dehiscence)
3. zygomaticomaxillary suture
4. zygomatic process of the maxillary bone
5. maxillary tuberosity
6. hamular process of the medial pterygoid plate
7. lateral pterygoid plate
8. maxilla serving as the anterolateral will of the maxillary sinus

FIGURE 7-9C

Part 1: Maxilla (anterior midline area)
Part 2: Buccal view

Part 3:
1. anterior nares (openings) of the nasal fossae
2. nasal septum
3. anterior nasal spine
4. diastema
5. crown, enamel
6. root, cementum
7. interproximal crestal alveolar bone
8. right and left nasal fossae
9. bony core of the inferior turbinate

FIGURE 7-10A

Part 1: Maxilla (anterior midline region)
Part 2: Palatal view
Part 3:
1. incisive foramen
2. median palatal suture
3. accessory foramina (many in the area)

FIGURE 7-10B

Part 1: Maxilla (anterior midline region)
Part 2: Palatal view
Part 3:
1. median maxillary suture
2. incisive foramen
3. edentulous ridge crest (crestal alveolar bone)

FIGURE 7-10C

Part 1: Maxilla (anterior midline region)
Part 2: Palatal view
Part 3:
1. median maxillary suture
2. view into the incisive canal through the incisive foramen
3. foramen of Stensen (usually lateral to the foramen of Scarpa)
4. Foramen of Scarpa (usually close to the midline)

FIGURE 7-11

Part 1: Maxilla and associated structures
Part 2: Palatal view
Part 3:
1. incisive foramen
2. median maxillary suture
3. palatomaxillary suture
4. greater palatine foramen
5. lesser palatine foramen
6. posterior border of the hard palate
7. hamular process of the medial pterygoid plate
8. zygomatic process of the maxilla
9. zygomatic process of the temporal bone
10. zygomaticotemporal suture
11. palatal process of the maxilla
12. palatal bone
13. lateral pterygoid plate
14. medial pterygoid plate

FIGURE 7-12A

Part 1: The structures in this 3-D CBCT reconstruction include the facial parts of the skull including the mandible, maxilla and orbits.

Part 2: The view is from the anterior straight on looking at the buccal
Part 3:
1. orbit with greater wing of the sphenoid bone behind it
2. inferior orbital rim
3. zygomatic process of the maxilla
4. zygomatic process of the temporal bone
5. zygomaticomaxillary suture
6. clivus in the middle cranial fossa
7. anterior nasal spine
8. bilateral impacted maxillary canines
9. fenestration
10. alveolar process of the maxilla
11. external oblique ridge
12. posterior border of the ramus of the mandible
13. angle of the mandible
14. body of the mandible
15. digastric fossa on lingual surface
16. mental foramen
17. retromolar trigone

FIGURE 7-12B

Part 1: The structures in this 3-D CBCT reconstruction of the left side of the skull are of the hyoid bone, mandible, maxilla, orbits, and spine
Part 2: The view is from the lateral looking at the lateral aspects of the skull
Part 3:
1. superior orbital rim
2. frontomaxillary suture
3. nasal bone
4. lamina papyracea is the medial wall of the orbit and is the lateral wall of the ethmoid sinuses
5. zygomatic process of the maxilla
6. U-shaped malar process, the "root" of the zygoma
7. alveolar process of the maxilla
8. orthodontic appliance
9. mental foramen
10. digastric fossa on lingual surface
11. body of the mandible
12. posterior clinoid process of the sella turcica
13. zygomaticomaxillary suture
14. zygomatic process of the temporal bone
15. mandibular condyle
16. coronoid process
17. anterior arch of C1, the atlas
18. odontoid process of C2, the axis
19. spinous process of C1, the atlas
20. pedicle of C2, the axis
21. body of C2, the axis
22. intervertebral disk space
23. body of C3
24. greater horn of the hyoid bone
25. body of the hyoid bone
26. body of C4

Note: The carotid bifurcation is located just medial to the intervertebral space between C3 and C4.

FIGURE 7-13A

Part 1: The structures in this 3-D CBCT reconstruction of the left side of the skull are of the hyoid bone, mandible, maxilla, orbits, and spine.

Part 2: The view is a cut away of the left side of the skull from the right buccal aspect.

Part 3:

1. orbit
2. nasal bone
3. "root" of the zygomatic or malar process
4. anterior nasal spine
5. palatal process of the maxilla
6. internal oblique ridge
7. buccal cortex of the mandible
8. lingual cortex of the mandible
9. body of the hyoid bone
10. body of C4
11. greater horn of the hyoid bone
12. vertebral body of C3
13. intervertebral space
14. body of C2, the axis
15. odontoid process of C2, the axis
16. pedicle of C1, the atlas
17. anterior arch of C1, the atlas
18. ramus of the mandible
19. clivus
20. pituitary fossa
21. posterior clinoid process of the sella turcica

FIGURE 7-13B

Part 1: The structures in this CBCT image include the base of the skull, mandible, and zygomatic arches.

Part 2: The view is from the inferior axial aspect.

Part 3:

1. orthodontic appliance
2. digastric fossa
3. genial tubercle; there may be four of these for the attachments of the genioglossus and geniohyoid muscles
4. inferior border of the body of the mandible
5. body of the hyoid bone
6. greater horn of the hyoid bone
7. mandibular condyle
8. vertebral foramen for vertebral artery
9. tip of the odontoid process of C2
10. pedicle area of the cervical "stacked-up" vertebrae
11. space for the spinal nerve
12. space for the cerebrospinal fluid (CSF)
13. lateral mass of the "stacked-up" cervical vertebrae
14. body of the cervical vertebrae
15. clivus, which is inferior and posterior to the pituitary fossa
16. temporal process of the zygomatic arch
17. zygomaticotemporal suture
18. temporal bone
19. coronoid process of the mandible
20. zygomatic process of the maxilla
21. root of the zygoma, the so-called malar process
22. maxillary bone

FIGURE 7-14

1. Accessory canals (from the inferior alveolar canal to the molar root apices containing the artery, vein, and nerve to the pulp)

FIGURE 7-15

1. inferior cortex of the mandible
2. inferior alveolar canal

3. lamina dura (radiopaque thin white line)
4. periodontal membrane space (radiolucent thin black line)
5. coronal pulp space (pulp chamber)
6. interproximal contact point
7. dentin
8. enamel
9. interseptal alveolar bone (interradicular alveolar bone)
10. crestal plate (thin white radiopaque line)
11. root canal space (containing the dental pulp)
12. cementum (frequently not distinguishable from the subadjacent dentin, unless hypercementosis is present)

FIGURE 7-16

1. soft tissue shadow of the upper lip
2. cervical margin (line) of the enamel
3. alveolar bone margin (dark band between 2 and 3 is the root)
4. median maxillary suture
5. soft tissue outline of the nose
6. incisive foramen

FIGURE 7-17

1. incisive foramen
2. median maxillary suture
3. incisive canal
4. superior foramen of the incisive canal (in floor of the nose)
5. bony margin of the nasal fossa
6. soft tissue of the nasal septum
7. nasal septum
8. air space of the common meatus

FIGURE 7-18

1. soft tissue outline of the nose
2. median maxillary suture
3. anterior nasal spine
4. bony margin of the nasal fossa
5. foramen of Scarpa
6. superior foramen of the incisive canal

FIGURE 7-19

1. foramen of Scarpa
2. foramen of Stensen
3. median maxillary suture

FIGURE 7-20

1. median maxillary suture
2. anterior nasal spine
3. bony margin of the nasal fossa
4. common meatus (air space in the nose) and part of the inferior meatus beneath turbinate
5. soft tissue lining of the septum
6. soft tissue of the inferior turbinate (thin turbinate bones can be seen within)

FIGURE 7-21

1. orifice of the nasolacrimal duct (at infundibulum of the inferior turbinate not seen)
2. bony margin of the nasal fossa
3. permanent canine
4. permanent 1st premolar
5. permanent 2nd premolar

6. permanent central incisor
7. permanent lateral incisor
8. primary canine
9. primary 1st molar
10. primary 2nd molar

FIGURE 7-22

1. soft tissue outline of the nose
2. lateral fossa
3. bony margin of the nasal fossa
4. anterior wall of the maxillary sinus (3 and 4 comprise the "inverted Y" landmark)
5. air space in the maxillary sinus
6. air space (common meatus) in the nasal fossa

FIGURE 7-23

1. soft tissue shadow of the gingiva
2. crest of the alveolar bone (alveolar crest)
3. soft tissue outline of ala of the nose
4. "inverted Y"
5. air space in the maxillary sinus
6. soft tissue of the nasal fossa (darker thin band just above is the inferior meatus)

FIGURE 7-24

1. soft tissue outline of the nose
2. columella
3. external (soft tissue) naris
4. cartilaginous septum
5. anterior nasal spine
6. nasal air space; superiorly is the common meatus (air space) and beneath the inferior turbinate is the inferior meatus
7. soft tissue of the inferior turbinate

FIGURE 7-25

1. embossed dot on all films (should be at occlusal)
2. soft tissue outline of the nasolabial fold
3. floor of the maxillary sinus
4. bony septum in the maxillary sinus
5. air space of the maxillary sinus
6. metal part in bite block

FIGURE 7-26

1. soft tissue shadow of the nasolabial fold
2. soft tissue shadow of the cheek (buccinator muscle and buccal mucosa)
3. mucosal (gingival) lining of an edentulous alveolar ridge
4. bone margin of an edentulous maxillary alveolar ridge
5. maxillary sinus

FIGURE 7-27

1. nasolabial fold
2. floor of the maxillary sinus
3. posterior superior alveolar canal (in lateral wall of the sinus)
4. sinus air space

FIGURE 7-28

1. bony margin of the nasal fossa
2. anterior wall of the maxillary sinus
3. "inverted Y" landmark
4. embossed dot on all films

FIGURE 7-29

1. metal and plastic parts of bite block
2. diastema
3. soft tissue outline of the nose
4. incisive foramen
5. anterior nasal spine
6. nasal fossa

FIGURE 7-30

1. mamelon
2. lingual pit
3. cervical enamel margin
4. crestal alveolar bone margin
5. anterior nasal spine
6. inferior meatus
7. soft tissue of the inferior turbinate
8. soft tissue of the bony septum
9. bony septum
10. common meatus

FIGURE 7-31

1. incisive foramen (This area is pear-shaped and darker in the radiograph.)
2. soft tissue outline of the nose
3. anterior nasal spine
4. soft tissue lining of the nose
5. nasal air space (common meatus)
6. bony nasal septum
7. soft tissue (mucosal) lining of the septum

FIGURE 7-32

1. mamelon
2. permanent central incisor
3. lingual pit
4. primary canine about to be exfoliated
5. primary 1st molar
6. soft tissue outline of the nose
7. permanent lateral incisor
8. developing permanent canine
9. developing permanent 1st premolar
10. developing 2nd permanent premolar
11. anterior wall of the maxillary sinus
12. bony wall of the nasal fossa

FIGURE 7-33

1. first premolar (note the usual buccal and palatal roots)
2. vestigial lingual cusp on canine
3. air space of the maxillary sinus
4. bony wall of the maxillary sinus

FIGURE 7-34

1. lingual pits in shovel-shaped incisors with heavy marginal ridges
2. lateral fossa
3. nasal fossa
4. maxillary sinus

COMMENT: The bony wall of the nose is generally smoother, straighter, thicker, and slightly more radiopaque than the sinus wall, which is thin and irregular or wavy. The two lines criss-cross to form an "X" (rather than a "Y") in some cases.

FIGURE 7-35

1. zygomatic process of the maxilla
2. hard palate/floor of the nose

3. nasal mucosa
4. nasal cavity
5. maxillary sinus air space
6. sinus septum
7. floor of the maxillary sinus
8. mucosa of the alveolar ridge
9. alveolar bone of the maxilla

COMMENT: Here we can see how the bony outlines of the nose and sinus criss-cross toward the anterior region. The thin dark lines superimposed on the canine are created by static electricity. There is caries on the distal aspect of the canine and mesial aspect of the premolar, which needs a post and a crown.

FIGURE 7-36

1. inferior meatus (above this line throughout its length is the soft tissue of the inferior turbinate in the nose)
2. posterior superior alveolar canal and branches in the lateral wall of the sinus (superimposed on the soft tissue of the turbinate)
3. nasal mucosa
4. floor of the nose/hard palate
5. floor of the maxillary sinus (which is at the alveolar crest because of pneumatization of the sinus whereby the sinus enlarges after adjacent teeth are extracted)
6. sinus air space
7. zygomatic process of the maxilla

FIGURE 7-37

1. sinus recess
2. wall of the nasal fossa
3. sinus septum
4. floor of the maxillary sinus
5. crimp mark and poor image in the area caused by film bending

FIGURE 7-38 (Same patient as in Figure 7-36B)

1. inferior meatus (above this is the soft tissue shadow of the inferior turbinate)
2. posterior superior alveolar canal and branches (in the lateral wall of the sinus)
3. nasal mucosa
4. hard palate/floor of the nose
5. maxillary sinus air space
6. U-shaped zygomatic process of the maxilla
7. inferior border of the zygomatic arch
8. lateral pterygoid plate margin
9. maxillary tuberosity

FIGURE 7-39

1. floor of the maxillary sinus
2. sinus air space
3. thickened sinus mucosa (maxillary sinusitis)
4. zygomatic process of the maxilla

FIGURE 7-40

1. sinus floor mucosa
2. floor of the maxillary sinus
3. zygomatic process of the maxilla
4. air space of the maxillary sinus
5. bony septum in the maxillary sinus
6. sinus mucosa on both sides of the septum
7. oral mucosa of the hard palate (below hard palate/floor of nose)
8. prominent soft tissue in the nasal fossa

FIGURE 7-41

1. upper mandibular ramus
2. margin of the maxillary tuberosity
3. enlarged (hyperplastic) coronoid process of the mandible (causing notch in zygomatic arch)
4. inferior border of the zygomatic arch
5. medial sigmoid depression
6. hamular process of the medial pterygoid plate
7. lateral pterygoid plate

FIGURE 7-42

1. maxillary sinus air space
2. zygomatic arch
3. medial pterygoid plate (anterior part of the lateral pterygoid plate is also superimposed here)
4. lateral pterygoid plate
5. hamular process of the medial pterygoid plate
6. maxillary tuberosity
7. floor of the maxillary sinus
8. coronoid process of the mandible
9. embossed dot in the film
10. "KS" marking indicating "D"-speed film
11. bite block

FIGURE 7-43

1. maxillary tuberosity
2. margin of the alveolar bone (buccal and lingual crestal margins superimposed)
3. floor of the maxillary sinus
4. interproximal alveolar bone margin (crestal margin)
5. bony septum in the sinus
6. margin of the zygomatic arch
7. thickened sinus mucosa
8. U-shaped zygomatic process of the maxilla
9. zygomatic arch

FIGURE 7-44

1. floor of the maxillary sinus
2. hard palate/floor of the nose
3. zygomatic process of the maxilla
4. follicular space inside bony crypt of the developing 3rd molar
5. hamular process of the medial pterygoid plate
6. lateral pterygoid plate
7. coronoid process of the mandible
8. oral mucosal soft tissue shadow

FIGURE 7-45

1. zygomatic process of the maxilla
2. hard palate/floor of the nose
3. sinus recess
4. sinus septum and soft tissue mucosa on both sides
5. anterior wall of the maxillary sinus (continuous with sinus floor)

FIGURE 7-46

1. lingual foramen
2. genial tubercles (In this view, individual genial tubercles are not usually seen; combined with the lingual foramen, you have the appearance of a donut.)
3. unusual accessory foramen with unusual cortication (There appears to be an accessory canal within the bone between this and the lingual foramen.)
4. accessory foramens (foramina) of nutrient canals

FIGURE 7-47
1. mental foramen (does not usually have a corticated margin)
2. inferior cortex of the mandible

FIGURE 7-48
1. relative radiolucency frequently seen in this area; possibly caused by thin cortical bone and/or large digastric fossa
2. inferior cortex of the mandible
3. margin of the inferior cortex

FIGURE 7-49
1. mamelons
2. dental papilla of developing teeth
3. genial tubercles
4. lingual foramen (Note that there appears to be a corticated accessory foramen below this area.)
5. inferior cortex
6. crimp mark caused by #2 film bending (For this reason, #1 film is often used in this location.)

FIGURE 7-50
1. margin of the inferior cortex
2. inferior cortex
3. canal space for accessory lingual artery and vein
4. corticated canal wall
5. genial tubercles
6. lingual foramen

FIGURE 7-51
1. inferior cortex
2. margin of the inferior cortex
3. genial tubercles
4. lingual foramen
5. canal space for accessory lingual artery and vein with corticated canal walls
6. mental ridge
7. soft tissue shadow of the lower lip

FIGURE 7-52
1. soft tissue shadow of the lower lip
2. atypical genial tubercles
3. nutrient canals in cross section and/or accessory foramens of nutrient canals

FIGURE 7-53
1. mamelons
2. developing permanent canine

FIGURE 7-54
1. genial tubercles
2. lingual foramen
3. inferior cortex
4. permanent central incisor
5. permanent lateral incisor
6. primary canine
7. primary 1st molar
8. developing permanent canine
9. developing 1st premolar
10. developing 2nd premolar

FIGURE 7-55
1. margin of the inferior cortex
2. inferior cortex
3. corticated wall of the inferior alveolar canal
4. inferior alveolar canal (mandibular canal)
5. mylohyoid ridge (internal oblique ridge)
6. submandibular fossa

FIGURE 7-56
1. external oblique ridge
2. internal oblique ridge
3. inferior alveolar canal
4. submandibular fossa
5. retromolar trigone

FIGURE 7-57
1. inferior alveolar canal
2. bony crypt wall of a developing tooth
3. follicular space of a developing 3rd molar; this space should not measure more than 2.5 mm on intraoral films or 3 mm on panoramic films. If the size of the follicular space is wider than these measurements, it should be considered as pathologically enlarged—usually caused by cyst formation (follicular or dentigerous cyst) or tumor induction. The maxillary canine follicular space is often larger.
   COMMENT: Notice root formation has barely begun. Much of the root formation occurs after the tooth first erupts into the oral cavity. When root length exceeds crown length and the tooth has not yet begun to erupt into the mouth, eruption is delayed. The usual reasons for delayed eruption are impaction as a result of a lack of space or the presence of a cyst or tumor.
4. developing 3rd molar
5. papilla of developing tooth
6. bulbous root shape (more difficult to extract)
7. tapered root shape (easer to extract)

FIGURE 7-58
1. internal oblique ridge
2. submandibular fossa
3. inferior alveolar canal (mandibular canal)
4. mental foramen
5. anterior branches of the inferior alveolar canal (incisive and possibly labial branches)

FIGURE 7-59
1. internal oblique ridge
2. mental foramen
3. submandibular fossa
4. inferior cortex
5. fixer stains (developer stains are radiolucent or dark marks)

FIGURE 7-60
1. Distal mandibular pseudo-hyperostosis
2. In situation A, a tooth is missing anterior to the tooth in question. The molar has tipped mesially and formed a pseudo-pocket on the mesial pressure side and a pseudo-hyperostosis on the distal tension side. In situation B, a tooth is missing distal to the tooth in question with no missing anterior tooth. Here the original crestal height has been maintained just distal of the tooth.

FIGURE 7-61

1. The radiolucent area is a developing tooth bud with just a hint of the "circumflex" (^) or "accent circonflexe en français" pattern of calcification of a mesial cusp tip.

FIGURE 7-62

1. The term is pneumatization. ("To pneumatize" means to fill with air… you can coin "pneumohead" if you want…it might just catch on!)

FIGURE 7-63

1. This is called a "stepladder" trabecular pattern (a variation of normal).
2. It is of no significance, though it was once thought to be related to marrow changes associated with sickle cell anemia.

FIGURE 7-64

1. Part A: loose trabecular pattern
2. Part B: dense trabecular pattern
3. The trabecular pattern is a feature of the cortex. You can hollow out all of the spongy bone in the marrow space without seeing any change in the trabecular pattern in a subsequent radiograph.

FIGURE 7-65

1. Lingual midline: two enlarged genial tubercles
2. They are significant in that they may prevent the proper seating of an old (or even new) denture.

   COMMENT: An old denture will impinge on this as the ridge slowly resorbs and the denture becomes more and more hyperextended at the flange or margin.

FIGURE 7-66

1. Arrow A: external oblique ridge
   Arrow B: inferior border of cortex
   Arrow C: internal oblique ridge

FIGURE 7-67

1. mandibular condyle
2. coronoid process
3. sigmoid notch
4. ramus of the mandible
5. body of the mandible
6. angle of the mandible
7. mental foramina
8. inferior cortex of the mandible
9. bite block
10. inferior alveolar canal
11. maxillary tuberosity
12. airway
13. air as tongue is not on the palate
14. posterior soft tissue wall of the airway
15. soft palate and uvula
16. zygomatic arch
17. articular eminence of the TMJ

FIGURE 7-68

1. anterior arch of C1, the atlas
2. vertebral body of C2, the axis
3. vertebral body of C3
4. vertebral body of C4
5. body of the hyoid bone
6. greater horn of the hyoid bone
7. calcifications at the carotid bifurcation between C3 and C4
8. styloid process
9. real shadow of the hard palate on the left side
10. ghost image of the hard palate on the right side
11. inferior orbital rim
12. panoramic innominate line composed of the lateral wall of the orbit superiorly and the malar process of the zygomatic arch
13. inferior orbital foramen
14. anterolateral wall of the maxillary sinus
15. posterolateral wall of the maxillary sinus
16. malar process of the zygomatic arch (root of the zygomatic arch)
17. lateral wall of the orbit
18. pterygomaxillary fissure
19. inferior turbinate of the nose
20. nasal septum
21. soft tissue outline of the nose
22. anterior nasal spine
23. medial sigmoid notch

FIGURE 7-69

1. external auditory meatus
2. glenoid fossa of the TMJ
3. space for the disk
4. articular eminence
5. mandibular condyle
6. mandibular foramen
7. inferior alveolar canal
8. mental foramen
9. incisive branch of the inferior alveolar canal
10. nutrient canals
11. zygomaticomaxillary suture
12. zygomatic process of the temporal bone
13. zygomatic process of the maxilla
14. soft tissue of the earlobe
15. maxillary tuberosity
16. maxilla
17. right and left inferior turbinates of the nose
18. outline of dorsum of the tongue
19. middle meatus
20. inferior meatus
21. common meatus
22. nasal septum
23. lateral pterygoid plate
24. external oblique ridge

FIGURE 7-70

1. soft tissue shadow of the lips, which are closed, indicating no bite block was used
2. mandibular foramen
3. bilateral ghost images of the contralateral inferior border of the ramus indicating the patient was positioned too far back
4. retained lamina dura residues indicating systemic disease, present or past, sometimes involving the kidneys or GI tract
5. bilateral soft tissue of the cheek
6. soft tissue outline of the upper and lower edentulous ridges
7. external oblique ridge
8. internal oblique (mylohyoid) ridge
9. inferior turbinate of the nose spread out across the maxillary sinus indicating the patient was positioned too far back

10. dome-shaped mucous retention cyst in sinus requiring no treatment; the term mucocele should not be used as this is a specific type of inflammatory cyst
11. bilateral ear lobes
12. bilateral soft tissue outline of the pharynx
13. double image of wishbone-like hyoid bone demonstrating the body and two greater horns (cornus)
14. soft tissue outline of the nose

FIGURE 7-71

1. lateral pterygoid plate
2. double image (bilateral of epiglottis with hyoid bone superimposed)
3. right styloid process
4. anterior arch of C1, the atlas
5. triangular bite block
6. air as lips were not fully closed
7. soft tissue of the inferior turbinate of the nose surrounded by the radiolucent air spaces of the inferior, common, and middle meatuses
8. right and left middle meatuses
9. nasal septum
10. inferior margin of the orbit
11. teardrop-shaped pterygomaxillary fissure
12. right and left mandibular condyles
13. right and left external auditory meatuses
14. bilateral airspace as tongue was not positioned against the palate
15. soft palate
16. "blunderbuss" or slightly open apices indicating both root formation and eruption are almost complete
17. root formation before eruption suggests possible delayed eruption in this case due to a lack of space
18. C2, the axis
19. C3
20. C4

FIGURE 7-72

1. This is a cone beam computed tomography (CBCT) screen as displayed on the computer.
2. The views are: axial (top L), sagittal (top R), coronal (bottom L), and 3D coronal

FIGURE 7-73 Axial view at the level of the maxillary sinus and TMJ

1. soft tissue outline of the nose
2. cartilaginous nasal septum
3. opening of the nasolacrimal duct beneath the inferior turbinate
4. inferior turbinate
5. bony nasal septum
6. choana (posterior opening of the nose into the nasopharynx)
7. acetabulum (articulates with the C1 vertebra)
8. medial pterygoid plate
9. head of the right condyle
10. lateral pterygoid plate
11. coronoid process of the mandible
12. maxillary portion of the zygomatic arch
13. maxillary sinus

FIGURE 7-74 Axial view at the level of the hard palate and C1

1. soft tissue at base of the nose
2. anterior nasal spine
3. incisive canal
4. hard palate
5. maxillary sinus
6. upper part of the oral pharynx
7. left styloid process
8. acetabulum at base of the skull
9. first cervical vertebra, the axis
10. tip of the odontoid process of the atlas the 2nd cervical vertebra
11. anterior arch of C1
12. right ramus of the mandible
13. lateral pterygoid plate
14. apices of the 1st or 2nd molar
15. apex of the canine tooth

FIGURE 7-75 Axial view at the level of the apices of the mandibular teeth and C3

1. soft tissue at the base of the lower lip
2. buccal cortex of the mandible
3. lower ramus just above the angle of the mandible
4. foramen for the vertebral artery
5. root of the pedicle of C3
6. space containing the spinal nerve and cerebrospinal fluid
7. vertebral body of C3
8. lower part of the oral pharynx
9. lower tip of the uvula
10. lingual cortex of the mandible
11. mandibular right canine tooth

FIGURE 7-76 Coronal view at the level of the drainage of the nose into the maxillary sinus

1. crista galli at the level of the tympanic plate containing fibers of cranial nerve II, the olfactory nerve
2. anterior ethmoid sinus air cells
3. ostiomeatal complex where the frontal, anterior ethmoid, and maxillary sinuses drain
4. infundibulum drains the maxillary sinus
5. uncinate process forms the lower part of the infundibulum
6. nasal septum slightly deviated with polypoid soft tissue indicating allergy
7. inferior turbinate
8. buccal cortex of the mandible
9. inferior alveolar canal
10. hard palate
11. inferior meatus air passage
12. common meatus air passage
13. middle meatus air passage
14. maxillary sinus
15. concha bullosa, is an anterior ethmoid air space in the middle turbinate
16. inferior medial wall of the orbit forms the upper part of the infundibulum

FIGURE 7-77 Coronal view at the level of the sphenoid sinuses and posterior orbit

1. posterior part of the orbit
2. tiny superior turbinate
3. zygomatic arch

4. maxillary sinus
5. lower left 2nd molar
6. lower left turbinate
7. lower right turbinate; the turbinate cycle involves them becoming engorged by blood as a part of temperature regulation; the right and left sides are not synchronized
8. coronoid process of the mandible
9. zygomatic arch
10. tiny right superior turbinate
11. right and left sphenoid sinuses just behind the posterior ethmoid

FIGURE 7-78 Sagittal view close to the level of the midline
1. frontal sinus
2. anterior ethmoid sinus air cells
3. nasal bone
4. inferior turbinate
5. hard palate
6. soft palate
7. uvula
8. chin rest of machine
9. body of the hyoid bone
10. C4 vertebral body
11. C3 vertebral body
12. C2-C3 intervertebral disk space
13. odontoid process of C2, the axis
14. oral pharynx
15. anterior arch of C1, the atlas
16. tonsillar tissue lining of the nasopharynx
17. clivus
18. sphenoid sinus
19. posterior ethmoid sinus air cells
20. pituitary fossa
21. prominent vertical plate of bone delineating the anterior and posterior ethmoid sinuses

MULTIPLE CHOICE QUESTIONS WITHOUT FIGURES

1. C
2. A
3. C
4. D
5. A
6. C
7. B
8. D
9. D
10. A
11. B
12. A
13. A
14. B
15. D

Chapter 8

SHORT ANSWER QUESTIONS WITH FIGURES

FIGURE 8-1
1. There are several possibilities:
   - amalgam
   - gold foil (this was a gold foil)
   - cast gold inlay
2. Old radiolucent tooth-colored restorative materials:
   - silicophosphate cement
   - acrylic
   - composite resin

COMMENT: When a tooth has been restored with a radiolucent material, it would have been done before about 1985. The distinguishing feature from caries is the sharp, smooth outline of the cavity preparation. Also, older cavity preparations are much larger than those of current practice.

FIGURE 8-2
1. Possible RPD materials:
   - chrome cobalt (or other alloy)
   - gold
2. Radiolucent acrylic
3. Radiopaque cement

FIGURE 8-3
1. Porcelain jacket crown
2. Radiopaque cement outlines the preparation

FIGURE 8-4
1. Lower 1st molar materials:
   - gutta percha and screw-in post in the distal canal
   - silver points and root canal sealer cement in the mesial canals
   - amalgam in the coronal portion

COMMENT: To complete the restoration of this tooth, a full crown offers the best long-term prognosis.
2. Distal of lower 1st molar: cervical burnout

COMMENT: The difference between this and root caries is that cervical burnout disappears when another bitewing is taken at a different horizontal angle. Common locations are the distal aspect of the lower canines and the distal aspect of the upper molars.

FIGURE 8-5
1. Leaded-glass fragment embedded in the lower lip
2. Other possibilities:
   - scratched emulsion
   - amalgam tattoo
   - metal fragment such as shrapnel

FIGURE 8-6
1. The two metallic objects are:
   - ivory #9 rubber dam clamp
   - root canal file

FIGURE 8-7
1. The x-ray related materials are:
   - cotton roll
   - acrylic of bite block
   - metal of bite block

FIGURE 8-8
1. Materials you can see:
   - all porcelain posterior denture teeth
   - porcelain anterior teeth with metal retention studs
   - wire mesh to reinforce and strengthen the denture
2. The denture acrylic is radiotransparent; therefore you cannot see it.

COMMENT: Some prosthodontists hesitate to make a complete upper denture against the natural lower dentition because of the possibility of accelerated resorption of the residual ridge. When they do make one, they often prefer acrylic teeth to prevent wear on the lower teeth by the porcelain and to better absorb the stress from the occlusion. When the acrylic denture base keeps breaking, a thin cast metallic palate usually solves the problem.

FIGURE 8-9

1. The radiopaque object is a wrought wire clasp to retain an acrylic transitional removable partial denture (in other words a "flipper").

FIGURE 8-10

1. The maxillary teeth are the porcelain teeth of a maxillary complete denture.

COMMENT: It is often desirable to leave in complete and partial dentures with all-acrylic bases because the acrylic is invisible and the prosthesis makes it easier to take the radiographs.

FIGURE 8-11

1. The premolars: radiopaque composite resin
2. The molar: amalgam

COMMENT: Note the difference in density between the two materials.

FIGURE 8-12   A space maintainer

FIGURE 8-13

1. Materials you can see:
   • fresh amalgam restoration on 1st molar
   • amalgam fragments
   • rubber dam clamp
2. Items you cannot see:
   • rubber dam
   • the restoration (if acrylic) in the 2nd premolar
   • the exact nature of the restoration in the 2nd molar

FIGURE 8-14

1. Materials in the upper 1st molar:
   • gutta percha
   • five screw-in retentive pins

FIGURE 8-15

1. Lingual pits were routinely filled with amalgam. The radiolucent restorations are most likely on the buccal aspect and consist of the older radiolucent composite material.

COMMENT: The author has included a number of these older radiolucent restorations because they are still to be found in many patients and nowadays students are prone to interpret these as caries, fractured teeth, and defects like enamel hypoplasia.

FIGURE 8-16

1. Okay, you wanted newer radiopaque anterior composites…you got it!

FIGURE 8-17   Notice that some fragments resembled rusted metal while others were completely blackened. Most likely there were two different metals here and unlike amalgam were not tissue compatible and over time probably contributed to the severe bone loss in the area. The patient would not speak about the possible source of these fragments.

FIGURE 8-18

1. Treatment and materials in primary 2nd molars:
   • Maxillary:
     —Pulpotomy and pulpotomy cement
     —Stainless steel crown
   • Mandibular:
     —Occlusal amalgam

FIGURE 8-19

1. These are implant-related materials:
   A: Implants have been placed within the maxillary alveolar bone such that they are covered by soft tissue. Healing caps are in place at the proximal or "business" end of the implant. Signs of osseous integration include a lack of significant radiolucent area(s) in the vicinity of the implant and evidence of bone that has grown in between the threads on the implant.
   B: Healing caps have been exposed surgically and replaced with the appliance that is screwed into the implant. The appliances have been prepared to receive crowns. Temporary acrylic crowns are in place but cannot be seen; however, the radiopaque cement holding them in place can be seen.
   C: Porcelain bonded to gold crowns is in place. These are often screwed into the proximal end of the appliance so that at any time the crown, appliance, and even the implant can be removed by unscrewing the desired part.

COMMENT: Notice the slight V-shaped bony defect in the collar area of the implant at the crest of the ridge. This is normal for implants; however, the depth of the V-shaped notch should not exceed 2 to 3 mm, and the bone in this area should not appear demineralized or more radiolucent than the remaining alveolar bone around the implant.

COMMENT: Smoking compromises the vasculature and oxygen supply to implant-related tissues and almost always results in implant failure.

FIGURE 8-20

1. The patient is wearing three earrings, probably diamond studs.
2. Circle A: ghost images of the two earrings on the left earlobe
3. Circle B: ghost images of the one earring on the right earlobe

FIGURE 8-21

1. The ghost image of the left earring in circle A is higher than the one in circle B because the patient's head was tipped toward the right causing the left earring image and its ghost to be higher up in the image.
2. The object in circle C is probably jewelry.
3. Extraoral jewelry probably pierces the skin and mucobuccal fold toward the right side in line with the lower canine.
4. Orthodontic treatment

FIGURE 8-22

1. Lower 1st molar restorations:
   A: This is a stainless steel crown. Notice that it is somewhat radiotransparent because you can see the outline of the tooth and possibly a restoration under the crown. Also note the marginal adaptation is pretty good but not perfect as is seen with stainless steel crowns.

      COMMENT: Notice the large pulps, spaces between the premolars and textbook-healthy crestal bone. All these indicate a young patient with newly erupted permanent teeth. At this age, stainless steel crowns are commonly used.

B: This is a cast gold inlay. Here the margins are more conservative, and there is less tooth coverage than a full gold crown. Here the margins are pretty good but slightly open at the mesial aspect. This area will need to be watched for redecay.

COMMENT: Notice the missing lower 2nd molar and the extruding maxillary 2nd molar. An undesirable collapse of the occlusion has begun. Compare the maxillary premolars with patient A. Note the smaller pulp chambers in patient B, who is in his early 30s.

2. Patient B has the amalgam tattoo. Note the amalgam fragments between the lower premolars. This is how you confirm the pigmented lesion in the mouth is a harmless amalgam tattoo vs. a pigmented nevus that should be removed and sent for histopathologic examination.

FIGURE 8-23

1. Prosthesis comparison:
   A: Fixed prosthesis (bridge) with porcelain bonded to metal
   B: Class VI removable partial denture (butterfly) made from cast chrome cobalt or similar material with an invisible acrylic tooth

COMMENT: In our dental school we will not treatment plan a butterfly partial because patients are known to have aspirated these. This can be life-threatening, and because of the clasps, they can be difficult to dislodge, even with the Heimlich maneuver.

FIGURE 8-24

1. Left upper central incisor materials:
   A: gutta percha in the apical ⅓ of the root canal, a puff of root canal cement beyond the apex, prefabricated screw-in post with cement or remaining gutta percha in the rest of the root canal, porcelain bonded to metal crown
   B: gutta percha at the apical end of the root canal; the apex has been sealed via surgical access with amalgam, a cast gold post in the remainder of the root canal, porcelain bonded to metal crown.

FIGURE 8-25

1. Both patients have a bonded lingual wire retainer.
2. Comparison of the two patients:
   A: The composite resin bonding material is an older radiopaque variety; thus it is less well seen; the bonding material cannot be seen on the centrals and is poorly seen on the laterals.
   B: Newer, more radiopaque, bonding material that is well visualized on all of the teeth

FIGURE 8-26

1. It is in the left orbit.
2. It is actually a prosthetic eyeball; most of the eyeball is made of radiotransparent plastic and part of the lens is glass.
3. The patient's lips are open as can be seen by the black oval-shaped air in rectangle A. The lips should be closed.
4. The two horizontal white shadows in rectangles B and C are the ghost images of the contralateral inferior cortex of the mandibular ramus because the patient was positioned to far back in the machine.

FIGURE 8-27

1. The small radiopaque calcifications on the patient's *left* are consistent with carotid artery calcifications at the bifurcation and appear to be above and below the C3-C4 area. The greater horn of the hyoid bone points to this location in the cervical spine when the spine is absent in the pan image. The intervertebral space between C3 and C4 on a panoramic image is the location of the carotid artery bifurcation. On the *right*, we see vascular clips from the surgery to remove the carotid arterial calcifications from the right carotid artery.

FIGURE 8-28

1. Part D is a radiograph of the left buccal mucosa. Place the film between the cheek and the teeth and expose with about 65 kV and about three or four impulses to get the soft tissue and any poorly mineralized bodies in the cheek.
2. Mystery solution: If you said a BB in the cheek, you were right once again.

FIGURE 8-29

1. Types of images: If you said the left is a periapical image of the upper anterior midline, that would be acceptable; it is actually a cropped panoramic image.
   Image B is a cropped #2 film placed in the mucobuccal fold at the anterior midline.
2. Note that several incisors are absent. There was a history of an auto accident whereby the anterior teeth were knocked out by contact with the steering wheel. Unbeknownst to the patient, a chip from a central incisor was embedded in the lip. The lip was bloody and swollen and was asymptomatic after healing. The fragment was discovered serendipitously on radiographic examination, and subsequently the patient divulged the history of the accident.

FIGURE 8-30

1. The cause of the bluish-black macule is an amalgam fragment embedded in the gingiva.
2. Unless there are clinical signs of infection, these fragments are usually well tolerated and do not require treatment. In some cases they may be removed for aesthetic reasons.

MULTIPLE CHOICE QUESTIONS WITHOUT FIGURES

1. B
2. D
3. D
4. A
5. B
6. B
7. D
8. E
9. D
10. A

Chapter 9

MULTIPLE CHOICE QUESTIONS WITH FIGURES

FIGURE 9-4

1. D
2. A

FIGURE 9-5
1. B
2. C

FIGURE 9-6
1. A
2. E

FIGURE 9-7
1. D
2. C

FIGURE 9-8
1. A

FIGURE 9-9
1. A

FIGURE 9-10
1. D

FIGURE 9-11
1. C

FIGURE 9-12
1. D

FIGURE 9-13
1. B

FIGURE 9-14
1. D

FIGURE 9-15
1. D

FIGURE 9-16
1. E

FIGURE 9-17
1. C

FIGURE 9-18
1. A

FIGURE 9-19
1. D

FIGURE 9-20
1. B

FIGURE 9-21
1. E

FIGURE 9-22
1. E

FIGURE 9-23
1. D

FIGURE 9-24
1. C

MULTIPLE CHOICE QUESTIONS WITHOUT FIGURES
1. B
2. D
3. D
4. A
5. D
6. C
7. A
8. A
9. D
10. E
11. A
12. D

Chapter 10

GENERAL CASES

CASE 10-1
1. Excessive orthodontic forces
2. Iatrogenic root resorption

CASE 10-2
1. Distal drift; the tooth is also tipped mesially.

CASE 10-3
1. Microdont and distomolar; however, it may also be said it is unerupted and impacted.

CASE 10-4
1. Taurodont (bull-like or like the ungulate's dentition; bulls have short legs and big bodies compared with cows).
2. The pulp chamber is usually elongated with parallel walls; the root canal does not taper from the floor of the pulp chamber. Compare with the adjacent 1st molar.
3. Taurodontism is usually a solitary finding. It may be seen in association with many syndromes and anomalies. Here is a partial list: amelogenesis imperfecta, Down syndrome, ectodermal disturbances, Mohr syndrome, osteoporosis, tricho-dento-osseous syndrome, and Klinefelter syndrome.
4. Yes, primary teeth can be affected.

CASE 10-5
1. Dentinogenesis imperfecta
2. Seen here: chipped enamel, bulbous crowns, obliteration of the pulp and root canal spaces; not seen here: tapering root form, root fracture
3. Osteogenesis imperfecta

CASE 10-6
1. Dilaceration
2. It got this way because of a tortuous or difficult path of eruption. Remember, the root forms as eruption progresses.

CASE 10-7
1. Image B—Billy has the problem.
2. You knew because of Billy's lack of interseptal bone in the anterior region.

3. Do a space analysis and initiate interceptive orthodontic therapy, or refer Billy to the orthodontist.

CASE 10-8
1. Differential diagnosis:
   - Abfraction
   - Toothbrush abrasion
   - Older radiolucent restoration or sealant
   - Cervical caries
   - Erosion
2. This was abfraction.
3. The cause is poorly understood, though it is seen in patients with occlusal trauma and bruxism. If occlusal abnormalities exist, they should be eliminated; the defects can be restored with bonded composite tooth-colored material. There is some question that restorations are not well retained in such teeth.

CASE 10-9
1. External root resorption
2. Prognosis is poor for the ultimate retention of avulsed and reimplanted teeth.
3. Bone quality and quantity, allowing and assuming the patient is not a smoker or has any other health impediment, this is an ideal case for an implant.

CASE 10-10
1. Microdont, peg lateral
2. Place a porcelain veneer. Denyse has one, and it looks great!

CASE 10-11
1. Dentin dysplasia O'Carroll type 1a; subtypes 1b and 1c have varying degrees of increased root formation and the presence of linear horizontal bands of pulpal remnants and periapical radiolucencies. Subtype 1d is different as the teeth are usually fully developed; they also have the horizontal bands of pulpal remnants and huge prominent pulp stones in the root areas.
2. Management involves meticulous home care, occlusal equilibration, and periodontal maintenance at accelerated intervals. In spite of this, type 1a—the most severe form—often leads to premature loss of the teeth.

CASE 10-12
1. Eruption sequestrum
2. This problem often resolves spontaneously. Sometimes the patient can feel the bone spicule and believes he has an embedded piece of chicken bone or the like. The pain is felt when there is slight infection associated with the sequestration of the spicule. With a little topical anesthetic and sterile cotton pliers, it can be removed.

CASE 10-13
1. Pulp stones; note that they are usually the same density as dentin.
2. The developmental anomaly is dentin dysplasia O'Carroll type 1d.
3. No, it is not present here. You will know it when you see it (I hope).
4. The significance is endodontic therapy. You can imagine that such cases might be best managed by the endodontist.

CASE 10-14
1. To begin, the 1st molar is supraerupted, probably because there is also a missing opposing tooth or teeth. Second, this has altered the contact area, which now favors food impaction. As a result, the patient picked up the habit of using a round toothpick several times a day, thus abrading the 1st molar (toothpick abrasion). The abraded area closely resembles root caries. This case demonstrates the importance of correlating the x-ray findings with a thorough clinical examination and history.
2. *Factitial* means a self-induced injury.

CASE 10-15
1. Transposition is the problem. The 1st premolar and canine have exchanged places.
2. The orthodontist will probably not be able to help at this point, though some realignment may be needed. Aesthetically, the two transposed teeth can be made to look like each other with porcelain veneers or full porcelain crowns.

CASE 10-16
1. Note the shovel-shaped incisors. The lingual pit centrally was filled prophylactically, but the lateral pit was not. The lateral pit has a dens in dente and invaginated enamel, and dentin can be seen. The prophylactic scaling of a tooth with a dens in dente prevents early carious pulpal involvement. In all probability, this patient did not receive a complete radiographic examination or the dens in dente was not recognized. The patient received a prolonged course of orthodontic therapy, which resulted in iatrogenic resorption of the root apices. *Iatrogenic* means an unintended ill effect as a result of dental treatment.

Did you see all that? If yes…you deserve a break.

CASE 10-17 Welcome back.
1. If you noticed there is a tooth there, you are right! If you said this is a migrated tooth, possibly a canine…even better. If you also noted the external resorption of the tooth, then you get full points.

CASE 10-18
1. The anomaly is a supernumerary tooth termed a *mesiodens*. It is the most common extra tooth.
2. It should be extracted immediately. Also, Dad should take another radiograph like an occlusal so he can see higher up. The mesiodens is often paired; when only one is seen to be heading south, the other may be heading north and sometimes erupts into the floor of the nose!

CASE 10-19
1. The pulps of the premolars are large, probably at the extreme of normal. There are conditions characterized by large pulps, but this patient is healthy. Should these teeth need restoration, iatrogenic pulp exposure is possible. The mesial pulp horn of the 1st molar has receded. Note the small radiopaque composite restoration on the mesial surface, which was probably placed as a pit just after the 2nd primary molar exfoliated. Note also the pulp stones in the distal part of the pulp chamber.

CASE 10-20
1. Congenitally missing 2nd mandibular premolar
2. The occlusal plane of the permanent dentition is higher up than that of the primary teeth. Thus when the 1st premolar and 1st

molar fully erupt, the retained 2nd primary molar will be below the occlusal plane. This can result in extrusion of the opposing molar. Therefore as soon as the plane of occlusion is established, the retained baby tooth will need a crown to restore the occlusion. In time the deciduous tooth may exfoliate, and then the best prosthesis would be an implant.

3. None. If there were multiple missing teeth affecting other family members, then familial hypodontia may be present. If, in addition to multiple missing teeth, the teeth are hypoplastic and misshapen, I would suspect hereditary hypohidrotic ectodermal dysplasia, chondroectodermal dysplasia, or incontinentia pigmenti—all of which may look similar with regard to the dentition.

CASE 10-21

1. Enamel hypoplasia, environmental type.
2. This happened during the first year of life. To figure this out, remember the "1-2-3 rule" for the permanent central incisors and molars: If the defect is on the incisal ⅓ or occlusal of the molar, the problem developed in the 1st year of life; the middle ⅓, the 2nd year of life; and the cervical ⅓, the 3rd year of life. This 1-2-3 rule will serve you well for your entire career.

CASE 10-22

1. Attrition; in such cases, look also for flattening of the interproximal contacts best seen here at the mesial aspect of the 2nd premolar. Here the contact has now been lost and may be the area of food impaction.

CASE 10-23

1. The anomalies are (1) a supernumerary lateral incisor, sometimes referred to as "twinning" in this presentation and (2) microdontia of at least one or both of the laterals, also known as "peg" laterals.

   COMMENT: Gemination occurs when one tooth bud attempts to divide; there are no extra teeth. Fusion is when two tooth buds fuse with an apparent missing tooth. Twinning is seen with an extra tooth, as this case illustrates.

CASE 10-24

1. The nonvital tooth is the canine.
2. Features: obliterated pulp space (pulp chamber and root canal) without any apparent cause. Most likely this tooth was traumatized at one time.
3. No treatment. Nature has done the job of filling the canal; the periapical area looks acceptable. Note that the apical lamina dura is absent, but this alone is not a reason to initiate a "mission impossible" in trying to do endodontic treatment on this tooth.

CASE 10-25

1. Ectopic eruption
2. Probably prophylactically seal the lingual pits of all the maxillary incisors because they are shovel shaped. However, the lateral definitely needs sealing because of the dens in dente there. Did you see that?

CASE 10-26

1. Anomaly: Dentin dysplasia Shields type II
   COMMENT: Shields was the one who first recognized that there are types I and II dentin dysplasia. O'Carroll classified the radiographic appearance as previously discussed.
2. Restorative material: amalgam; UGH!

CASE 10-27

1. Treatment: Endodontics and a stainless steel crown
2. Enamel hypoplasia, Turner environmental type
3. The connection: Turner type enamel hypoplasia occurs in the developing enamel of the permanent tooth replacing a primary tooth that has abscessed or has been intruded or devitalized as a result of trauma. In this case the primary molar was abscessed, but the damage occurred before treatment could be initiated. This underlines the need for frequent dental checkups in children and the need for radiographs when indicated.

CASE 10-28

1. The anomaly is fusion between the developing left incisors; the clue is that no teeth have been extracted.
2. Clinically, you would call this an example of macrodontia, which means "a big tooth" but does not specify the exact cause.
3. Fusion is a single enlarged, joined, or double-appearing tooth, and when this tooth is counted as one, there is a missing tooth.
   COMMENT: If an incisor had been extracted, then gemination would be the answer; that is to say, it could have been gemination of the central and extraction of the lateral. Thus it is history and tooth number rather than appearance that distinguish fusion and gemination. Even then, it is hard to identify fusion between a tooth of the normal complement and a supernumerary tooth from gemination of a tooth of the normal complement in the presence of a supernumerary tooth.

CASE 10-29

1. The clinical appearance suggests the lateral incisor is nonvital, though this should be confirmed with pulp tests. If it is nonvital, the periapical lesion can be referred to radiologically as a periapical radiolucency of pulpal origin associated with external resorption of the root apex.
   COMMENT: This lesion consists of one of the following: periapical abscess, periapical cyst, or periapical granuloma; and all are periapical responses to pulpal inflammation or infection. Radiologically, this looks like a periapical granuloma because the apex is resorbed, and the lesion does not exceed 1 cm in diameter. But the lesion is not densely radiolucent as it would be for a granuloma, and there is a hint of a thin sclerotic margin as would be seen in a radicular cyst. Periapical lesions of pulpal origin may abscess, then granulate in, and finally become cystic, thus alternating histologically over time. It is for this reason it is imprudent to be too assertive clinically about the specific pathologic process and why features of transition between one reaction and another can sometimes be seen, as in this case. Radiologically, it would be accurate to say the lesion appears to be a periapical radiolucency of pulpal origin.
2. Treatment would be to get the periodontal disease under control as the crown-root ratio of this tooth is diminished. An occlusal analysis should be initiated to rule out occlusal trauma. Then the tooth is treated endodontically, followed by internal bleaching, and ultimately with one or more porcelain veneers, depending on whether the patient wants to eliminate the diastemata.

CASE 10-30

1. The tooth is ankylosed as evidenced by the lack of any visible periodontal membrane space. Ankylosis involves fusion of the cementum of the root with alveolar bone. Extraction will be difficult.

2. On percussion, such teeth are said to make a different kind of a sound, such as a hollow or "thunking" sound. In any case it is different from adjacent nonankylosed teeth.

CASE 10-31

1. The problem is a supernumerary incisor or mesiodens impeding the eruption of the central incisor.
2. Treatment involves removal of the primary central and probably the lateral as well as the supernumerary tooth.
3. The eruptive potential of the central incisor is excellent because the apex is wide open and root formation is less than the length of the crown. With about three or so weeks to go before Christmas, I wouldn't make any promises, but I would assure Mom the tooth should be well on its way and certainly visibly catching up to its mate by Christmas.

CASE 10-32

1. There is a supernumerary cusp or tubercle on the occlusal aspect of the 2nd premolar. This is called dens evaginatus or Leong's premolar.
2. These tubercles can result in a pulp exposure as there may be a pulp horn within the tubercle. Pulp exposures may occur from wear or iatrogenically when preparing the tooth for a restoration.

CASE 10-33

1. The best terms are supraeruption and extrusion.
2. The generalized condition is attrition, easily seen on the occlusal surfaces and is caused by physiologic wear.

CASE 10-34

1. This is dentin dysplasia type 1d. That is to say, Shields type I and O'Carroll subtype 1d with the prominent pulp stones and signs of pulp obliteration in several teeth.

CASE 10-35

1. So-called internal resorption; the problem is that there is no way to determine that the resorption is not external without physically examining the tooth.
2. This must be managed by endodontic therapy, even if the tooth tests vital. Once the canal has been prepared thoroughly, the dentist can look for a perforation in which an area on the canal wall bleeds. If there is no perforation, the prognosis is relatively good. If there is perforation, the tooth must be exposed surgically and the perforation sealed with amalgam while still maintaining the root canal space, which must be filled. The prognosis here is guarded but worth a try.

CASE 10-36

1. These teeth are microdonts and appear somewhat hypoplastic because of radiation stunting.
2. Teeth in a field of radiation treatment have been known to erupt, though it is often delayed. In this case root formation appears complete; thus eruption is not expected.
3. The maxillary irradiated bone is subject to complications of osteoradionecrosis. When oral microflora are allowed to enter into the bone, unmanageable infection can result. Thus orthodontic traction and oral surgery should be avoided.

CASE 10-37

1. There is a supernumerary tooth, called a paramolar, either buccal or lingual to the 2nd molar. Note the dark lines representing the follicular sac and root canal spaces outlining the little microdont.

CASE 10-38

1. It looks like an enamel pearl, not a pulp stone, because it is both in and out of the pulp cavity, and pulp stones tend to remain within the confines of the radiographic pulp space.
2. We can call this a "faux pearl," like real-life faux pearls and furs. Faux simply means "false" in French. So what happened? The angulation of the x-ray beam causes overlapping of portions of the mesial and distal roots above the furca, creating the illusion of a faux pearl. Look closely and you will also note the interradicular bone and furcal area of the tooth are somewhat obscured by the improper horizontal angulation of the beam.
3. The significance is that this is important to anyone responsible for management of a furcal problem and thinking it might be associated with an enamel pearl. Imagine initiating a surgical or curettement procedure and finding nothing!

CASE 10-39

1. The generalized pulp obliteration in an older individual with otherwise unremarkable teeth is a normal part of the aging process.

CASE 10-40

1. The problem is called ectopic root resorption. The distal root of the maxillary 2nd primary molar should not be resorbed in association with the eruption of the permanent 1st molar. Compare with the lower molar, which is okay.
2. The significance is that this person is probably going to have crowding of his permanent teeth and should be followed closely to confirm this.

CASE 10-41

1. The problem is erosion, which is a loss of tooth structure caused by chemicals.
2. This patient was actually bulimic. Her behavior was characterized by periodic bouts of binge feeding followed by vomiting.

    Erosion caused by exposure of the teeth to the gastric acids is called perimolysis. Common causes of perimolysis are anorexia nervosa, vomiting associated with chronic alcohol abuse, hiatal hernia, or gastrointestinal reflux.
3. Aside from the medical and psychologic help available, the dental hygienist can suggest to bulimics and anorexics that they rinse thoroughly with antacids or bicarbonate of soda as a mouth rinse after vomiting; and make them aware of the damage the habit is causing.

CASE 10-42

1. The anomaly is a supernumerary 4th molar that has erupted. Don't tell me you missed that!

    Okay, time for a break. When fatigue sets in, you start missing the easy things!

CASE 10-43

1. The mandibular lateral incisor, canine, and 1st premolar all have at least a bifurcated root canal space. The main sign of this is a sudden narrowing of the root canal space. This is seen in all three teeth. Second, the root canal can be seen to bifurcate or branch right where the narrow part starts, as can be seen in the canine. Third, you can sometimes see a double periodontal

membrane space down one or both sides of the root, indicating a bell-shaped root that is seen on the distal aspect of the lateral. Last, you can actually see a second root as is seen in the canine.

CASE 10-44
1. Macrodontia
2. Gemination
3. Gemination is a single, large, joined or double tooth in which the tooth count is normal when the large tooth is counted as one.

CASE 10-45
1. The primary 2nd molar is submerged and ankylosed.
2. There appears to be a periodontal defect developing distal to the primary tooth and possible root caries on the mesial aspect of the 1st permanent molar. Rule out cervical burnout with a bite-wing or physical probing of the area if accessible.
3. The treatment is to crown the primary molar to reestablish the plane of occlusion and to restore proper interproximal contact. The 2nd premolar will probably need orthodontic uprighting. The 2nd molar may also need ortho.

CASE 10-46
1. This is the typical collapse of the occlusion caused by not replacing the missing 1st molar. The maxillary 1st molar has supraerupted; sometimes there are associated root caries and a periodontal defect. The lower 2nd and 3rd molars are tipped mesially.
2. Treatment involves extraction of the lower 3rd molar if it is not needed; uprighting the 2nd molar; root canal therapy on the upper 1st molar followed by a reestablishment of the maxillary plane of occlusion with a crown and then a bridge or implant to replace the original missing molar.

CASE 10-47
1. This patient is about 16 to 18 years old.
2. There is diffuse calcification of the pulp.
3. There is no significance, except when endodontic therapy is needed. Notice that this finding does not appear to be age related or to represent any type of reactive response of the pulp.

CASE 10-48
1. The sign of future crowding is a lack of resorption of the primary incisor root in association with the eruption of the lateral incisor.

CASE 10-49
1. The anomaly looks like fusion of two supernumerary teeth, mostly because it almost looks like there are two roots and separate pulp and root canal chambers.

CASE 10-50
1. The condition is cleidocranial dysplasia.
2. The clavicle or collar bone; this allows the shoulders to be brought together in front of the patient.
3. Hypertelorism is when the eyes are far apart. Specific measurements are when: the distance between the inner canthi exceeds 45 mm, the interpupillary distance exceeds 75 mm, and the distance between the outer canthi exceeds 95 mm.

CASE 10-51
1. There are abnormally large pulps for his age. Note the more densely radiopaque band of dentin surrounding the pulps, giving a "tooth within a tooth" appearance. This is a very rare example of this latter finding. Note also the osteoporotic and even "burnt out" appearance of the alveolar bone characterized by enlarged marrow spaces and thickened, poorly mineralized trabeculae.
2. The patient has vitamin D–resistant rickets (hereditary hypophosphatemia).

CASE 10-52
1. The entity is an impacted, ankylosed mandibular molar, probably a 3rd molar, with no evidence of associated inflammation or connection to the oral environment.
2. This is a "leave me alone" situation. Embedded teeth under dentures may be left in if there is no associated pathology.

In this case the ankylosis may require a lot of bone removal to get the tooth out, which can only diminish the support for the denture. All edentulous patients should be examined periodically and receive a panoramic radiograph if indicated by the dentist.

CASE 10-53
1. Dentinogenesis imperfecta (A)
2. Osteogenesis imperfecta (B); note the current fracture of the tibia and the deformity at the distal end of this bone from previous fractures.
3. Blue sclera of the eyes. The sclera of the eyes is the part we know as the white part. Remember the expression from the civil war: "Don't shoot till you see the whites of their eyes!" The white, or sclera, of the eye surrounds the colored iris. The sclera sometimes appears blue because it is thinned by a disease process.

CASE 10-54
1. A single unerupted supernumerary premolar in each quadrant
2. Because these teeth will most likely attempt to erupt, the erupted teeth may become displaced. At this stage of development, they often shell out easily, and their removal is recommended.
3. The most common supernumerary tooth is the maxillary mesiodens, followed by the upper 4th molars, mandibular 4th molars, premolars, canines, and lateral incisors, in descending order of prevalence.

CASE 10-55
1. Ghost teeth
2. Focal dermal hypoplasia syndrome
   (Goltz-Gorlin syndrome); the jaw cyst–basal cell nevus syndrome is also known as the Gorlin-Goltz syndrome.

CASE 10-56
1. If you said concrescence…right on!
2. The joining of two teeth by cementum; thus they are united to each other by their roots.

CASE 10-57
1. Two microdontic supernumerary teeth in the maxillary left anterior area
2. Multiple endosteal and parosteal osteomas
3. Gardner's syndrome
4. Malignant polyposis mainly affecting the large bowel and rectum. I would strongly recommend prophylactic removal of these structures as the polyposis begins at about age 30 and affects virtually all patients by age 50.

CASE 10-58

1. Technically you could call this hereditary (vs. environmental) enamel hypoplasia, and specifically, amelogenesis imperfecta hypoplastic subtype.

COMMENT: There are four basic types of amelogenesis imperfecta: type I hypoplastic, type II hypomature, type III hypocalcified, and type IV combined variants of hypoplastic and hypomature with taurodontism. To date there are some 15 variants among the four subtypes with clinically smooth, pitted, rough, stained or discolored, and snow-capped presentations. The patterns of inheritance include autosomal dominant, some of which are X-linked, and autosomal recessive, some of which are X-linked. The least severe cases tend to be the dominant ones, and the most severe are the recessive cases.

CASE 10-59

1. Microdontia of the incisors, canines, and premolars characterized mainly by shortened roots and shovel-shaped incisors, which are susceptible to lingual pit and interproximal caries
2. This is known as the "shovel-shaped incisor syndrome."
3. Pits at the cusp tips, which tend to develop class VI caries

COMMENT: This syndrome is not yet well recognized but is seen very frequently in regions where the Hispanic population is high. Recognition is important because these patients are more susceptible to certain types of caries and early tooth loss should periodontal disease develop. When tooth loss occurs for any reason, the remaining affected teeth are poor abutments for prosthetic appliances because of the poor crown-root ratio. For these reasons and perhaps others as yet unknown, this syndrome needs to be recognized by dentists and learned by students so patients like Henry and his parents can have important counseling from the hygienist so that his teeth can be retained for a lifetime.

CASE 10-60

1. This patient has numerous enamel pearls.

COMMENT: These are known more broadly as ectopic enamel and subdivided into enamel pearls and cervical enamel extensions, which are sometimes associated with the buccal bifurcation cyst. Enamel pearls are sometimes removed because they may become associated with furcal periodontitis when located here. Enamel pearls may consist entirely of enamel; however, they may also include dentin and a pulpal extension. The latter possibility should be evaluated and endodontic treatment considered and presented to the patient if the pearl is to be removed. Ultimately, pearlectomy may be needed for the best periodontal prognosis of affected teeth. Each case must be considered individually, and the role of the hygienist and patient compliance must be part of the consideration.

2. The author has never seen so many enamel pearls in one patient. The author has counted 11 pearls and possibly as many as 16 or more, though several may not show up in the printed version. This case may represent a record for the most enamel pearls in a single patient. Here's the author's score sheet:
- Maxillary left 3rd molar: maybe at mesial developing apex
- Maxillary left 2nd molar: one distal
- Maxillary left 1st molar: one furcal
- Maxillary right 1st molar: maybe one mesial and one furcal
- Maxillary right 2nd molar: one mesial and one distal
- Maxillary right 3rd molar: maybe at distal developing apex
- Mandibular right 3rd molar: one or two at developing apex
- Mandibular right 1st molar: one or two furcal
- Mandibular left 1st molar: one, two, or three furcal
- Mandibular left 2nd molar: two furcal
- Mandibular left 3rd molar: one or two at developing apex

3. Other anomalies include: malformed maxillary incisors; apparently three erupted maxillary premolars bilaterally or the canines have supernumerary lingual cusps; bulbous crowns with shortened roots; some dilacerated roots and pulp calcifications.

CASE 10-61

1. Ectodermal dysplasia; there are a number of variants; this one probably represents hereditary hypohidrotic ectodermal dysplasia.

CASE 10-62

1. Amelogenesis imperfecta type III, hypocalcified, and it is probably a recessive subtype based on the expression, though this cannot be known without a genetic workup.

COMMENT: Note that the developing 3rd molars appear normal; however, the enamel chips off the teeth soon after eruption.

CASE 10-63

1. This question involves an assessment of eruptive potential. When the wide-open "blunderbuss" apex is seen, the root is still developing; thus there is some eruptive potential. However, if the crown length exceeds root length, eruption can be considered delayed, and in this case the delay is because the lower 3rd molars appear impacted. The uppers look like they will erupt. If a tooth has not erupted and root formation is complete, further eruption is unlikely. The lower and upper 3rd molars should be extracted. The uppers should be extracted also because they can extrude, resulting in a periodontal defect distal to the 2nd molar and distal root caries on the 2nd molar may develop.
2. The extraction of 3rd molars to avoid orthodontic regression is controversial. In theory (growth and development of the mandible) and in the orthodontic literature, this should not be expected.

SPECIAL SECTION ON 3RD MOLAR IMPACTIONS

CASE 10-64 Class 1, position C, vertical

CASE 10-65 Class 1, position C, horizontal

CASE 10-66 Class 2, position A, mesioangular

CASE 10-67 Class 2, position B, horizontal

CASE 10-68 Mandibular: Class 1, position B, mesioangular
Maxillary: Class C, mesioangular, NSA

CASE 10-69 Mandibular: Class 2, position B, mesioangular
Maxillary: Class C, mesioangular, SA

SPECIAL SECTION ON LOCALIZATION

CASE 10-70

1. A and B—the impacted 3rd molar is toward the buccal.

COMMENT: Remember, the lingual object including the lingual cusp is usually a little more radiopaque than the buccal cusp because it is closest to the film. The lingual cusp is also usually a little more inferior and a little flatter. Now in part A, look at the mesiobuccal cusp of the 2nd molar. It is less radiopaque and a little higher than the mesiolingual cusp. So now you have the known object, the mesiobuccal cusp of the 2nd molar (is on the buccal, right?). Okay, now look at this same cusp in part B. Which way did it move? It moved mesially with respect to the lingual cusp, right? Now look at the unknown object, the 3rd molar. It moved mesially as it is now superimposed on the distal aspect of the 2nd molar, right? So the 3rd molar moved in the same direction as the known object (the buccal cusp of the 2nd molar); therefore the impacted 3rd molar is also toward the buccal. You can reverse A and B and the rule still works.

CASE 10-71

1. A and B—the enamel pearl is toward the lingual.

COMMENT: In this case we have two known object locations: the malar process of the maxilla and coronoid process of the mandible are both buccal to the 2nd molar. In part A, note the position of the enamel pearl superimposed on the mesial root of the 2nd molar and the positions of the known buccal objects. In part B, the known buccal objects have both moved toward the distal with the coronoid process moving right out of the image. However, the enamel pearl moved mesially—the opposite direction of the two known objects. Therefore the enamel pearl is toward the lingual. You can reverse A and B and the rule still works.

SPECIAL SECTION ON PERIODONTAL ASSESSMENT

CASE 10-72

1. Canine: Horizontal bone loss; moat periodontal defect (three-walled infrabony pocket); prominent periodontal membrane space, loss of lamina dura, and adjacent reactive sclerotic bone consistent with periodontitis and unrelated pulp calcification
2. First premolar: Horizontal bone loss; moat periodontal defect; prominent periodontal membrane space and a zone of adjacent reactive sclerotic bone consistent with periodontitis; a horizontal radiolucent line indicating toothbrush abrasion or abfraction; class VI cusp tip enamel caries; distal drift and unrelated pulp calcification

CASE 10-73

1. Supragingival calculus
2. Calculus bridge or calculus splint
3. Individual tooth mobility
4. Vertical and horizontal bone loss
5. Periodontitis; note prominent periodontal membrane space, loss of lamina dura, and the more radiopaque reactive bone in the area.
6. The soft tissue outline of the floor of the mouth as the film has been superimposed over this area; if it were the tongue, the shadow would be convex.

CASE 10-74

1. "Floating tooth"
2. Malignant disease can cause a floating tooth appearance; this possibility must be ruled out as part of the clinical assessment of the patient.
3. The defect completely surrounds the tooth. There is a thin remaining wall of bone either on the buccal or lingual side of the apical ⅓ of the root. The slight jog in the distal root contour may be a root fracture, which may be the cause of the problem. A wide zone of sclerotic reactive alveolar bone surrounds the defect, strongly suggesting an inflammatory process rather than a malignant one.

4. Long-term mobility is indicated by the flattened contact point between the two molars; this is a form of attrition.
5. The cause of the mobility may be associated with the flattened mesial cusp tips of the 2nd molar caused by hyperocclusion, which may have been the earliest finding in the chain of events leading to the present condition.
6. Note the thickened periodontal membrane space; this may represent the early signs of a class 1 furcal involvement, which must be localized and confirmed by the clinical examination with a periodontal probe.

CASE 10-75

1. First molar:
   - Leaky restoration margin distally, indicated by a step defect and the softened dentin made radiopaque by the leaching of tin (Sn) from the amalgam into the dentinal tubules; this more radiopaque dentin is usually flame shaped, with the tip of the flame pointing into the pulp.
   - Vertical and horizontal bone loss with a lack of trabecular pattern at the cervical third of the root, indicating a loss of alveolar bone in this area
   - Periodontitis, as suggested by the loss of the lamina dura
   - Focally thickened periodontal membrane space at the mesial furcal area and centered on an unusually high lateral root canal and may represent the beginning of a periodontal abscess of pulpal origin
   - Pulp calcifications that may affect access to the root canal space needed for endodontic treatment

   A 1-cm diffuse, radiolucent area at the mesial apex, indicating a nonvital pulp representing a periapical abscess, cyst, or granuloma; however, tooth vitality must be confirmed by clinical pulp tests such as electrical, hot, cold, and percussion.
2. Second molar:
   - Redecay at the mesial and distal margins of the restoration
   - Vertical and horizontal bone loss with a lack of trabecular pattern at the cervical third of the root, indicating a loss of alveolar bone in this area
   - Periodontitis as suggested by the loss of the lamina dura
   - The tooth appears to be vital radiographically.

CASE 10-76

1. Three posterior teeth findings:
   - The 2nd premolar: rough contour and overhang, both of which can discourage flossing. Probe the area beneath the restoration for soft redecay, which is most likely present, and compare with the bitewing findings; in this situation the best treatment is to redo the restoration.
   - The 1st molar: Between the 1st and 2nd molar there is evidence of ramping at the crestal bone; this is a type of vertical defect and is often a single-walled infrabony defect.
   - The 2nd molar: Look at the dome-shaped radiopaque band of soft tissue within the sinus at the apex. This is known as periapical mucositis. It is often caused by either pulp infection or periodontal disease. In this case I would suspect a deep bony defect along the buccal aspect of this tooth secondary to calculus formation adjacent to the opening of Stensen's duct of the parotid gland. This impression must be confirmed with a clinical examination. In the absence of an odontogenic origin, the soft tissue in the sinus may represent polyp formation secondary to especially allergies and sometimes chronic sinus infection.

CASE 10-77

1. Take a look at these two molars:
    - In the 1st molar there is a poor distal contour to the restoration and a poorly adapted distal margin of the restoration; mild-to-moderate horizontal bone loss; a suggestion of a class 1 furcal involvement; and possible ankylosis as a result of the missing periodontal membrane space around most of the root.
    - For the 2nd molar there is moderate horizontal bone loss with an apparent class 3 (through and through) furcal defect, which must be confirmed clinically; there is a suggestion of partial ankylosis.

    COMMENT: Ankylosis can be further assessed by the dull wooden sound of such teeth on percussion compared with other teeth. With auscultation (listening with the blood pressure diaphragm) of the jaw during percussion, a louder sound can be heard when ankylosed teeth are percussed and compared with normal adjacent teeth.

CASE 10-78

1. A vertical lingual groove is often found here and results in an associated infrabony defect. Sometimes the groove can be seen on the lingual enamel running from the central pit area vertically onto the root. Radiographically, this is suggested by the prominent lingual groove in the lateral and the vertical faint hairline radiolucency in the same area of the central incisor. A developing palatal (lingual) periodontal defect may be indicated by the focal loss of the lamina dura around this tooth.

CASE 10-79

1. Defective restorations, description, and management:
    - Maxillary 1st molar: Very tiny amalgam fragment on distal and two more almost invisible fragments on mesial; correlate with clinical finding of amalgam tattoo.
    - Maxillary 2nd premolar: Overhang on distal; remove with hand instruments or redo restoration.
    - Mandibular 2nd molar: Overhang and redecay on distal and poorly contoured mesial; redo restoration.
    - Mandibular 1st molar: Rough contour and overhang on distal; poor contour, inadequate contact, and overhang on mesial; correct with hand instruments and abrasive strips or redo restoration.
    - Mandibular 1st premolar: Poor contour, poor contact on distal; poor marginal fill on mesial; redo restoration.

CASE 10-80

1. Periodontally significant findings:
    - Calculus, especially in association with molars
    - Molar hyperocclusion, as indicated by the grossly widened periodontal membrane space and widened lamina dura around both molars; needs to be confirmed clinically.
    - Second premolar extrusion; note the altered and deficient contact points, which often encourage food impaction.
    - Second premolar ankylosis; note the almost absent periodontal membrane space and lamina dura.
    - Horizontal bone loss associated with all three teeth, especially the molars; the calculus and hyperocclusion may be etiologic factors.
    - The external resorption at the distal apices of the 1st and 2nd molar roots may represent iatrogenic effects of previous orthodontic treatment and may be the root cause of the ongoing hyperocclusion.

SPECIAL SECTION ON CARIES AND CARIES SEQUELAE

CASE 10-81

1. Caries classification:
    - The 1st primary molar: Distal class II deep dentinal caries with pulpal recession; possible pulp exposure
    - The 2nd primary molar: Mesial class II deep dentinal caries with probable pulpal involvement

    COMMENT: Actual caries progression is usually more advanced clinically than what is seen on radiographs.
2. Turner's enamel hypoplasia should one or both of these teeth become abscessed. Primary teeth often abscess at the furcation area, causing a "gum boil" (parulis) clinically and damage to the enamel of the subadjacent developing premolar.
3. These teeth will exfoliate between the ages of 10 and 12 years.
4. The 1st molar may not have a pulp exposure, and if so, may be restored with an amalgam restoration; the 2nd molar probably has a pulp exposure and will need a pulpotomy and a stainless steel crown. There are many other approaches to the restoration of primary teeth; however, their preservation is important especially to the proper maintenance of space for the permanent dentition.

CASE 10-82

1. The 3rd molar is partially erupted with a mesial pseudopocket and significant calculus formation; a moat defect appears to surround the tooth.
2. Root caries, distal aspect of the 2nd molar with probable pulpal involvement. This is based on the symptoms associated with irreversible pulpitis and the widened periodontal membrane space at the apex of both roots—a sign of early abscess formation.

CASE 10-83

1. The one surface not to be sealed would be the lower 1st molar because there are occlusal caries into dentin. In such cases, combinations of sealant, fissurotomy, and caries removal and restoration can be used.
2. Cervical burnout can be seen on the mesial and distal aspects of the mandibular 2nd premolar.

CASE 10-84

1. Arrested caries
2. Cervical burnout
3. There are occlusal caries on the lower 1st premolar.
4. Class II more than halfway through the enamel; for some clinicians this indicates the surface should be restored rather than be remineralized. However, diligent probing could prove this to be arrested caries as with the molars. Arrested caries may need restoration for aesthetics or function.

CASE 10-85

1. Class III dentinal caries
2. Radiolucent tooth-colored filling material
3. Amalgam

CASE 10-86

1. Classification of caries:
    - Maxilla:
        —The 1st premolar: Distal class II full-thickness enamel caries; note typical V shape

—The 2nd premolar: Mesial superficial class II enamel caries; distal class II full-thickness enamel caries

—The 2nd molar: This was a large buccal caries involving the buccal cusp and wrapping around to the distal surface.

- Mandible:

—The 1st molar: Mesial class II full-thickness enamel caries; occlusal class I pit

—The 2nd molar: Early occlusal caries spreading horizontally at the DEJ just beneath the occlusal enamel. Look for the horizontal radiolucent band at the cervical of the lower 2nd molar; this was arrested buccal subgingival caries that were not seen in the clinical examination of this patient until the radiograph was studied.

—The 3rd molar: Occlusal redecay or recurrent caries.

2. Cervical burnout can be seen on the distal aspect of the lower 1st molar.

CASE 10-87

1. These are both relatively deep root caries, especially the molar.
2. The etiology for the lower molar is extrusion with the altered contact, probable food impaction, and development of the distal root caries. The etiology for the lesion on the distal aspect of the maxillary 1st premolar is not obvious but may be associated with a clasp of a maxillary removable partial denture, though the patient was obviously edentulous in the area for a long time for the extrusion of the lower molar to have occurred.

CASE 10-88

1. Recurrent caries: distal maxillary canine, distal mandibular 1st molar, mesial mandibular 2nd molar

CASE 10-89

1. The patient has a fractured mesiolingual cusp.
2. Restore with an amalgam or composite buildup and a crown.
COMMENT: Note the poor margins and contour on the adjacent crown, which should be replaced.

CASE 10-90

1. Take a look at the mesial aspect of the maxillary 2nd premolar. Can you see it now? Note the flame-shaped radiopaque area beneath the restoration, with the tip of the flame pointing toward the pulp. Note also the very slight radiolucent shadow at the gingival margin of the restoration. Note also the open contact. Thus the cause is a leaky margin and redecay associated with demineralized dentin with radiopaque tin ions leached into the dentinal tubules from the amalgam in association with the leaky margin. This finding has been confirmed in the literature with the use of spectroscopic analysis of the affected dentin. Note the caries on the distal of the maxillary 2nd premolar.

COMMENT: A very slight similar finding appears to be present beneath the restoration on the distal aspect of the maxillary 1st premolar. It is probably not yet symptomatic, though both restorations need replacement and the caries removed.

CASE 10-91

1. We wish to prevent the development of Turner enamel hypoplasia in the developing 2nd premolar.
2. Because the infection is persistent, the 2nd primary molar should be extracted and a space maintainer placed. The 1st primary molar should normally be restored now with a permanent material to help support the space maintainer. However, there are deep root caries on the mesial aspect and deep caries

on the distal aspect with a caries control temporary restoration. If this tooth is nonrestorable, it also should be extracted and the additional space incorporated into the space maintainer design.

CASE 10-92

1. The 2nd molar shows deep caries that may be arrested. However, there is evidence of early abscess formation at the apices of both roots. Note the widened periodontal membrane space and loss of the lamina dura in the apical areas. There is also a suggestion of pulp calcification.
2. The 2nd molar needs endodontic treatment, a buildup, and a crown. If an implant or implants cannot be used to fill the space, the molar may serve as a distal abutment for a fixed bridge as is or the 3rd molar may be extracted and the 2nd molar uprighted before making the bridge.

CASE 10-93

1. There is no problem. Though traumatized teeth can become nonvital and abscess, in this case we are looking at the air space within the nares of the nose at the apices of the central incisors. Also, it is the soft tissue outline of the nose crossing the roots of the central incisors—not a fracture line.

CASE 10-94

1. This tooth appears to be nonvital.
2. Because of its location to the side of the apex of the tooth, it is referred to as a lateral apical periodontal cyst, abscess, or granuloma (you cannot with certainty distinguish these radiographically). The granuloma is usually densely radiolucent with a punched-out look, less than 1 cm in diameter, and may have resorbed the apex. The cyst usually is delineated by a thin radiopaque line and may be small or fill an entire jaw. The abscess has diffuse margins with evidence of reactive bone at the periphery. All will resolve with successful endodontic treatment.
3. Stainless steel crown
4. Taurodontism

CASE 10-95

1. Caries: Mesial class II involving the pulp
2. Root shape: Bulbous caused by the presence of hypercementosis at the apical $\frac{1}{3}$; note the dentinal outline within the cementum.
3. Periapical reaction: Periapical mucositis secondary to pulpal infection
4. Management: Check occlusion because hypercementosis sometimes develops in association with tooth mobility. Caries removal, endodontics, a cast or manufactured post, buildup, and an aesthetic crown. Extraction: The now bulbous root shape makes extraction more difficult than normal.

SPECIAL SECTION ON THIRD MOLAR RELATIONSHIP TO THE MANDIBULAR CANAL

CASE 10-96

1. Yes, in all three instances a close relationship is suspected.

CASE 10-97

1. The superior wall of the inferior alveolar canal cannot be seen as it crosses the 3rd molar.
2. Figure 10-96A matches Figure 10-97B. Features: This characteristic feature, which indicates a close relationship between the inferior canal wall and the roots of the impacted 3rd molar,

is an interruption of the inferior alveolar canal wall. As the canal wall passes over the roots of the impacted 3rd molar it may be interrupted superiorly, inferiorly, or both superiorly and inferiorly. In this case the interruption in the canal wall is on the superior aspect as it passes across the roots of the 3rd molar.

Figure 10-96B matches 10-97A. Features: this characteristic feature, which indicates a close relationship between the inferior canal wall and the roots of the impacted 3rd molar is a dark band superimposed on the root of the tooth limited to the area of the canal as it passes over the roots. This means that in this area the canal is thinner because where the canal passes the root, the area within the canal is more radiolucent. This corresponds to a notch or groove on the surface of the root within which the canal rests. Rocking the tooth back and forth during the extraction may cause a severance of the canal wall and damage to the blood vessels and nerve within it.

Figure 10-96C matches Figure 10-97C. Features: classically this characteristic feature, which indicates a close relationship between the inferior canal wall and the roots of the impacted 3rd molar, is a narrowing of the canal as it passes over the roots of the impacted 3rd molar. In this case we see an interruption of the superior wall, a more radiolucent band which crosses the distal root indicating a notch in the root. In this case the canal may or may not be narrowed. Recognition of these features is important because when such an impacted 3rd molar is extracted surgically, manipulation of the tooth may impinge on the inferior alveolar canal and its contents consisting of the inferior alveolar artery, vein, and nerve. This may cause excessive bleeding or later paresthesia, often in the lower lip on the same side. The paresthesia (feeling of tingling or numbness) may be temporary or, less often, permanent.

COMMENT: These appearances suggest a very close relationship between the roots of the 3rd molar and the canal. In such cases it is best to acquire a CBCT scan either in the dental office or by referral to a CBCT imaging facility. The CBCT images will allow an exact analysis of the case such that the best treatment plan can be formulated and executed.

CASE 10-98

1. Radiolucent band on mesial and distal roots where the canal crosses the roots; slight interruption of the superior canal wall where the canal crosses the dilacerated mesial root; possible slight narrowing of the canal just anterior to the mesial root.

   First, we see two vertical fracture lines superiorly; these fracture lines seem to merge for the lower half of the fracture line.

   Second, we can see an interruption of the superior canal wall as it crosses the roots of the developing and erupting 3rd molar. This indicates a close relationship of the canal with the 3rd molar.

   Third, look at the apices of the developing roots. The mesial apex is normal and root formation is almost complete, but the distal apex has a radiolucent area within which the mesial upper fracture line passes. The crestal bone on the distal aspect of the tooth seems somewhat resorbed and radiolucent, indicating possible low-grade infection at the distal aspect of the erupting 3rd molar, which is not unusual. The fracture allowed the infection to migrate inferiorly along the fracture line and infect the pulp at the distal apex, which ultimately caused the toothache.

2. Final diagnosis: complex fracture of the left mandibular body and pulpitis of the left 3rd molar.

SPECIAL SECTION ON SINUS PNEUMATIZATION

CASE 10-99

1. Pneumatization seen on radiograph: yes

CASE 10-100

1. As is, things look bad for implants.
2. There is a retained root tip; notice the root canal and periodontal membrane space. Other possibilities for similar radiopacities include antrolith, antral exostosis, small antral osteoma, and foreign body or object.
3. Pneumatization
4. A sinus floor lift can be done by transplanting autogenous bone from a donor site such as the iliac crest (hip). Some patients undergo repneumatization failure of the implants. A fixed bridge would be an alternate choice.

Chapter 11

CASE INTERPRETATION

CASE 11-1

1. Left side
2. Sublingual salivary gland depression
3. No treatment is necessary; biopsy or an oral and maxillofacial radiologist's report may be needed to rule out other conditions if the radiologic diagnosis is uncertain.

CASE 11-2

1. Differential diagnosis:
   - Lateral periodontal cyst (developmental)
   - Lateral radicular cyst (inflammatory, in this case from periodontal disease)
   - Odontogenic keratocyst
2. Lateral periodontal cyst
3. Surgical removal and biopsy; because the patient has obvious periodontal disease, the lateral radicular cyst resembling a lateral periodontal cyst and occasional odontogenic keratocyst cannot be ruled out. All three conditions are histologically distinct.

   COMMENT: This was a lateral periodontal cyst.

CASE 11-3

1. Ground-glass alveolar bone pattern; loss of lamina dura; probable extension into the maxillary sinus
2. Fibrous dysplasia (craniofacial type based on involvement of zygoma)

   Paget's disease (alkaline phosphatase is very elevated, especially before treatment)

   Hyperparathyroidism (serum calcium is elevated in the primary type; urinary calcium is elevated in the secondary type)
3. Fibrous dysplasia (craniofacial type)
4. Some patients receive surgical reduction of the fibro-osseous mass for aesthetic reasons.

CASE 11-4

1. The radiolucent lesion is about 2 cm in diameter and is surrounded by a thin, well-corticated, radiopaque margin. The inferior margin is interrupted with a somewhat more diffuse radiopaque margin, indicating inflammation in this area. The mylohyoid ridge is superimposed on the lesion horizontally,

and there is a 3-mm roundish radiopacity in the center of the lesion.

2. Because of the history, and ascribing to the adage that "common things occur commonly," residual periapical cyst (residual cyst) with slight infection is the diagnosis; the central radiopacity is seen with some frequency with this cyst.

3. Other possibilities in this age group include calcified odontogenic cyst (Gorlin cyst) and calcifying epithelial odontogenic tumor (Pindborg tumor).

4. Biopsy and follow-up

CASE 11-5

1. There is a torus palatinus, which will probably need to be removed before denture construction.

CASE 11-6

1. The pain is probably caused by trauma of the soft tissue of the lower ridge from the cusp of the upper 1st molar.

2. The cause of the pain is a radiopaque pericoronal mass about 2 cm in diameter surrounded by a thin radiolucent band that is delineated by a diffusely thickened radiopaque zone of reactive bone. The mass consists of areas of radiopaque and radiolucent zones of varying density. The soft tissue overlying the lesion appears thickened and in contact with a cusp of the maxillary molar. The reactive bone surrounding the lesion is an indication of infection within the lesion.

3. Differential diagnosis:
   • Complex odontoma
   • Dentinoma
   • Ameloblastic fibro-odontoma
   • Odontoameloblastoma

4. Complex odontoma with secondary infection was the diagnosis.

5. Yes, assuming treatment is not delayed, the eruptive potential of the 1st molar is excellent because root formation does not exceed crown length.

CASE 11-7

1. African American

2. Periapical cemento-osseous dysplasia (one of several cemento-osseous dysplasias; the other two are focal and florid).

3. The teeth are vital.

4. The stages consist of: early osteoporotic stage, wherein the area becomes slightly more radiolucent with diminished and sometimes prominent trabeculae; and the second osteolytic stage, with little evidence of the formation of a cemental mass.

COMMENT: These two radiologically distinct stages are often combined into a single osteolytic stage. In this case a slight rim of sclerotic bone is associated with the right canine, indicating the lesion is active in this area, and absence of the sclerotic rim indicates dormancy in the other areas.

5. No treatment is needed, although periodic observation is recommended.

COMMENT: There are now three recognized subtypes of cemento-osseous dysplasias—focal, seen mostly in whites; periapical, seen mostly in blacks; and florid (multiple quadrants of involvement), seen mostly in blacks.

CASE 11-8

1. Well…if you said bilateral mandibular torus removal, you would be right on! Note the several round radiopaque lobes on this left side, and yes, the condition is almost always bilateral.

Regarding prognosis, they may occasionally recur, especially if teeth are still present in the area.

CASE 11-9

1. A large multilocular radiolucency extending from the left 1st molar crossing the midline to the right canine area; there is one large crenation at the inferior margin and several wispy trabeculae within the lesion. There is multiplanar root resorption of many of the adjacent teeth, and the thin radiopaque line superimposed on several teeth indicates expansion to the lingual on a panoramic radiograph.

2. Differential diagnosis:
   • Central giant cell granuloma
   • Central odontogenic fibroma
   • Ameloblastoma
   • Odontogenic myxoma
   • Odontogenic keratocyst

3. Diagnostic impression: This was a central giant cell granuloma.

4. Prognosis:
   • Central giant cell granuloma: Probability of this diagnosis is high because of age, sex, location, and radiographic appearance. Probability of recurrence is highest when the age is younger than 17 years and when there is pain, rapid growth, evidence of perforation, and the size is more than 2 cm.
   • Odontogenic fibroma: Has a predilection for females; may occur in young persons, but mean age is in 40s; is multilocular when large; and may resorb and displace teeth. Recurrence is rare.
   • Ameloblastoma: More common in males; may occur in young persons, but mean age is in late 30s; many in mandible with sparing of the posterior angle area; larger lesions are multilocular with well defined, rounded loculi; knife-edge pattern of root resorption; may displace teeth. Recurrence of multilocular lesions is high. Multiple re-treatment may rarely result in metastasis of histologically benign tumors.
   • Odontogenic myxoma: Equal sex predilection; average age is 20s and 30s; septa forming the loculi; loculi are straight and often at right angles to each other and form geometric shapes like squares, rectangles, diamonds, and triangles; may displace teeth. Recurs most frequently in larger multilocular lesions breaking out into the soft tissues (fish skeleton pattern).
   • Odontogenic keratocyst: May be seen in younger persons; slightly favors males; more scalloped at the margins rather than multilocular; rarely expands bone or resorbs teeth; mostly in the posterior mandible and ramus. About one-third will recur, and higher if associated with the basal cell nevus syndrome.

COMMENT: Any radiologically multilocular lesion must be considered benign but locally aggressive with a marked tendency to recur.

CASE 11-10

1. This lesion is classified as a pericoronal radiolucency with radiopaque flecks. The lesion is large, extending from the mandibular right 1st molar up into the ramus, almost to the level of the coronoid process. There is buccal expansion as indicated by the downward projection of the inferior margin and lingual expansion with trauma from the maxillary 2nd molar. The lesion contains dense, rounded radiopaque flecks with a radiolucent component, resorption of the distal root of the 1st molar, and downward displacement of the inferior alveolar canal, indicating the lesion may be odontogenic.

2. Differential diagnosis:
   - Ameloblastic fibro-odontoma
   - Developing odontoma
   - Cystic odontoma
   - Odontoameloblastoma
   - Calcifying odontogenic cyst
   - Calcifying epithelial odontogenic tumor
   - Ameloblastic fibrodentinoma
3. The diagnosis was ameloblastic fibro-odontoma.
4. Treatment is surgical removal; recurrence is rare.

CASE 11-11

1. Surgical ciliated cyst of the maxilla (postoperative maxillary cyst)
2. Variations in presentation:
   - Entirely within the maxillary sinus
   - Entirely within the maxilla, just beneath the sinus
   - Partly in the sinus and in the maxilla

   COMMENT: Lesions may be less than 1 cm in size or large enough to fill the entire sinus.

CASE 11-12

1. Reactive subpontine exostosis (subpontic hyperostosis)
2. Surgical removal, but may recur after a time. Removal of the bridge may result in spontaneous regression.

CASE 11-13

1. Hypercementosis
2. The radiology consists of a dense material that partially or completely surrounds the root(s) of a tooth through which the dentinal outline can be seen. The periodontal membrane space and lamina dura are usually seen, and either or both may be slightly thickened on one side of the tooth. The cementum may display denser cemental spikes, especially at the apex. Overall, the appearance is that of an enlarged bulbous root. Rarely it appears as a localized ball-like density at the apex of the root.
3. Paget's disease of bone (specify "of bone" because there is also Paget's disease of the breast). This case is unlikely to be associated with the disease because Paget's is most frequently seen with generalized hypercementosis.
4. One etiologic factor in hypercementosis is reported to be traumatic occlusion. In this case we see two possibilities. First, the 1st premolar is splinted to the canine, probably because the root is short and would make a poor distal abutment. Second, the splinted tooth probably serves for the clasp that helps retain and stabilize the partial denture, which is old and may be unstable. Thickening of the periodontal membrane space and/or lamina dura is further evidence of traumatic occlusion; the lamina dura appears thickened on the distal side of the root.
5. No, the dilacerated root is developmental and is an indication of an obstructed or altered path of eruption.

CASE 11-14

1. The right mandibular body appears somewhat rarefied with several crisscrossing radiolucent tracts, two of which terminate at the inferior cortex. There is a small bony sequestrum at the 3rd molar alveolar crest. A small, densely radiopaque area in the 2nd molar area may also be a sequestrum. There is a V-shaped notch in the inferior cortex, and the diffusely denser bone above this may represent a partially healed fracture site or infarcted nonviable bone. Recent extraction sockets are in evidence throughout.
2. The diagnosis was chronic rarefying osteomyelitis.
3. The lamina dura is resorbed in 4 to 6 weeks.
4. Prescribe clindamycin *stat* and obtain aerobic and anaerobic culture and sensitivity tests, including clindamycin, from the pus or exudate or from curetted material from within the bone such as a fistulous tract. Upon receipt of the test results, modify the antibiotic regimen if necessary.

CASE 11-15

1. The mandibular right 1st molar has deep occlusal caries with evidence of abscess and reactive bone formation at both root apices. An apparent through-and-through class 3 furcal defect indicates a probable coronal fracture line (which may be visible in this case) terminating in the floor of the pulp chamber above the furca. Apical to the 1st molar, the cortex is thinned but somewhat more opaque with a radiolucent line within which an "onion skin–pattern" periosteal reaction occurs. This consists of several alternating radiolucent and radiopaque bands of reactive new bone formation beneath and probably buccal (remember the bony hard clinical swelling) to the cortex.
2. Osteomyelitis with proliferative periostitis (periostitis ossificans; Garrè's osteomyelitis).
3. In this case, extract the tooth because of the fracture. In a sound tooth, endodontic therapy will bring about resolution.
4. Resolution of the swelling takes as little as 2 to 6 months and up to 1 year. Thus patience, parental reassurance, and radiographic evidence of resolution are key to the follow-up plan.
5. In resolution, the laminations first become indistinct; the subperiosteal new bone blends with the inferior border of the mandible. This is followed by remodeling, which produces regression of the bony enlargement and a return of the normal appearance of the cortex and bone in the region.

CASE 11-16

1. Pulp test both teeth adjacent to the radiolucency. The lateral incisor was nonvital.
2. The so-called "globulomaxillary cyst" is not a diagnosis but is a clinical term for this often pear-shaped lesion causing divergence of the adjacent roots and occurring in this location only. Most cases are a radicular cyst of an adjacent nonvital tooth, followed in frequency by lateral periodontal cyst, odontogenic keratocyst, or a number of other rarer cysts or solid lesions like calcifying odontogenic cyst, adenomatoid odontogenic tumor, and giant cell granuloma.
3. Good question! The lateral will receive endodontic treatment. The tooth may return to its normal position without orthodontic treatment. However, orthodontic treatment may be needed.

CASE 11-17

1. Stafne defect (submandibular salivary gland depression) is the diagnosis.
2. No treatment is necessary.
3. Tooth parallelism assessments are relatively accurate with panoramic radiographs. This is a basic physical principle of the geometry of panoramic imaging.

   COMMENT: Salivary gland depressions are now reported in association with all three major salivary glands, and all are on the lingual or medial side of the mandible. Thus the associated gland should be specified as part of an accurate radiologic diagnosis.

CASE 11-18

1. There is a multilocular radiolucent lesion in the mandibular right posterior quadrant at the crest of the edentulous ridge. The inferior margin blends with the adjacent host bone with a broad but distinct 1-cm transitional zone; the superior margin appears to be perforated with a peripheral cuff of bone at the mesial margin. Within the lesion there are wispy trabeculae of bone.

2. This was a peripheral giant cell granuloma.

3. Surgical removal; radiographic follow-up because about 1 in 10 recur; obtain serum calcium tests to rule out the brown tumor of hyperparathyroidism, which is histologically identical and which can, on rare occasions, present as a peripheral lesion; reline, rebase, or fabricate a new denture once healing is complete.

CASE 11-19

1. This lesion is a pericoronal radiolucency. It is large, extending from the left 1st molar area to the upper ramus. The fully developed 2nd molar is displaced mesially and inferiorly to an area apical to the 1st molar, and the developing 3rd molar is displaced posteriorly and superiorly to the upper posterior ramus. The 1st molar displays a pattern of knife-edge root resorption. The inferior margin consists of a thickened, sclerotic, smoothly curved line; the remaining margins are corticated but less distinct. The extended superior margin represents lingual expansion on a panoramic radiograph; a buccal component of expansion cannot be discerned here. Within the lesion there are several faint trabeculae; the inferior alveolar canal appears to be displaced inferiorly, indicating a possible odontogenic origin. There is soft tissue swelling at the superior margin, which appears to contact the maxillary 2nd molar.

2. Differential diagnosis:
   - Unicystic ameloblastoma
   - Ameloblastic fibroma
   - Calcifying epithelial odontogenic tumor
   - Odontogenic keratocyst
   - Atypical dentigerous cyst

3. Diagnosis: This was a unicystic or mural ameloblastoma.

4. Surgical excision and follow-up.

COMMENT: Here the surgical and pathology findings are important as well as the preoperative radiologist's report. If the lesion separates easily at surgery and if histopathologically the mural nodule does not extend much into the connective tissue wall of the original dentigerous cyst, probability of recurrence is very low. If, however, the lesion separates with difficulty from the adjacent bone, and if the ameloblastomatous proliferation extends into the adjacent bone histologically, higher recurrence rates, up to 25%, have been reported. Suspecting the nature of the lesion presurgically with the aid of an oral and maxillofacial radiologist's report can lead to more aggressive surgery in areas of bony adherence and ultimately improve the prognosis. Radiologic signs of transcapular penetration might include knife-edge root resorption, both buccal and lingual expansion, perforation of a thinned expanded margin, and the appearance of trabeculae within the lesion and/or scalloping at the margin.

CASE 11-20

1. The lesion is a large radiolucency with radiopaque foci in the right posterior mandible. It extends from the 2nd premolar to the angle area with posterior displacement of the developing 2nd and 3rd molars. On this panoramic radiograph there is a characteristic downward bowing of the inferior cortex, indicating inferior and buccal components of expansion, and an upward projection of the crest of the ridge, indicating both lingual and superior expansion; thus the three-dimensional shape of the lesion would be "ball-like." At the crest of the ridge there is soft tissue swelling that appears to contact the erupting maxillary 2nd molar. Within the lesion, the mineralized component appears to consist of an admixture of both a spicular osseous component and smooth, rounded, calcific spherules of cementoid-like material, the latter tending to clump toward the center of the lesion. There is a downward bowing of the inferior alveolar canal, and the distal root of the 1st molar appears to project into the lesion. Interestingly, there is a single, thin, radiopaque margin of condensed bone bisecting the lesion at the distal 3rd forming a second lacuna beyond which there is little indication of a distal margin; the remaining margin appears thinly radiopaque.

2. Differential diagnosis:
   - Ossifying fibroma (cemento-ossifying fibroma)
   - Juvenile ossifying fibroma (aggressive ossifying fibroma)
   - Ameloblastic fibro-odontoma
   - Ameloblastic odontoma
   - Cystic odontoma
   - Calcifying odontogenic cyst
   - Calcifying epithelial odontogenic tumor

3. The diagnosis was an ossifying fibroma.

4. Management consists of surgical removal with radiographic follow-up. Recurrence is not anticipated; however, if the lesion is aggressive, rapid regrowth would be observed.

COMMENT: This lesion is radiographically characteristic of ossifying fibroma with the exception of the distal indistinct margin. Loculation has been seen in several large lesions. The concern is the possibility that this could be a juvenile ossifying fibroma with both trabecular and psammomatoid patterns radiographically. The most typical juvenile ossifying fibroma would be seen in the first or second decade, be fast growing, be painful, be located in the maxilla, and have histologic signs including lack of a significant capsule and specific cellular components. This case did not, to our knowledge, recur; however, one of our most aggressive juvenile cases was in this location in the mandible of a boy the same age.

CASE 11-21

1. The pathognomonic radiographic sign that strongly suggests the diagnosis is the "fingerprint pattern" observed within an area of ground-glass bone replacement and enlargement. If you spotted this…bravo!

2. The diagnosis is fibrous dysplasia. If you knew this too, you have serious potential!

COMMENT: There are three types of fibrous dysplasia—monostotic, occurring in one bone only; craniofacial, affecting the maxilla and one or more facial bones; and polyostotic, affecting two or more bones. There are two subtypes of polyostotic fibrous dysplasia: the Jaffe-Lichtenstein syndrome, having irregularly outlined "coast of Maine" café au lait skin pigmentations; and the McCune-Albright syndrome with the skin pigmentations and endocrinopathies.

CASE 11-22

1. Diagnoses:
   - Socket sclerosis
   - Stafne defect (parotid salivary gland depression; round radiolucency in upper ramus)

2. Significance:
   - Socket sclerosis indicates continuing or past systemic disease at the time of the tooth extraction, especially gastrointestinal or renal disease; we have frequently observed this finding in diabetes. Significantly, it is important to find out if these systemic problems are of a continuing nature because they may have an impact on patient management.
   - Parotid Stafne defect is recognized for what it is; there is no other significance.
3. Male

COMMENT: Both of these findings can be helpful in forensic cases seeking to identify an unknown victim, because they suggest systemic disease and gender (most salivary gland depressions are in males and increase in size with age).

COMMENT: There are three types of Stafne defects. These are depressions on the lingual side of the mandible made by each of the major salivary glands—submandibular, sublingual, and parotid. These depressions are associated with resorption of the lingual cortex adjacent to a lobe of the associated salivary gland.

CASE 11-23

1. Radiologic pattern: multilocular
2. Most significantly, the small, well-defined, very round radiolucent areas, some of which are outlined by a thin, distinct, radiopaque margin in the area of the 1st molar; these represent corticated vascular canals seen in cross section and suggest some type of vascular lesion. In addition, the lesion is multilocular and almost displays the typical "ballooned-out" appearance. The history of a 20-year-old with rapid growth, pain, and a "welling up" of blood at surgery is typical. Finally, the patient's name "Sang" is the simple common French word for "blood"! The English word sanguinous means "blood-associated."
3. Diagnostic impression: aneurysmal bone cyst

COMMENT: Vascular lesions are perhaps the most important category of jaw pathology to clinically suspect radiographically because perioperative bleeding can lead to exsanguination and death. This is not a common sequel of aneurysmal bone cysts; however, the risk increases with some hemangiomas and especially arteriovenous malformations. Preoperative recognition of vascular lesions leads to a thorough workup and preparedness for all possible eventualities, thus greatly improving the prognosis.

CASE 11-24

1. Overall pattern: multilocular
2. Clinically, this pattern suggests a locally aggressive benign lesion having a significant propensity to recur.
3. The multilocular radiolucent lesion is large, extending from the mandibular left 2nd premolar region into the upper ramus. The superior margin is expanded, indicating superior and lingual expansion of the lesion, and this margin also appears perforated. Internally, two patterns are seen: first, the loculi form angular or geometric shapes such as rectangles, triangles, squares, and diamonds. Second, in the more mesial, less-loculated part of the lesion, faint thin bony septa can be seen at right angles to a more prominent septum (fish skeleton appearance), indicating the lesion is breaking out of the bone and extending into the soft tissue. The angle area is involved.
4. Differential diagnosis:
   - Odontogenic myxoma
   - Ameloblastoma
   - Central odontogenic fibroma
   - Desmoplastic fibroma
   - Hemangioma
   - Arteriovenous malformation
   - Aneurysmal bone cyst
5. Diagnosis: Odontogenic myxoma
6. The 2nd premolar is extruded and appears to have eroded the opposing maxillary ridge.

COMMENT: Odontogenic myxomas have linear trabeculae that meet at right or sharp angles, unlike any other lesion. Second, if the "fish skeleton" pattern can be seen, it can help. Finally, when treated, the lesion consists of a pale, brownish "gelatinous mass," which further helps suggest the specific diagnosis at surgery. These are characteristic clues.

CASE 11-25

1. Radiographic pattern: interradicular radiolucency
2. The lesion is large, extending from the canine to the 3rd molar area in the left body of the mandible. Superiorly, the lesion scallops up in between the roots of the posterior teeth with resorption of the lamina dura and possibly slight root resorption of the mesial root of the 1st molar; inferiorly, there is resorption of the endosteal surface of the mandibular cortex. The margin appears well defined in most areas but is less well defined mesially and is noncorticated in most areas. The lesion is wider mesiodistally than it is superior-inferiorly. The teeth appear vital.
3. Diagnosis: This was a simple bone cyst (traumatic cyst, solitary bone cyst).

COMMENT: This is a typical example. However, the recently reported cone shape, whereby one or more margins are very straight and linear, sometimes forming a cone shape, is absent in this case. The greater width mesiodistally is also a new finding for jaw lesions. The history of trauma, although helpful, is frequently impossible to confirm because of the active lifestyle of most kids and is not necessary for this diagnosis.

CASE 11-26

1. Same condition? No
2. If you said yes, you probably thought this is a case of periapical cemento-osseous dysplasia—one area being in the lytic stage and the other in the mature phase.
3. If you said no, you probably said the 2nd premolar radiolucency represents the mental foramen. The lesion apical to the 1st premolar is a case of focal cemento-osseous dysplasia.

COMMENT: In the cemento-osseous dysplasias, any single individual lesion resembles the others; the specific diagnosis is a radiographic one but must also be correlated with location, sex, and race. The focal variant may be solitary, and the vast majority are in white women in their 30s and 40s. This case demonstrates the mature stage characterized by a crescent-shaped radiopaque mass at the root apex; surrounding this is a mixed radiolucent area within which are characteristic tiny, rounded, calcific spherules, and at the periphery there is an irregular band of reactive sclerotic bone, indicating the lesion is active. No treatment is normally recommended.

CASE 11-27

1. Differential diagnosis:
   - Cystic odontoma
   - Calcifying epithelial odontogenic tumor (Pindborg tumor)
   - Calcifying odontogenic cyst (Gorlin cyst)
   - Odontoameloblastoma
   - Adenomatoid odontogenic tumor

2. Root resorption: There are two things to know about root resorption—first, it is usually associated with a slow-growing benign lesion such as a tumor, cyst, or reactive lesion. Root resorption is rare in malignant lesions, though it can be seen, especially in chondrosarcoma and osteosarcoma. Second, roots (resorbed or not) tend to straddle cysts and penetrate into tumors, though this is not a hard and fast rule.

3. The diagnosis was calcifying odontogenic cyst. Note the resorbed root of the central incisor straddles the lesion. The only other cystic lesion on our list, the cystic odontoma, is seen in much younger persons. Odontoma can also be associated with the calcifying odontogenic cyst. Confused? In the calcifying odontogenic cyst the mineralized material can be clumps of dentinoid or an odontoma.

COMMENT: There was a big hint once again in the name of the patient! M. Phantome in French means "Mr. Ghost"…and in English a phantom is an elusive apparition like a ghost…still mystified? The Gorlin cyst is also referred to as the odontogenic ghost cell tumor, and the characteristic cells in all Gorlin cysts are called ghost cells.

CASE 11-28

1. Radiographic pattern: pericoronal radiolucency with radiopaque flecks

2. Differential diagnosis:
   - Calcifying epithelial odontogenic tumor (Pindborg tumor)
   - Calcifying odontogenic cyst (Gorlin cyst)
   - Ameloblastic fibro-odontoma
   - Ameloblastic odontoma
   - Odontoameloblastoma
   - Adenomatoid odontogenic tumor

3. Diagnosis: Calcifying epithelial odontogenic tumor

COMMENT: The features of Pindborg tumor demonstrated in this case include—an expansion pattern in the occlusal view characterized by buttress formation—i.e., the expanded margin is thicker distally, suggesting a solid lesion; the associated tooth is a molar that is not usually impacted; there is occlusal or coronal clustering of the calcified material also seen in the Gorlin cyst; there is a knife-edge pattern of root resorption sometimes seen in the Pindborg tumor; the impacted tooth has been pushed down into the inferior cortex, a characteristic of the Pindborg tumor; possibly the calcified material can be seen to be small, smoothly rounded clumps corresponding to the calcified amyloid.

The Gorlin cyst shows a hydraulic effect at the expanded margin—i.e., the expanded bone is the same thickness throughout and meets the bone at an equal angle both mesially and distally. The Gorlin cyst is rarely associated with an unerupted molar. The root resorption in a Gorlin cyst is not of the knife-edge pattern.

CASE 11-29

1. Radiographic appearance: interradicular multilocular radiolucency

2. Differential diagnosis:
   - Botryoid odontogenic cyst (botryoid lateral periodontal cyst)
   - Odontogenic keratocyst
   - Ameloblastoma
   - Central giant cell granuloma

3. Diagnosis: Botryoid odontogenic cyst

4. Surgical excision; recurrence 8 to 10 years after excision is possible. Thus long-term radiographic follow-up is in order.

COMMENT: The developmental lateral periodontal cyst has three subtypes. First is the soft tissue variant called the gingival cyst of the adult and can erode the outer cortex and present as a faintly radiolucent lesion with trabeculation in the lumen. Second is the lateral periodontal cyst. Third is the botryoid odontogenic cyst, which is grossly like a cluster of grapes and often, but not always, multilocular radiologically. All three variants may present as interradicular radiolucencies in the lower canine-premolar area. All three are similar histologically and are characterized by the presence of epithelial plaques on the cyst wall.

CASE 11-30

1. Diagnosis: If you said nasopalatine duct cyst (incisive canal cyst)…great!

2. Radiographically, we can see the corticated margin is quite a bit thicker than what we see in a normal cyst. This is reactive bone secondary to infection, which may occur when there is a connection to the mouth and explains the salty taste and discomfort. Second, there is no inferior corticated margin at all; this is a characteristic sign of a nasopalatine duct cyst when the duct diameter is relatively wide compared with the cyst.

3. Anatomic structure: incisive foramen; it is radiolucent but without a corticated margin; its maximum diameter is 5 to 6 mm.

4. Several old tooth-colored restorations; old because for the past 10 to 15 years these restorative materials are radiopaque. Second, orthodontic treatment with excessive force as noted by the shortening and blunting of the root tips of the laterals; in addition, they seem to have rotated back to the classic position in a class 2, division 1 malocclusion.

CASE 11-31

1. Diagnosis: Condensing osteitis (focal sclerosing osteomyelitis); pulp tests consisting of hot, cold, percussion, electrical, or a test preparation with the handpiece (with no anesthesia as routine pulp tests are difficult with crowns and large deep restorations) would indicate the tooth is nonvital.

2. Root canal therapy or tooth extraction; approximately 75% of the cases will regress to a normal appearance, and they will not progress with successful treatment. (Progression may be an indicator of unsuccessful treatment, or more important, a misdiagnosis. See the next case.) In cases that do not regress (but have healed), the remaining periapical radiopacity is referred to as bone scar.

3. Lower 3rd molar caries: occlusal caries that need restoration

CASE 11-32

1. Diagnosis: Idiopathic osteosclerosis; though there are no caries, pulp testing might still reveal the tooth to be nonvital as a result of trauma, factitial exposure of the pulp caused by excessive tooth brushing, or a cracked tooth. In idiopathic osteosclerosis the tooth is vital.

2. No treatment is needed. Once discovered, the condition does not tend to progress or regress.

3. Lower 3rd molar caries: There are probably root caries on the distal aspect of the 2nd molar. This is a common sequela of food impaction and chronic infection is associated with this type of 3rd molar impaction. Rule out eburnation (cervical burnout) by

confirming the presence of root caries with a bitewing radiograph and clinical probing. The impaction according to the classification in this text: mesioangular (tooth orientation); class I (space from distal of 2nd molar to ramus is equal or larger than the mesiodistal diameter of the 3rd molar); position A (the most superior aspect of the 3rd molar is level with or above the occlusal plane of the 2nd molar).

CASE 11-33

1. Diagnostic impression: Malignant disease either primary to the site or metastatic such as in breast cancer.
   - Signs of malignancy include widened periodontal membrane space along one side of a tooth, in this case the mesial of the 2nd premolar and 1st molar; bonelike material extending beyond the normal crestal height of the alveolar bone; and the clumping effect as seen on the occlusal image.
   - Signs of slow growth (unusual for a malignant disease) include mesiodistal displacement of teeth and lingual displacement of the 2nd premolar. The 1-year-old bridge occludes with the lingually displaced 2nd premolar.
   - Features indicating the nature of the abnormal radiopaque tissue can best be seen in the periapical radiograph. Benign cartilaginous lesions demonstrate a pattern of small round dots, referred to as calcific foci, which appear to be interconnected with fine trabecula-like lines to give an overall pattern of a snowflake. Malignant cartilaginous disease can be similar or so bizarre as to be unrecognizable. In this case you could easily make out the rounded, flocculent, calcific foci, and with a little imagination one or two snowflakes can be seen. This indicated the malignant tissue might be pretty well-differentiated cartilaginous tissue.
   - Ultimately a biopsy of the area was taken and proved to be well-differentiated chondrosarcoma, which can be slow growing and was the radiologic diagnostic impression. Ultimately the patient's toothache, the alert oral and maxillofacial radiologist, and the skilled surgical team may have greatly extended the patient's life as she is still alive today.
2. The 2nd premolar is not being pushed up by the tumor. It is projected upward because of its lingual position within the layer and the negative (−4 to −7 degrees) projection angle of the panoramic beam.

CASE 11-34

1. There is an increased density of the right mandibular body. The lower 1st molar demonstrates an increase in the width of the periodontal membrane space along one side (mesial) of the root; there is also a class 2 furcal involvement, possibly as a result of the increased mobility. Notice the pathologic fracture of the mandible just distal to the 3rd molar. In the occlusal view there is a "sunburst" periosteal reaction.
2. Diagnosis: Osteosarcoma (osteogenic sarcoma); this case is classic for the disease, though in the jaws many patients are around 20 years of age. If you saw the features and got it right, bravo!

CASE 11-35

1. Radiographic pattern: floating tooth
   COMMENT: As soon as you say "floating tooth," you must then determine whether it is of the benign type caused by periodontal disease or the malignant type caused by primary or metastatic disease.

2. The radiolucent lesion surrounds the root of the left central incisor; throughout the lesion, trabecular remnants can be seen; though well demarcated, there is no evidence of reactive bone at the periphery.
3. Diagnosis: If you said malignant disease, that would be as good as you can do because the hot spot on the technetium scan does not help us in this case. The inflammation of a periodontally involved floating tooth would also give a similar hot spot. So it's back to the radiograph, and the findings as described in answer 2 are classic for the malignant type of floating tooth pattern, especially the trabecular remnants whereby the bone destruction is so rapid that some bone is left behind.
   Final diagnosis: Metastatic adenocarcinoma of the lung, which did show up on the lung scan

CASE 11-36

1. Radiologic pattern: Multilocular radiolucency
2. On the panoramic radiograph alone the lesion resembles many of the multilocular radiolucencies. However, when the axial CT image is added, we see minimal expansion, which significantly reduces our choices. So now the radiologic pattern must be modified to multilocular radiolucency with minimal expansion.
3. Differential diagnosis: The author can think of only one lesion that is multilocular but without appreciable expansion and that is an odontogenic keratocyst.
4. Diagnosis: Odontogenic keratocyst (keratocystic odontogenic tumor)
   COMMENT: Feel bad?…Don't…The author was given a variation of a case like this to present as an unknown to the rest of the radiologists at the 2002 annual meeting and guess what? I blew it!

CASE 11-37

1. Radiographic findings: There is a geographic area of bone destruction within which permeative changes consisting of small punctate radiolucencies without a radiopaque margin can be seen distal to the 2nd molar. On the CT, note the demineralization of the buccal cortex and slight expansion.
2. Diagnosis: Permeative change within a larger area of geographic bone destruction is always malignant. If you got this far, then you get almost full points. However, the slight expansion would make the malignant lesion slow growing, since expansion is not a feature of malignant disease. One malignant central lesion in this area of the mandible that behaves this way is central mucoepidermoid carcinoma. Though there is nothing pathognomonic about this lesion in this location, remember that this is a favorite location for central mucoepidermoid carcinoma.
   Final Diagnosis: Central mucoepidermoid carcinoma

CASE 11-38

1. Radiology: Within a broad geographic area of bone effacement, small punctate permeative changes can be seen. There are two radiopaque lesions at the apices of the 2nd premolar and mesial root of the 1st molar.
2. Diagnosis so far: Permeative changes are ominous and indicate rapidly destructive malignant disease. Note the similarity to vascular channels; however, permeative changes are not well rounded, the margins can be blending, and there is no well-defined cortical margin. The radiopaque areas may in this case represent blastic malignant disease.
3. In B, you can see "hot spots" in the neck, superior cranial vault, and mandible. These correspond to sites of metastases to bone.

Lesser hot spots can be seen in the frontal and maxillary sinuses and probably are caused by sinus infection (sinusitis).

4. Diagnosis: Metastatic prostate carcinoma

CASE 11-39

1. Panoramic radiograph (A): The mandibular left 1st molar is impacted, and the distal root of the primary 2nd molar has been resorbed. Surrounding much of the impacted 1st molar is a radiolucent area bounded inferiorly by a thin but distinct radiopaque line. There may be slight posterior displacement of the developing 2nd molar and resorption of the mesial occlusal portion of the bony crypt wall. A slightly more radiopaque area can be seen at the bifurcation of the 1st molar and may represent a cervical enamel extension with which this lesion is believed to be associated in some cases.

2. Eruptive potential: The 1st molar can still erupt because the apices are open; however, as root length begins to exceed crown length, the eruptive potential diminishes.

3. Occlusal radiograph (B): There is lingual displacement of the roots of the 1st molar and a burnt-out radiolucent area buccal to this tooth corresponding to the lesion. The presence of a periosteal reaction cannot be determined from this occlusal, though the radiopaque line in the panoramic view may suggest the presence of this reaction, which is sometimes present.

4. Differential diagnosis:
   • Buccal bifurcation cyst (inflammatory paradental cyst)
   • Eruption cyst
   • Ameloblastic fibroma
   • Unicystic ameloblastoma

5. Diagnosis: Buccal bifurcation cyst

COMMENT: The unerupted 1st molar, possible cervical enamel extension, and various features of this case, especially the lingual displacement of the involved tooth, are typical. The lesion seems to be well recognized in Canada and Europe because many of the reports come from there.

6. Treatment: Extract the 2nd primary molar, curette out the cyst and associated granulation tissue, smooth off the enamel extension, and observe the tooth for eruption. If the tooth does not erupt within a month or two, initiate orthodontic traction. In either case, maintain the position of the 1st molar after eruption and until the premolars have erupted.

CASE 11-40

1. Diagnosis: Calcified acne scars
   COMMENT: Similar lesions include miliary osteomas and small phleboliths.

CASE 11-41

1. Diagnosis: The original diagnosis was cementifying fibroma. Currently this diagnosis would be ossifying fibroma. The "coiled worm" pattern, though rare, is suggestive and should be distinguished from the "fingerprint" pattern we saw for fibrous dysplasia.

CASE 11-42

1. First molar pattern: Floating tooth; this is either malignant disease like gingival carcinoma or advanced periodontitis.

2. The floating tooth appears to have developed from the long-standing open contact on the mesial aspect. Calculus can be seen on the mesial root. The distal root is fractured and may be a contributing factor. The floor of the maxillary sinus appears inverted in the apical region of the tooth. The sinus is cloudy, indicating a sinusitis probably of reactive odontogenic origin. There are also small radiopacities within the radiolucent zone different from trabecular remnants but noteworthy just the same. This case appears inflammatory in origin and represents advanced chronic periodontitis. It is possible that the tiny radiopaque flecks represent dystrophic calcification much like those seen within long-standing residual radicular cysts.

3. The unerupted tooth is the 2nd premolar. It appears to have migrated mesially. There appears to be internal resorption within this tooth. There may be an additional pulpitis resulting from exposure of the apex to the periodontal defect.

4. Management involves extraction of the molar and the impacted premolar, followed by keen observation of healing. In this situation it is appropriate for the dentist to treat the sinusitis with an antibiotic, such as amoxicillin, and a decongestant.

CASE 11-43

1. The 1st premolar exhibits distal drift, the root apex appears resorbed with hypercementosis, and there is redecay beneath the amalgam restoration.

2. The 2nd molar is impacted and appears to be associated with a pericoronal radiolucency containing a radiopacity consisting probably of a complex odontoma but possibly a calcifying odontogenic cyst or a calcifying epithelial odontogenic tumor.

3. Immediately above this area there is a thickening of the sinus mucosa that may be of odontogenic origin, but the cause is not obvious in this radiograph.

CASE 11-44

1. The lesion is a periapical radiopacity. It is approximately 2 cm in diameter and is round in shape. The lesion is intimately associated with the apices of the 1st molar with about one half of the root length obscured by the lesion. The lesion is mainly radiopaque with small radiolucent foci throughout. Surrounding the lesion is a thick radiolucent band. The roots of the adjacent teeth appear to be displaced by the lesion.

2. Diagnosis: Cementoblastoma

3. Mandibular left 2nd molar: Reactive periapical radiolucent lesion with resorption of both root apices; class 3 furcal involvement associated with probable tooth fracture and secondary carious destruction. The periapical lesion is a radicular cyst, granuloma, or abscess. The infection appears to have caused rarefaction of the bone between the cementoblastoma and the reactive periapical lesion; the infection may be associated with an unusually wide radiolucent zone circumscribing the cementoblastoma.

4. Maxillary teeth are obscured because the tongue was not against the palate when the radiograph was taken.

CASE 11-45

1. Diagnosis: Cherubism

2. Note the involvement of the sinus and the apparent extension beyond the infraorbital rim. The roof of the sinus is the orbital floor; pressure and upward expansion of the orbital floor cause the eyes to appear to look upward in some cases. The normal position of the lower eyelid is that it should be just touching the limbus, which is the margin of the colored iris (covered by the transparent cornea) and the white sclera.

3. Simple observation; the swollen cherubic appearance and radiographic changes usually regress spontaneously around age 20 to 30 years.

CASE 11-46

1. Diagnosis: Adenomatoid odontogenic tumor.

COMMENT: In this age group, sex, and location, especially with the radiopaque flecks looking like figures such as snowflakes, paw prints, or donuts, and the thick radiolucent rim representing the thick capsule found with this lesion, this diagnosis is strongly suggested. Also in this location, the lesion tends to grow inward and occupy the sinus rather than cause significant facial swelling. In other locations, the lesion may resemble a number of conditions, and the radiologic diagnosis is much less certain.

2. Management is by surgical removal; the lesion shells out easily and does not tend to recur.

CASE 11-47

1. Primordial cyst; it would be hard to miss this diagnosis once you discover one of the 3rd molars is missing. Remember, a primordial cyst develops instead of a tooth.

2. Odontogenic keratocyst (OKC); just about all primordial cysts are OKCs.

3. Case management; remember that these cysts recur in about 10% to 50%, usually within 2 to 5 years after treatment. However, some have suggested radiographic follow-up should be for at least 10 years.

COMMENT: The following features may be helpful in predicting OKC recurrence:

- Clinical findings:
  —Cysts are a component of the jaw cyst basal cell nevus syndrome
- Radiographic findings:
  —Radiologically, if the cyst is large and multilocular with internal spiculation
  —Radiologically, if there is evidence of perforation
- Surgical findings:
  —Surgically, when separation from the bony wall is difficult
- Pathologic findings:
  —Histologically, if "abtropfung" or a "dropping down" of epithelial cells in the connective tissue capsule is present
  —Histologically, if "daughter cysts" are seen in the connective tissue capsule
  —Histologically, if the epithelium is separated from the connective tissue cyst wall

CASE 11-48

1. Diagnosis: Osteoporosis
2. Radiologic features:
   - Thinning of the inferior cortex and adjacent lamellations with endosteal detachment in the premolar region
   - Markedly thinned cortex at the angles of the mandible
   - The alveolar bone is more radiolucent than normal.
   - The trabeculae are coarser, less numerous, and not as radiopaque as normal.

COMMENT: The observation of osteoporotic change in the mandible is not seen in the early stages and is more suggestive of well-established disease.

CASE 11-49

1. The diagnosis is florid cemento-osseous dysplasia.

2. There are two complications of this condition. One is secondary infection and sequestration of a cemento-osseous mass, as can be seen here in the mandibular left premolar area. The second complication is the development of associated simple (traumatic) bone cysts, which may be multiple and tend to recur after surgical curettage (not present here).

CASE 11-50

1. Café au lait is a French expression for "coffee with milk."
2. Polyostotic fibrous dysplasia, Jaffe-Lichtenstein type

COMMENT: The history of pain in the hip is a typical presenting complaint because the disease in the polyostotic form often affects the femoral neck, which becomes weakened and subject to weight-bearing pathologic fracture. Also, the café au lait skin pigmentations with an irregular outline are associated with this type. Last, the patient's last name J-L was a clue…did you miss that one? It is also for these reasons that this would not be a case of craniofacial fibrous dysplasia, which only affects the maxilla and facial bones with no other stigmata.

3. The lesions in the jaws demonstrate the full range of densities seen in fibrous dysplasia:
   - Radiolucent, lower right quadrant
   - Mixed radiolucent-radiopaque, lower left quadrant
   - Radiopaque ground-glass pattern with areas of increased density, upper right quadrant
   - Radiopaque-hyperostotic pattern, upper left quadrant

4. If you thought this is the ghost image of the spine caused by slumping of the patient, you would have made a good effort. Actually, this is standard on the old Panorex-brand machine, in which the radiation was turned off so the patient would receive less radiation while the chair shifted for the other half of the exposure.

CASE 11-51

1. Diagnosis: Dentigerous cyst (follicular cyst)

COMMENT: Note how the cyst has pushed the floor of the maxillary sinus in a superior direction. This folding-back phenomenon can be seen at the apex of the 1st premolar and corresponds to the thin black line in the CT image of the left sinus. This is all that remains of the original sinus space. The remainder of the sinus is occupied by the cyst, with the 3rd molar in the center.

2. The 3rd molar is positioned lingual to the center of the layer of the panoramic radiograph; therefore it is projected upward with respect to other structures in the center of the layer or buccal to this position.

CASE 11-52

1. Diagnosis: Osteopetrosis, malignant infantile form; the "bone-in-a-bone" feature and generalized increased bone density producing an amorphous, structureless appearance are highly suggestive. In fact, osteopetrosis is frequently a radiologic diagnosis.

COMMENT: The "petros" part of the disease nomenclature is from the Greek word meaning "rock" or "stone," reflecting the rock-like increased density of the bone. This is caused by a failure of osteoclastic resorption of bone with a resulting imbalance between bone formation and bone resorption; thus the name Peter, which also means "rock." One of the synonyms for Peter is Rock. Did you get the clue?

2. Case management: In a nutshell, these patients have difficulty with any bone infection, mostly because the marrow, which is the source of the blood cells necessary to fight the infection,

is greatly reduced or obliterated by the excessive deposition of bone. Thus this child must have the very best preventive dentistry the profession can offer. Also, these patients are more prone to bone fractures. Jaw fractures from boisterous play can be very troublesome to manage.

CASE 11-53

1. Diagnosis: Florid cemento-osseous dysplasia complicated by multiple traumatic cysts

   COMMENT: In this case the one cyst previously operated on filled in with abnormal-appearing bone. The middle radiolucency may be an extension of the mesial traumatic cyst, which enlarged after surgery, and the most distal corticated traumatic cyst appears to be the most recent. This is the typical behavior of the most severe manifestation of this complication of florid osseous dysplasia. Remember that the other complication was local infection and sequestration of the cemento-osseous mass and the reminder about the traumatic cysts with that case…oh, NOW you remember!

2. Management consists of thorough curettage of the traumatic cyst cavities and the removal of all the cemento-osseous material; several re-treatments may be necessary to induce healing.

CASE 11-54   Jaw lesions:

1. Diagnosis: Multiple odontogenic keratocysts. Odontogenic keratocysts (OKCs) are known to imitate many other cysts, such as dentigerous, lateral periodontal, residual, periapical, and "globulomaxillary"; in this case they resemble dentigerous cysts because of their association with unerupted displaced teeth.

2. Radiopaque material: Desquamated keratin, which gives the "cloudy lumen" appearance of some OKCs and is the whitish, cheesy, curdlike material noted at surgery or upon aspiration.

3. Management: Surgical removal of the cysts and close follow-up, because recurrence is high—up to 60% 3 to 5 years after enucleation. In fact, two of these OKCs recurred. However, because of the close follow-up, they were noted as small 1- to 2-cm lesions and were easily removed.

4. Rib deformities:
   - Bifid rib just below the right clavicle
   - Bridging of ribs between the bifid rib and the one superior to it
   - Hypoplastic ribs affecting the two ribs inferior to the bifid rib

5. Skin lesions: Basal cell nevi (basal cell skin carcinomas)

6. Diagnostic impression: Nevoid basal cell carcinoma syndrome (Gorlin or Gorlin-Goltz syndrome); other features include a broad bridge of the nose and hypertelorism, palmar and plantar pits, calcification of the falx cerebri, and multiple other anomalies, especially skeletal problems like kyphoscoliosis and spina bifida occulta.

   Bonus questions:

   Forget about the details of this case for a moment. What if, in another patient, the skeletal finding was hypoplastic or missing clavicles:

7. Name of condition: cleidocranial dysplasia

8. In the jaws, look for numerous unerupted permanent teeth with retained or missing primary teeth.

CASE 11-55

1. Radiology: In the maxillary posterior regions there are multiple radiopaque masses surrounded by a variable radiolucent zone.

In the anterior maxilla, especially on the right side, the alveolar bone appears less dense and somewhat amorphous (lacking morphology or details), possibly corresponding to a ground-glass pattern, within which small radiopaque foci can be seen. Several teeth display a widened periodontal membrane space, and the lamina dura appears absent throughout the maxilla. The mandible appears normal and lacks all of the features seen in the maxilla.

2. Diagnosis: Paget's disease of bone (involvement of the maxilla only is the clue, if you called this florid cemento-osseous dysplasia; plus this patient is white).

3. Dental anomaly: generalized hypercementosis

4. Removable partial denture loosens over time? Possibly; however, Paget's disease is slowly progressive and typically, like the hat size, dentures become too tight. In a partial denture, the base area may become too tight; however, the teeth may make poor abutments and loosen because of the bone disease.

5. Long-term: A few patients may develop osteosarcoma and both benign and malignant giant cell lesions (central giant cell granuloma in the jaws and giant cell tumor in the remainder of the skeleton) in the bones affected by the disease.

CASE 11-56

1. Panoramic radiology (A): There is a generalized demineralization of the alveolar bone, creating a ground-glass pattern with a generalized loss of the lamina dura. There is a loss of cortication outlining the inferior alveolar canal bilaterally. Associated with the left 3rd molar is a more circumscribed radiolucent area with displacement of the 3rd molar into the mid-ramus, thought to be consistent with a "brown tumor."

2. Skull (B): There is a generalized demineralization of the skull, complete effacement of the outer table, demineralization and thinning of the inner table, and a granular appearance of the rest of the skull. In the frontal area there is a 1-cm, round, radiolucent area thought to represent a "brown tumor."

3. Hands (C): In this disease the characteristic very early finding is subperiosteal erosion along the radial margin (toward the thumb) of the middle phalanges. (The three bones in each of the fingers consist of distal, middle, and proximal phalanges; next are the metacarpals, then the carpals, and the bigger radius and smaller ulna on the side of the little finger.) In this case of more advanced disease, all of the phalanges are affected.

4. Diagnosis: Hyperparathyroidism secondary to renal disease (renal osteodystrophy)

5. Tetrad of features:
   - Bones (demineralization, brown tumors)
   - Stones (kidney stones)
   - Abdominal groans (nausea, vomiting, anorexia, stomach ulcers, pancreatitis)
   - Psychic moans with fatigue overtones (mild personality change to severe psychosis; weak muscles)

6. Management: Dietary factors such as a low-phosphate diet and vitamin D supplements; however, renal transplant brings about resolution and regression of the signs and symptoms. Delay orthodontic treatment until after complete resolution, and remember that the cyclosporin antirejection drug suppresses the immune system; therefore immaculate home care will be needed.

COMMENT 1: Differential diagnosis for ground-glass appearance and loss of lamina dura:

- Fibrous dysplasia
- Paget's disease of bone
- Hyperparathyroidism

COMMENT 2: Upon resolution, what happens to the brown tumors that are histologically identical to central giant cell granulomas? They generally fill in with dense sclerotic bone, especially in the skull.

FINAL COMMENT: Remember the name Rene P and the clue of organ (renal or kidney) and gland (parathyroids)? Did you catch that one? This is how some students develop that syndrome characterized by hunched shoulders and a flat forehead…you know, when asked a question, the student hunches the shoulders and says, "I don't know," and when told the answer responds by palm-slapping the forehead saying, "I knew that!" Okay, back to work!

CASE 11-57

1. There are multiple radiopacities consistent with endosteal and periosteal osteomas. There are several unerupted and displaced teeth. Some of the unerupted teeth may be supernumerary teeth; no odontomas can be seen in this case.
2. Diagnosis: Gardner's syndrome
3. Malignant intestinal polyposis is associated with this syndrome. It usually begins at age 30, and by age 50 most patients are affected. Resection of the colon and rectum is the only way to survive.

COMMENT: Did you get the clue? How does your garden grow? Yes, Mary was a "gardener"!

CASE 11-58

1. Jaws (A): In the right ramus, in and below the coronoid process and in the upper left ramus, there are multilocular radiolucent lesions with apparent cortication at the margins. The remainder of the mandible demonstrates diffuse osteoporotic change. (These are typical features of jaw involvement.)
2. Skull (B): Multiple "punched out" radiolucent lesions; these are classic and almost pathognomonic.
3. Diagnosis: Multiple myeloma

CASE 11-59

1. A radiolucent area extends from the right 1st molar to the left 2nd molar. Within this area there are multiple noncorticated and several corticated foramen-like radiolucent areas. Within the radiolucent area and beyond it into the left ramus, fine radiopaque striae are arranged in a parallel fashion to form straight and curved canal-like structures, some of which have the foramen-like areas interspersed. The left inferior alveolar canal cannot be seen, and the right canal appears to first widen in the molar area and then become indistinct with the appearance of the multiple smaller canals. There is associated resorption of the inferior cortex, especially on the left side, and resorption of several root tips and root displacement on the left side. It is not known whether the most distal left mandibular tooth is a 2nd or 3rd molar. If, however, it is the 3rd molar, its position and development compared with the other 3rd molars are significant. However, where did the 2nd molar go? It is rarely congenitally missing, and the author cannot answer this. Faster development and advanced eruption can be seen in teeth developing in the presence of a central vascular lesion.

2. Diagnostic impression: Central vascular lesion of bone

COMMENT: Nowadays most central vascular lesions seen in the jaws are believed to represent arterial or venous malformations, and probably the diagnosis of a central "hemangioma" is inappropriate for some pathologists.

Preoperative recognition of a vascular lesion is important because there have been reports of a dozen or more deaths in association with the treatment of central vascular lesions, even when the nature of the lesion was known preoperatively. The patient seen here did not survive the procedure though all possible precautions were taken before and during the surgery.

Simple extraction of a tooth associated with a central vascular lesion can lead to exsanguination of the patient before the bleeding can be stopped.

Compressibility or pulsation of a tooth in the socket and perisulcular bleeding are further signs of an underlying vascular lesion.

CASE 11-60

1. This radiopaque body represents a calcified cervical lymph node.

CASE 11-61

1. The lower 3rd molar is extruded and mesial root caries are present.
2. Because of the typical location of the carotid artery bifurcation between C3 and C4, this represents carotid arterial plaque.
3. While the nonfunctional symptomatic 3rd molar needs extraction, most importantly, the patient should be advised to see his physician as carotid calcification is associated with and can be a contributing cause of a stroke.

CASE 11-62

1. The radiopacity indicated by the yellow arrow measures about 2 cm in diameter, is ovoid in shape, and consists of several visible radiopaque concentric rings that encompass a small radiopaque central mass, which is surrounded by a radiolucent zone. The peripheral outline appears to be scalloped.
2. The yellow lymph node is most likely associated with a long-standing low-grade, chronic infection. The radiopacity as indicated by the orange arrow most likely represents an enlarged submandibular lymph node that may or may not be calcified and is most likely a sublingual lymph node.
3. Look closely at the angle of the mandible and just apical to the mandibular implants. These might also represent enlarged lymph nodes, which require further investigation. Because of the size and number of these other lymph nodes, it would be prudent to see if there is a history of cancer; and even if there is no such history, these may represent signs of metastatic disease.

CASE 11-63

1. At the red arrow there is a cluster of multiple round radiopacities from about 1 to 6 mm in size, of which, the larger ones appear more radiopaque. These appear to be located in the anterior portion of the upper pharyngeal airway, which has a dark outline in the radiograph.
2. The orange arrow points to several pinpoint- to small-sized ovoid radiopacities located within the shadow of the posterior airway and between the C3 and C4 cervical vertebrae and are closely associated with the peripheral tip of the greater wing of the hyoid bone.
3. From an assessment standpoint, it would be important to point these out to the doctor. Diagnostically, the upper cluster of

radiopacities represents calcifications within the crypts of the pharyngeal tonsils and may be associated with chronic ear, nose, and throat infections. The small, easy-to-miss calcifications at the level of the C3 and C4 vertebrae represent calcifications within the carotid artery at the bifurcation. These calcifications indicate a potential for stroke at a later age and thus a discussion regarding treatment options with the patient's physician.

Chapter 12

SHORT ANSWER QUESTIONS WITH FIGURES

FIGURE 12-15
1. This image was captured on a cone beam computed tomography (CBCT) machine.
2. Image A: coronal; image B: axial; image C: sagittal
3. The incisive canal; if you said incisive foramen that would be acceptable too due to the position of the crosshairs.
4. The incisive canal runs from the incisive foramen in the maxilla to the superior foremen of the incisive canal in the floor of the nose.
5. No one knows what function the incisive canal serves; perhaps in an earlier age (many, many thousands of years ago) there was a function.

FIGURE 12-16
1. Figure A is a cone beam computed tomography (CBCT) 2D panoramic reconstruction.
2. Figure B is a CBCT image.
3. In Figure B, we see the axial view of the case in Figure A.
4. The green line is the operator-drawn central plane from which the software will reconstruct the 2D panoramic view seen in Figure A.
5. The area outlined in yellow is the operator-selected thickness of the layer for the 2D panoramic reconstruction seen in Figure A.
6. In Figure B we see the extent of the periodontal defect affecting the upper left 1st molar, which almost completely surrounds the palatal root and which cannot be seen in Figure A, the panoramic reconstruction.

FIGURE 12-17
1. This is a digital periapical image taken with a #1-size sensor.
2. The radiolucent area was thought to represent internal resorption, but during the instrumentation of the canal, there was resistance on the file right to the apex, which would not be expected if there was internal resorption.
3. Image B is a CBCT scan, sagittal view.
4. The final diagnosis was superimposition of the incisive canal on the root of the central incisor. In this case the CBCT image resulted in the correct diagnosis, which could not be determined by the intraoral image.

FIGURE 12-18
1. Figures A and B are small-volume CBCT images.
2. Figure A is the axial view whereas Figure B is the coronal view of the 2nd molar at the level of the furcation.
3. The cause of the patient's pain on probing of the furcation was the infection associated with advanced furcal bone loss.
4. The 2nd molar crown is made of metal, most likely cast gold.
5. The black shadow adjacent to the crown is a CBCT artifact, which is termed "beam hardening" and is usually associated with dense materials such as metal or gutta percha.

6. The whitish horizontal blur is also a CBCT artifact associated with metals and is termed "spray" or "star" artifact.

FIGURE 12-19
1. Figure A is an occlusal radiograph of the maxillary anterior region.
2. Figure A demonstrates the classic signs of this diagnosis, though they are subtle: Look at the apical region of the right central incisor, which is seen to the left here. The distance between the apex and the wall of the nasal fossa is enlarged; the wall of the nasal fossa has a reverse convexity; the wall of the nasal fossa is somewhat thickened and irregular; and finally the bone in the area is more radiolucent. These are the classic signs of a nasoalveolar cyst.
3. Figures B, C, and D are CBCT images; B is the axial view of the bony depression made by the cyst, C is a sagittal view of the depression, and D is a 3D reconstruction of the depression within which the cyst was located. The CBCT images helped to confirm the diagnosis and the extent of the cyst.
4. The CBCT images helped to confirm the diagnosis of nasoalveolar cyst and the extent of the cystic erosion of the maxilla at the base of the nose.

FIGURE 12-20
1. Part A is a portion of a panoramic image of the right maxillary sinus area.
2. The landmark is the posterior superior alveolar canal.
3. Starting at the upper left, image B is a coronal view of the nose and lower turbinate, the maxillary sinus and its lateral wall, and the posterior edentulous ridge as well as the oral cavity.
4. Actually the posterior superior alveolar canal is often in the lateral wall of the maxillary sinus, and infiltration of local anesthetic in the area produces anesthesia of the teeth in the area.
5. The significance of this landmark is in Le Fort fractures of the face, particularly Le Fort 1 osteotomy in maxillofacial reconstruction surgery.

FIGURE 12-21
1. Image A is a cropped panoramic image; image B is a digital intraoral periapical image, and image C is a CBCT sagittal view of the area in question.
2. Because of the nonresolution of the periapical lesion, my best bet would be to redo the endo, and this was done but to no avail.
3. Image C is the diagnostic image. Look again, if you can find the problem. Okay here goes:
   The thing you note first is the destruction of the alveolar plate on both the buccal and lingual sides of the tooth. This is the first clue because when a fracture happens, the tooth is invariably going to have a crack in it. Now look really closely at the thin black line extending from the lingual side and vertically downward at an angle toward the buccal side. This line is the fracture and could only have been seen with a CBCT scan. In such a case the tooth must probably be sacrificed and CBCT can be used to calculate the volume of bone grafting material which will be needed and can also monitor the integration of the graft over time. Because there is probably severe destruction of the periosteum in the area, some sliding flaps will be needed as well as other advanced periodontal procedures to ensure the success of the graft.

FIGURE 12-22

1. The CBCT views are as follows: Figure B, sagittal; Figure C, coronal.
2. Electric pulp testing was not carried out because of the metallic crown on the suspected tooth, which was the 2nd premolar, due to the reaction at the apex.
3. The reaction at the apex of the 2nd premolar is termed "periapical mucositis of the maxillary sinus." This reaction is characterized by a radiolucent area bounded by a thin, dense radiopaque line termed a "periapical halo," and beyond this thin radiopaque line is a focal soft tissue swelling of the sinus mucosa.
4. The differential diagnosis for the soft tissue density in the maxillary sinus would at first glance be that of a mucous retention cyst which is innocuous and does not require treatment. The second possibility is periapical mucositis, which is confirmed by the periapical radiolucency surrounded by a thin "halo" of bone; this appearance is associated with advanced pulpitis and/or pulp necrosis.
5. The CBCT was taken after the endo was done, but the root canal appears unfilled. This could only be because a rare palatal root was present and not filled in the first root canal treatment.
6. While there was no doubt the 2nd premolar needed root canal treatment due to the periapical findings, this appearance is often seen in association with a nonvital or partially vital tooth. Sensitivity to sweets as well as to hot and cold are symptoms associated with a carious tooth, which can in fact be seen at the mesial aspect of the 1st molar in Figure A. In addition, there is a very slight thickening of the periapical periodontal membrane space of the elongated palatal root apex, and the apical lamina dura may or may not be resorbed. The 1st molar should have also been suspected as the cause of the patient's symptoms and should have been pulp tested and either treated with a sedative dressing or endodontic treatment, depending on the results of the pulp testing.

FIGURE 12-23

1. The yellow arrows point to a depression on the medial side of the upper ramus, near the base of the coronoid process within which fibers of the temporalis muscle insert. The depression is not always deep enough to be seen. This depression was discovered by Drs. Steven Bricker and Birgit Glass and Dr. Langlais, fortunate enough to be able to work with them, and we ultimately gave a name to this depression, which had never been recognized and named. We called it the medial (because it is on the medial side) sigmoid (because it is just below the sigmoid notch) depression because it is a depression in the base of the coronoid process. So we have: medial sigmoid depression. And now you know the whole story!
2. The green arrow points to an area of apical osteosclerosis. It is innocuous and probably located there just by chance as these areas can be seen anywhere in the jaws.
3. The orange arrow points to a fairly new diagnosis which is focal cemento-osseous dysplasia. The lesion is in every way like an ordinary cementoma (periapical cemental dysplasia), except it has no racial predilection with many patients being White and is usually seen on only one tooth. No treatment is needed.

FIGURE 12-24

1. On the patient's left side, there seems to be a round radiolucent lesion that we missed until the CBCT scans were taken. The CBCT scans were done to measure the space available for the implants.
2. Figure B is a CBCT set of images with the coronal view (looking from the front of the patient) on the left and sagittal view on the right (looking at the patient or volume from the side).
3. The diagnosis was a residual cyst. A residual cyst occurs when a nonvital tooth has a periapical cyst at the apex that stays in after the extraction. These usually resolve spontaneously, but occasionally, one of these continues to grow very slowly after the extraction. A newly reported sign of a long-standing residual cyst is the presence of calcifications in it, which we can see here. The cyst was simply curetted out and sent to pathology for analysis, which confirmed the clinical diagnosis. Healing was uneventful, which is what you want.

FIGURE 12-25

1. Figure A: Sagittal (looking from the side); Figure B, coronal (looking from the front or back); Figure C, axial (looking from the top or bottom).
2. The jaw cyst is at the angle of the mandible area, more toward the retromolar pad, and it extends up into the ramus, to the area of the lingual foramen, as can be seen in Figure B, the coronal view.
3. It is not very expansile, and there is a "cloudy" lumen. All this adds up to the presence of an odontogenic keratocyst, now renamed odontogenic keratocystic tumor because of its great tendency to recur, no matter how carefully the surgery is done, i.e., even with marginal osteotomy, there is still a recurrence rate somewhere in the 20% to 35% range. It is also associated with a syndrome that includes many other characteristic findings like bifid ribs, basal cell carcinomas of the skin, and other anomalies. Here the recurrence rate is as high as 80%.
4. In the sinus, there is a mucous retention cyst. These are innocuous and are self-limiting.

MULTIPLE CHOICE QUESTIONS WITH FIGURES

1. B
2. D
3. A
4. D
5. D
6. C
7. D
8. C
9. C
10. A
11. D
12. B
13. E
14. C
15. E
16. D

MULTIPLE CHOICE QUESTIONS WITHOUT FIGURES

1. B
2. E
3. A
4. D
5. A
6. E
7. E
8. D
9. A
10. C
11. A
12. D
13. B
14. C
15. A

Chapter 13

SHORT ANSWER QUESTIONS WITH FIGURES

FIGURE 13-12
1. The volume is the area within the yellow circle.
2. The rotation pattern is termed "symmetric."
3. The dose increases with volume size.

FIGURE 13-13
1. The area within the yellow circle
2. The rotation pattern is "asymmetric."
3. The larger volume has a lower dose than the dose would be with a symmetric rotation pattern because only part of the volume is within the beam during the rotation cycle.

FIGURE 13-14
1. The "X" plane is coronal.
2. The "Y" plane is sagittal.
3. The "Z" plane is axial.
4. The shape of the volume is cylindrical.
5. In CBCT, the linear, volumetric, and angular measurements are accurate.

FIGURE 13-15
1. This is an axial view.
2. The restorative device is a metallic implant; a second implant appears to be mesial to this one.
3. The anatomic structure is the mandible.
4. The anatomic level of this image is just superior to (above) the apices of the teeth.
5. The implant appears to be located outside of the mandibular bone, on the lingual side.
6. The green line depicts the coronal view with respect to the intersection point of the two planes and which will be displayed in the same window of the software; the blue line depicts the sagittal view with respect to the intersection point of the two planes and which will be displayed in the same window of the software. This allows the clinician to look at the object in the volume in all three dimensions.
7. The blue and green lines have been so placed because the clinician wants to observe the exact location of the implant at this level in all three dimensions.

FIGURE 13-16
1. This is the coronal view; this is labeled in green at the top of the image.
2. The right mandible, maxilla, maxillary sinus, right and left nose, and medial and lateral pterygoid plates just lateral to the nose on the left side; we know the right and left sides due to the labeling in Figure 13-15, which is the same case.
3. The level of this image is approximately the 1st or 2nd right molar area. This is best seen in Figure 13-15.
4. The orange hash marks each represent a measurement of one-half of a centimeter (0.5 cm) or 5 millimeters (5 mm).
5. The object, an implant, appears to be located within the mandible at the medial (inner) portion; however, due to a faulty trajectory during placement, the apical part and lateral parts of the implant are outside of the mandibular bone.
6. The blue line is still the sagittal plane; however, since this is the coronal view, the red line represents the level of the axial view that was seen in Figure 12-15.

FIGURE 13-17
1. This is a sagittal view, and the label can be seen in the upper middle part of the image.
2. In this plane and at this level, we see parts of the right mandible, maxilla, and maxillary sinus.
3. The anatomic level is through the mandible at an angle that intersects with both implants and which can be seen in the axial view.
4. In this view, the apical part of the implant appears to be outside of the mandibular bone.
5. The planes corresponding to the colors of the lines do not change from view to view or from level to level. Therefore the green line is the coronal cut, and the red line is the axial cut, both of which are also displayed on the monitor as a set of three images; one image depicts the actual plane; the other two lines depict the level of the other two dimensions. All three of these last three images were all displayed at the same time so as to be able to see a chosen anatomic location in all three dimensions.
6. The prognosis of this implant is poor. The use of an imaging guide, which can become the surgical guide, helps greatly to ensure proper placement of the implant.
7. The polypoid pattern of the sinus mucosa suggests a mild allergic sinusitis in the right maxillary sinus.

FIGURE 13-18
1. These are "cross-sectional" cuts and are selected at a plane at right angles to the area of interest, in this case possibly the mandible or the maxilla each of which may have a slightly different clinician-selectable cross-sectional profile.
2. The volume size would be about 2 to 4 cm × 2 to 4 cm. As a reference, a volume size of 8 cm × 8 cm will cover most of the dentate parts of the maxilla and mandible in the volume.
3. The "rule" on selectable volume size is simple: Select the smallest volume that will satisfy the purpose for which the CBCT scan was taken.

FIGURE 13-19
1. This is a cross-sectional view.
2. The location is in the maxillary canine—1st premolar location; the low-density (radiolucent) shadow in the upper right-hand corner of the image is possibly the maxillary sinus. With this small a volume and no prior knowledge about the case, the exact location is hard to determine with certainty.
3. As always with this particular software, the red line is the axial plane with respect to this view.
4. The green line is the sagittal plane with respect to this view.
5. The radiopaque material is part of an imaging guider. Minimally, it represents the planned location of the implant; maximally some imaging guides can have the gutta percha drilled out for use as a drilling guide.
6. In this case the guide is excellent as an imaging guide, but as a drilling guide it would result in gross misplacement of the implant.

7. The blue and green lines were so placed because the clinician wished to see exactly where the intersection point of the lines is not only located anatomically but will be depicted by an image through this plane.
8. The patient's left inferior turbinate of the nose (right side of the image) is "polypoid" in its outline. This is a sign of allergy.

FIGURE 13-20A

1. The left view is a cross-sectional (right angle) view of the posterior mandibular body.
2. The right view corresponds to the green line on the left view.
3. The high-density object is a manufactured combined imaging and drill (surgical) guide embedded in a plastic wafer on which an occlusal index has been taken in the laboratory on mounted models or in the mouth while the plastic is warm.
4. These images represent the mandibular 2nd premolar and 1st molar location.

FIGURE 13-20B

1. To make the determination as to which radiolucency is which, we lowered the red line to where it intersects with the inferior alveolar canal on the right side sagittal view. On the left cross-sectional, view we now see the red line passing through the lower radiolucency, confirming this as the inferior alveolar canal.
2. The crest of the ridge is well healed. However, there are several socket areas that are still apparent, not completely filled with bone, and there is persistence of the lamina dura in the implant area. The differential diagnosis would include bone graft material or socket sclerosis. In normal healing, the lamina dura disappears in about 6 weeks, i.e., long before the crest of the ridge heals over the socket and before the deposition of visible bone. This is therefore an example of socket sclerosis, which has been associated with some systemic diseases, principally kidney and intestinal disorders.
3. This is not the most ideal implant site for the aforementioned reasons. It is possible that there could be healing problems in association with the implant placement; however, the authors are not aware that the finding in this case is an absolute contraindication to implant placement. Rather, it means it might be fruitful to investigate the patient's current health status and determine whether there is any contraindication to implant placement. Absolutely, this imaging guide can be used as a drilling guide, and in fact, this product was designed for these two purposes.

FIGURE 13-21

1. This image is a colorized 3D reconstruction.
2. The general purpose of this type of reconstruction is that it can serve as a set of models as part of the record as well to plan treatment. Remember these models can be rotated around by the software and can be viewed from any angle in conjunction with the three standard axial, sagittal, and axial views. Therefore space and other measurements can be made for orthodontics or implants or 3rd molar removal or for the localization of impacted unerupted teeth, all of which may be seen or required by this patient.

FIGURE 13-22

1. Movement artifact is characterized by a generalized blurriness of the image as well as a ghostlike faint outline of some structures.
2. Movement by the patient during the scan causes either a focal blurriness of a part of the image from the top to the bottom or a more generalized lack of definition and detail if the patient has moved constantly throughout the exposure. One reason for this effect is if the machine rubs against the patient's head or neck during the exposure causing the patient to move. In other instances, the movement by the patient may have been due to a failure to properly instruct the patient before the exposure. In other instances, the patient may be subject to medical conditions or medications causing a lack of concentration. Finally, the patient may have uncontrollable tremors, which prevent him or her from remaining still during the exposure. However, movement is a rare artifact in CBCT imaging.

FIGURE 13-23

1. The appliance is an imaging guide which cannot be used as a drilling guide because it is not aligned with the proper drilling trajectory.
2. The CBCT image is a coronal view.
3. The artifacts in the CBCT image are beam hardening and spray artifacts due to the presence of metallic restorative materials in the maxillary fixed partial denture (bridge).
4. The anatomic structure is the maxillary sinus.
5. The patient's pain is due to the presence of a knife-edge edentulous ridge crest in the left mandible.
6. Preimplant treatment would include resection of the knife-edge ridge crest and possibly a buildup of the implant site with bone graft material.

FIGURE 13-24

1. Cephalometric (ceph) on the left and panoramic (pan) on the right
2. There was a lead apron worn for the ceph image as indicated by the half-moon shape at the lower middle margin of the image; the pan image does not usually indicate the presence or absence of the lead apron. The lead apron is no longer required but may be worn should it be requested by the patient. In children, the lead apron is still recommended.
3. The object appears to be of a metallic nature.
4. The metallic object was slightly below the ridge crest in the ceph image; however, though the ceph suggests the true shape of the object, it does not indicate a buccal mucosal (cheek) location, or a lingual (tongue) position or possibly a location in the alveolar bone, just beneath the gingiva of the edentulous ridge. In the panoramic image, however, the object is widened and projected upward from the ridge crest. This confirms a position lingual to the ridge crest, probably in the tongue.

FIGURE 13-25

1. Top left quadrant view: axial
2. Top right quadrant view: cross-sectional; check the blue line in the top left quadrant, which indicates the exact angle of the cross-sectional view (cut).
3. Bottom left quadrant view: panoramic 2D reconstruction
4. Bottom right quadrant view: 3D reconstruction of the volume
5. The general type of software is an implant planning program.
6. The patient is wearing an imaging guide, which is aligned a little too much to the buccal side for use as an implant guide. This also shows how difficult it is to judge clinically, even with the aid of 2D imaging, the proper implant drilling trajectory.
7. A new surgical guide needs to be constructed with the aid of the CBCT information before a proper drilling trajectory can be achieved.

FIGURE 13-26

1. On the left, we see a 2D panoramic image; this is not a 2D panoramic reconstruction as can be done using the software.

2. On the right, we see a CBCT cross-sectional view of the planned implant.
3. The radiopaque object is an implant imaging guide consisting of gutta percha embedded in acrylic.
4. In this case the drilling trajectory appears to be good. However, the available bone thickness will require a bone graft buildup to create an adequate width of the bone at the planned implant site.

FIGURE 13-27
1. This is a CBCT image.
2. The view is a cross-sectional view of the posterior mandible.
3. The object in the bone is an implant with a healing abutment attached.
4. The implant looks to be a little wide for the available bone; failure may start on the buccal side (left in the image) because the superior part of the implant does not appear to be embedded in bone. The implant could not go any deeper as there are only several millimeters of space between the end of the implant and the inferior alveolar canal.

FIGURE 13-28
1. This is a linear tomogram with a cross-sectional view of the posterior mandible.

2. Even if properly placed, this implant would impinge on the inferior alveolar canal, which is probably the upper of the two round radiolucent areas with an apparent thin cortical outline.
3. At a minimum, a periapical image may be taken; however, a CBCT scan would not only confirm the location the inferior alveolar canal, but also the proper dimensions of the planned implant could be measured accurately as was seen in Questions 9 and 10.
4. As a patient becomes edentulous in the posterior mandible, the orientation of the bone cannot be assumed to be perfectly vertical. Without proper imaging, this can lead to placement of an implant incorrectly and a perforation by the implant on the lingual side, as was illustrated in Figure 13-16.

MULTIPLE CHOICE QUESTIONS WITHOUT FIGURES

1.	D	6.	E
2.	C	7.	C
3.	D	8.	D
4.	D	9.	A
5.	B	10.	D

PART 2

Section 1

MULTIPLE CHOICE QUESTIONS WITHOUT FIGURES

1.	C	58.	D	115.	C	172.	D
2.	B	59.	B	116.	A	173.	D
3.	B	60.	B	117.	C	174.	D
4.	D	61.	B	118.	A	175.	A
5.	A	62.	C	119.	E	176.	B
6.	C	63.	B	120.	A	177.	A
7.	C	64.	B	121.	C	178.	E
8.	E	65.	C	122.	A	179.	D
9.	A	66.	C	123.	B	180.	C
10.	B	67.	C	124.	D	181.	D
11.	C	68.	D	125.	B	182.	D
12.	D	69.	B	126.	B	183.	D
13.	A	70.	D	127.	C	184.	A
14.	A	71.	C	128.	C	185.	C
15.	D	72.	E	129.	B	186.	D
16.	B	73.	A	130.	B	187.	C
17.	C	74.	E	131.	A	188.	B
18.	B	75.	A	132.	A	189.	E
19.	D	76.	B	133.	D	190.	A
20.	A	77.	A	134.	A	191.	A
21.	B	78.	A	135.	A	192.	D
22.	D	79.	B	136.	A	193.	A
23.	D	80.	E	137.	D	194.	D
24.	C	81.	C	138.	A	195.	B
25.	D	82.	C	139.	D	196.	A
26.	D	83.	D	140.	B	197.	C
27.	B	84.	B	141.	D	198.	D
28.	D	85.	C	142.	D	199.	B
29.	B	86.	D	143.	C	200.	E
30.	C	87.	C	144.	C	201.	A
31.	A	88.	B	145.	A	202.	A
32.	D	89.	D	146.	A	203.	D
33.	C	90.	D	147.	B	204.	A
34.	B	91.	B	148.	A	205.	D
35.	D	92.	C	149.	D	206.	E
36.	E	93.	D	150.	A	207.	D
37.	B	94.	E	151.	B	208.	E
38.	C	95.	B	152.	D	209.	E
39.	C	96.	D	153.	A	210.	B
40.	C	97.	B	154.	A	211.	C
41.	A	98.	E	155.	C	212.	E
42.	B	99.	E	156.	D	213.	C
43.	A	100.	B	157.	C	214.	A
44.	D	101.	B	158.	C	215.	B
45.	B	102.	B	159.	E	216.	C
46.	B	103.	C	160.	B	217.	A
47.	B	104.	D	161.	D	218.	C
48.	C	105.	E	162.	A	219.	A
49.	C	106.	A	163.	A	220.	D
50.	E	107.	C	164.	C	221.	C
51.	D	108.	C	165.	D	222.	C
52.	A	109.	C	166.	D	223.	E
53.	A	110.	B	167.	C	224.	C
54.	D	111.	C	168.	A	225.	B
55.	C	112.	C	169.	A	226.	B
56.	D	113.	B	170.	A	227.	D
57.	E	114.	D	171.	B	228.	E

229.	C	256.	D	283.	C	310.	D
230.	D	257.	C	284.	D	311.	D
231.	B	258.	D	285.	E	312.	B
232.	E	259.	A	286.	A	313.	B
233.	C	260.	B	287.	A	314.	D
234.	C	261.	A	288.	B	315.	B
235.	A	262.	D	289.	E	316.	C
236.	E	263.	B	290.	E	317.	C
237.	C	264.	D	291.	D	318.	A
238.	A	265.	D	292.	C	319.	D
239.	E	266.	E	293.	D	320.	A
240.	D	267.	A	294.	D	321.	D
241.	B	268.	D	295.	D	322.	B
242.	A	269.	B	296.	C	323.	D
243.	B	270.	B	297.	B	324.	E
244.	D	271.	D	298.	A	325.	E
245.	E	272.	C	299.	E	326.	C
246.	B	273.	A	300.	C	327.	D
247.	A	274.	D	301.	C	328.	E
248.	A	275.	B	302.	A	329.	A
249.	B	276.	C	303.	B	330.	A
250.	A	277.	D	304.	D	331.	B
251.	E	278.	B	305.	A	332.	D
252.	E	279.	D	306.	A	333.	A
253.	B	280.	A	307.	C	334.	E
254.	B	281.	D	308.	A	335.	B
255.	B	282.	B	309.	D		

Section 2

MULTIPLE CHOICE QUESTIONS WITH FIGURES

1.	C	33.	C	65.	C	97.	B
2.	A	34.	D	66.	A	98.	D
3.	D	35.	A	67.	B	99.	D
4.	D	36.	B	68.	D	100.	D
5.	B	37.	B	69.	D	101.	C
6.	D	38.	C	70.	E	102.	B
7.	C	39.	D	71.	B	103.	E
8.	A	40.	A	72.	A	104.	E
9.	D	41.	A	73.	C	105.	E
10.	C	42.	C	74.	B	106.	D
11.	D	43.	D	75.	D	107.	C
12.	A	44.	D	76.	C	108.	D
13.	C	45.	A	77.	D	109.	A
14.	C	46.	C	78.	B	110.	E
15.	B	47.	B	79.	B	111.	C
16.	D	48.	C	80.	A	112.	A
17.	B	49.	D	81.	B	113.	E
18.	A	50.	B	82.	C	114.	B
19.	D	51.	D	83.	B	115.	A
20.	D	52.	B	84.	C	116.	D
21.	C	53.	D	85.	A	117.	B
22.	A	54.	A	86.	D	118.	C
23.	E	55.	C	87.	C	119.	C
24.	D	56.	C	88.	A	120.	C
25.	B	57.	D	89.	D	121.	B
26.	D	58.	A	90.	B	122.	A
27.	D	59.	D	91.	A	123.	C
28.	D	60.	D	92.	D	124.	C
29.	D	61.	A	93.	C	125.	D
30.	B	62.	B	94.	C		
31.	A	63.	C	95.	A		
32.	A	64.	C	96.	D		

MULTIPLE CHOICE QUESTIONS WITHOUT FIGURES

126.	B	139.	A	152.	A	165.	E
127.	C	140.	B	153.	D	166.	A
128.	A	141.	A	154.	D	167.	B
129.	B	142.	C	155.	E	168.	D
130.	C	143.	A	156.	B	169.	B
131.	D	144.	D	157.	E	170.	A
132.	C	145.	C	158.	C	171.	E
133.	B	146.	C	159.	E	172.	D
134.	A	147.	D	160.	A	173.	A
135.	C	148.	B	161.	B	174.	D
136.	A	149.	A	162.	C	175.	A
137.	D	150.	E	163.	E		
138.	C	151.	C	164.	D		

GLOSSARY

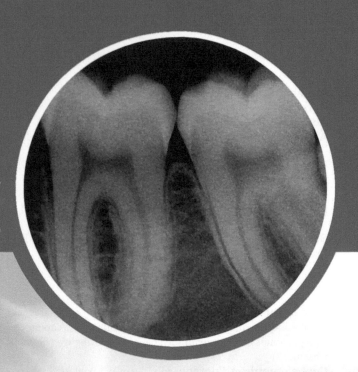

A

Abfraction tooth loss not caused by tooth decay (10)
Abrasion wearing away of tooth structure (10)
Adumbration cervical burnout (10)
Arrested caries the decay process becomes inactive and stops progressing (10)

B

Blooming digital artifact characterized by a blackening of all or parts of an image (1)
Bottle caries decay seen in children who are fed liquid with high sugar content in bottles (10)

C

Centers for Disease Control and Prevention a federal agency that conducts and supports health promotion, prevention, and preparedness activities with the goal of improving overall public health (3)
Cephalometric radiograph an x-ray of the skull used to assess the relationships of the teeth to the upper and lower jaws and to the facial skeleton (4)
Charge coupled device a light-sensitive circuit that stores and displays data for an image (5)
Complementary Metal Oxide Sensors (COMS) a battery-powered chip inside a sensor that stores a digital image (5)
Cone Beam Computed Tomography (CBCT) a specialized technology that produces 3D images of the teeth, soft tissues, and bone in a single scan (3)
Cone cutting the improper aim of the x-ray beam resulting in a missing image (5)

D

Dentition the existing teeth in the oral cavity (6)
Diagnostic coverage term meaning all needed structures for an accurate diagnosis are able to be seen on the film (9)
Diagnostic quality accuracy of films to properly define results (9)
Diagnostic sensitivity periapical pathology or other lesions that can be visible on an x-ray (9)
Double image an additional layer within which structures appear in the image (6)

E

Elongation the result of under-angulation of the x-ray beam (5)
Enamel hypoplasia caused by defective enamel matrix formation with a deficiency of vitamin D in the body; enamel is hard but thin (10)
Erosion when acids wear way the enamel of the teeth (10)

F

Focal trough a three-dimensional zone where images are sharp (6)
Foreshortening the result of over-angulation of the x-ray beam (5)

G

Ghost image an image opposite or slightly above its real counterpart (6)
Gray scale resolution the number of gray shades in an image (4)

H

Health Insurance Portability and Accountability Act passed by the legislature in 1996, it provides data privacy and security provisions for safeguarding medical information (4)
Hyoid bone a U-shaped bone that is located at the base of the mandible (6)

I

Image processing used to enhance the appearance of a digital image to augment patient education (4)
Image quality the overall sharpness of a digital film (9)
Image viewing methods by which an image can be displayed for viewing (4)
Imaging software computer software that is used in digital radiography (4)
Incipient lesions the earliest stage of cavity development in which the cavity is less than halfway through the enamel (9)
Intraoral bitewings x-rays that are taken inside the mouth to display the interproximal contacts (1)
Intraoral radiographs x-rays that are taken inside of the oral cavity (3)

L

Low radiation dose using specific techniques such as "F"-speed film or a long, rectangular cone to reduce radiation exposure (9)

M

Mandibular canal a canal within the mandible that contains the inferior alveolar nerve, inferior alveolar artery, and inferior alveolar vein (10)

O

Occupational Safety and Health Administration a federal organization that ensures safe and healthy working conditions by enforcing standards and providing workplace safety training (3)

P

Panoramic bitewing machine a panoramic machine designed and programmed to open the posterior contacts when in a bitewing mode (9)
Panoramic radiograph an x-ray that captures the entire mouth in a single image. The image contains the teeth, upper and lower jaws, and surrounding tissues and structures (4)
Parotid salivary glands a pair of major salivary glands located above the inferior border of the mandible and in front of each ear (9)

Periapical imaging x-rays that are taken inside the mouth to display the periapical regions of involved teeth (1)

Personal protective equipment equipment that is designed to protect workers from contact with infectious material (4)

Photostimulable phosphor plate technology a method used to obtain digital x-ray images (3)

Pixel the smallest element of an image that can be processed on a digital x-ray (12)

R

Radiation caries decay that has developed in a patient after radiation therapy (10)

Rampant caries decay that advances at a rapid rate (10)

Ramus a branch of the mandible (6)

Real image an image that is located in the plane of convergence for the light rays that originate from a given object (6)

Recurrent caries decay that occurs under or around an existing restoration (10)

Root caries decay that is on the root surface of the tooth (10)

S

Saturation relevant area on an x-ray has a maximum pixel content (9)

Scanner used to scan sensors into the computer system (4)

Sensor a piece of equipment used to transfer images into a computer (4)

Sensor reuse the process of repeated use of digital sensors over time, although some may need to be erased (4)

Spatial resolution refers to the number of pixels used in the creation of a digital image (4)

T

Temporomandibular joint a hinge joint that connects the jaw to the temporal bones of the skull (6)

Tomography a technique for displaying a layer of tissue containing teeth (9)

Tomosynthesis a tomographic panoramic can be further subdivided into multiple thin layers (9)

Toothbrush abrasion wearing down of the enamel and receding gums that can result from over-brushing (10)

X

Xerostomia caries decay that is associated with dry mouth, secondary to drugs and age (10)

X-ray equipment equipment used to produce x-radiation for the production of radiographs (4)

INDEX

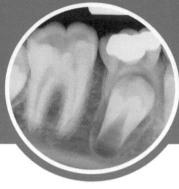